Hepatology:
Diagnosis and
Clinical Management

T0200763

Hepatology: Diagnosis and Clinical Management

Edited by

E. Jenny Heathcote MB, BS, MD, FRCP, FRCP(C)

Francis Family Chair in Hepatology Research
Professor of Medicine, University of Toronto
Head, Patient Based Clinical Research Division
Toronto Western Research Institute
University Health Network/Toronto Western Hospital
Toronto, Ontario, Canada

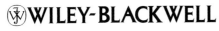

A John Wiley & Sons, Ltd., Publication

Library of Congress Cataloging-in-Publication Data

Hepatology : diagnosis and clinical management / edited by E. Jenny Heathcote.
        p. ; cm.
    Includes bibliographical references and index.
    ISBN 978-0-470-65617-4 (pbk. : alk. paper)
    I. Heathcote, Jenny.
    [DNLM: 1. Liver Diseases–diagnosis.   2. Liver Diseases–therapy.   WI 700]
    616.3'62–dc23
                        2012002557

A catalogue record for this book is available from the British Library.

Wiley also publishes its books in a variety of electronic formats. Some content that appears in print may not be available in electronic books.

Set in 9/12pt Palatino by Toppan Best-set Premedia Limited, Hong Kong
Printed in Singapore by Ho Printing Singapore Pte Ltd

2   2014

Contents

Contributors

Jordan J. Feld MD MPH
Assistant Professor of Medicine, University of Toronto
Staff Physician, Liver Centre
Division of Gastroenterology
Toronto Western Hospital
University Health Network
Toronto, Ontario, Canada

Scott K. Fung MD FRCPC
Assistant Professor of Medicine, University of Toronto
Toronto General Hospital
University Health Network
Division of Gastroenterology
Department of Medicine
University of Toronto
Toronto, Ontario, Canada

Anthony E. Hanbidge MB BCh FRCP(C)
Associate Professor, Department of Medical Imaging
University of Toronto
Site Director Abdominal Imaging, Toronto Western Hospital
Joint Department of Medical Imaging
University Health Network
Mount Sinai Hospital
and
Women's College Hospital
Toronto, Ontario, Canada

Gideon M. Hirschfield MB, BChir, MRCP, PhD
Assistant Professor of Medicine, University of Toronto
Staff Physician, Liver Centre
Division of Gastroenterology
Toronto Western Hospital
University Health Network
Toronto, Ontario, Canada
and
Centre for Liver Research
University of Birmingham
Birmingham, UK

Binita M. Kamath MBBChir, MRCP, MTR
Assistant Professor, University of Toronto
Staff Physician, Division of Gastroenterology, Hepatology and Nutrition
The Hospital for Sick Children
Toronto, Ontario, Canada

Korosh Khalili MD, FRCPC
Assistant Professor, Department of Medical Imaging
University of Toronto
Toronto, Ontario, Canada

Leslie B. Lilly MD, MSc, FRCPC
Assistant Professor of Medicine, University of Toronto
Multi Organ Transplant Program
Toronto General Hospital
University Health Network
Toronto, Ontario, Canada

Simon Ling MB, ChB, MRCP
Professor of Pediatrics, University of Toronto
Division of Gastroenterology, Hepatology and Nutrition
The Hospital for Sick Children
University Health Network
University of Toronto
Toronto, Ontario, Canada

Vicky L. Ng MD, FRCPC
Associate Professor of Paediatrics, University of Toronto
Staff Physician, Division of Gastroenterology, Hepatology, and Nutrition
Medical Director, Liver Transplant Program
Sick Kids Transplant Center
The Hospital for Sick Children
Toronto, Ontario, Canada

Eberhard L. Renner MD, FRCP(C)
Professor of Medicine, Director GI Transplantation
Toronto General Hospital
University Health Network
University of Toronto
Toronto, Ontario, Canada

Eve A. Roberts MD, MA, FRCPC
Adjunct Professor of Paediatrics, Medicine, and Pharmacology
University of Toronto
Associate, Division of Gastroenterology,
Hepatology and Nutrition
The Hospital for Sick Children
Toronto, Ontario, Canada

Nazia Selzner MD, PhD
Assistant Professor of Medicine, Multi Organ Transplant Program
Staff Physician, Division of Gastroenterology
Toronto General Hospital
University Health Network
University of Toronto
Toronto, Ontario, Canada

Hemant A. Shah MD, FRCP(C)
Assistant Professor of Medicine, University of Toronto
Staff Physician, Liver Centre
Division of Gastroenterology
Toronto Western Hospital
University Health Network
Toronto, Ontario, Canada

Morris Sherman MB, BCh, PhD, FRCP(C)
Associate Professor of Medicine, Department of Medicine
University of Toronto
Toronto General Hospital
University Health Network
Toronto, Ontario, Canada

David K.H. Wong MD FRCPC
Assistant Professor of Medicine, University of Toronto
Staff Physician, Liver Centre
Division of Gastroenterology
Toronto Western Hospital
University Health Network
Toronto, Ontario, Canada

Foreword

In this brand new textbook, *Hepatology: Diagnosis and Clinical Management,* editor Jenny Heathcote, The Francis Family Chair in Hepatology Research and Professor of Medicine at the University of Toronto, has assembled twenty-six chapters which comprehensively address the topic. This book is targeted at those physicians who have never received advanced training in Gastroenterology or Hepatology, and yet are faced on a very regular basis both in the emergency room or on the general medicine ward with patients who appear to have something wrong with their liver. It offers a highly practical approach.

Hepatology represents a close collaboration between experts in liver disease in both internal medicine and paediatrics, comparing and contrasting the causes, course and complications of liver across the age spectrum. Furthermore, the chapters are all written by hepatology experts across the University of Toronto, some internists others paediatricians; the result is a superb book that is practical and academic and unlocks the mysteries of diseases of the liver.

The chapters provide significant insights into pathophysiology of diseases of the liver, their diagnosis and likely outcomes. Starting with the assessment of liver disease in adults, then contrasting this with the evaluation of hepatic disease in children and youth, the book addresses all of the major disease categories in the field. The final chapter focuses attention on the radiologic examination of the liver.

The contributors constitute an impressive group of highly accomplished hepatologists, all committed to enhancing the knowledge base in liver disease of their colleagues in general internal and paediatric medicine. The result is a tour de force, a volume that rightly deserves its place on the shelves of generalists in these specialties as well as in Family and Community Medicine.

As Chairs, respectively, of the Departments of Internal Medicine and Paediatrics, we wholeheartedly endorse this book and recommend it as a first line source of information in enhancing the complex world of hepatology.

Wendy Levinson and Denis Daneman
Professor and Chair Professor and Chair
Department of Medicine Department of Paediatrics
Lady Eaton Chair in Internal Medicine RS McLaughlin Foundation Chair in Paediatrics
The University of Toronto Faculty of Medicine

Preface

Hepatology is a rapidly growing specialty, particularly since the discovery of hepatitis A, B, C, D, and E and the development of liver transplantation, i.e. in the last 40 years. Unfortunately, training in this field has not kept pace with these scientific breakthroughs and thus there are many who have received little or no teaching from well-trained hepatologists.

The function of the liver is very complex yet most liver disease is asymptomatic for many years; sadly it is often missed at a stage when prevention, control, or cure is possible.

It is perhaps in part the "international scene" in Toronto (52% of its citizens were not born in Canada) that has favored the development of a comprehensive adult and pediatric program at the University of Toronto—almost all members of which have contributed to this book. We hope that we have covered most of the hepatic diseases seen by emergency room physicians and internists. We have tried to put this first edition together in a concise manner that is easy to use and comprehend, by covering both academic and practical aspects of the topics chosen. The overall aim of this book is to facilitate the recognition, diagnosis, and management of suspected liver disease.

E. Jenny Heathcote
Toronto

Acknowledgements

I am indebted to Dr. Telisha Smith-Gorvie (Emergency Room physician at University Health Network, Toronto) for reading and critiquing each chapter of this book and making sure that the content is clear and helpful for the physicians for whom it is intended.

I would like to take the opportunity to say how lucky I was to have trained with the late Dame Professor Sheila Sherlock as it was she who inspired, encouraged and supported me throughout my training and subsequently once a staff physician. I also want to thank the University of Toronto for all the support they have given me since my appointment in 1979. I am also very fortunate to have worked alongside a superb team of both adult and paediatric hepatologists at the Univesity of Toronto who have greatly contributed to this book.

Last but not least I would like to take this opportunity to thank both my secretary, Geraldine Karkada, who has been so patient and helpful during the preparation of the manuscripts and to Wiley-Blackwell who invited me to put this book together.

Clinical assessment of the adult patient with possible liver disease: history and physical examination

CHAPTER 1

Eberhard L. Renner

University of Toronto, and GI Transplantation, Toronto General Hospital, University Health Network, Toronto, Ontario, Canada

---

Key points

- A thorough history and physical examination must always be the starting point in the approach to the patient with possible liver disease.
- Many individuals with chronic liver disease are asymptomatic. Except for pruritus, when symptoms are present they tend to be non-specific.
- A detailed history regarding use of prescription, non-prescription, and alternative medicines, as well as risk factors for liver disease such as obesity, high-risk sexual behavior, alcohol and illicit drug use, transfusions, piercings, tattoos, and travel, deserve special attention. Family history is essential.
- The physical examination in patients with possible liver disease requires a full routine internal medicine physical, inclusive of a search for signs compatible with cirrhosis and portal hypertension such as ascites, jaundice, hepatic encephalopathy (flapping tremor), a firm liver (normal, large, or small size), splenomegaly, spider nevi, and palmar erythema.

Introduction

The liver has an enormous functional reserve, a unique potential to regenerate, and, except for its capsule, no sensory innervation. It is therefore not surprising that symptoms and signs of both acute and chronic liver disease are only apparent when function is severely compromised.

History

When taking a history, it is important to gather information regarding symptoms and signs related to the current illness, both those specific to liver disease

Hepatology: Diagnosis and Clinical Management, First Edition. Edited by E. Jenny Heathcote.
© 2012 John Wiley & Sons, Ltd. Published 2012 by John Wiley & Sons, Ltd.

and including those that may well have occurred in the decades past. Complications of other medical issues may have occurred entirely in the past, not extending to the present. For example, in a patient presenting with new-onset ascites, who had a variceal bleed 3 years ago, and who experimented with illicit drugs 25 years ago, all these facts really belong in the history of "current" illness.

The following reviews the key elements in the history of patients with suspected liver disease.

Overt symptoms/signs of liver disease
Jaundice

Hyperbilirubinemia becomes noticeable as scleral icterus when the serum bilirubin exceeds approximately 50 μmol/L. Bilirubin is deposited in tissues including the skin. The degree of skin pigmentation, that is the ethnicity, makes skin icterus more (e.g. African American) or less (Caucasian) difficult to detect. Jaundice (hyperbilirubinemia) may be a consequence of the liver's inability to efficiently conjugate and/or excrete bilirubin into bile, or due to extrahepatic biliary obstruction, for example choledochlithiasis or pancreatic cancer. As conjugation of bilirubin is possible even when the liver is failing, the conjugated fraction predominates unless the cause is hemolysis, in which case this rarely results in visible jaundice. Hyperbilirubinemia does not allow one to discriminate between hepatocyte dysfunction and biliary obstruction.

Ascites and peripheral edema

Fluid retention with increasing abdominal girth due to ascites and/or swollen lower extremities (feet and ankles) secondary to peripheral edema is the most frequent presenting symptom of patients with cirrhosis, whereas acute liver disorders, such as hepatic vein obstruction (Budd–Chiari syndrome or right-sided heart failure), usually causes just ascites initially. Many patients will not interpret this as such, but state that their pants and shoes no longer fit and/or complain about weight gain. Fluid retention with ascites and peripheral edema is not specific for liver disease; the differential includes congestive cardiac or renal failure. In the context of liver disease, fluid retention with ascites and peripheral edema does not indicate etiology, but rather the presence of portal hypertension. Fluid retention is typically associated with processes impairing portal venous flow at the sinusoidal (cirrhosis) or postsinusoidal level (Budd–Chiari syndrome, veno-occlusive disease), but only very rarely with presinusoidal processes such as portal vein thrombosis or chronic biliary disease.

Acute liver diseases, including fulminant hepatic failure, are, at least in their initial phase, not associated with portal hypertension and are therefore not typically associated with fluid retention. Having said that, rapid onset of massive ascites, right upper quadrant pain, and mild jaundice is the classic triad of acute hepatic outflow obstruction, such as in acute Budd–Chiari syndrome, or sinusoidal obstruction syndrome following a bone marrow transplant.

Hematemesis and melena
Massive vomiting of blood is the most dramatic presenting symptom of cirrhosis. This may be a consequence of bleeding lesions in the upper GI tract secondary to portal hypertension, including esophageal or gastric varices, or less frequently portal hypertensive gastropathy or duodenal varices. In children, portal vein thrombosis is a more frequent cause of portal hypertensive bleeding than in adults. A massive portal hypertensive upper GI bleed can also lead to loss of red blood per rectum. Such massive bleeds are typically associated with hemodynamic instability and represent a serious emergency as they carry a high mortality (around 30%, depending on the severity of the underlying liver disease). Slower GI transit times and/or slower bleeds allow for (partial) degradation of hemoglobin to hematin and may present as vomiting of "coffee grounds" and/or melena. Varices are portosystemic collaterals. Less frequently, they are found in the rectum. Dilatation of small intramucosal vessels, the correlate of portal hypertensive gastropathy, can also occur in the distal colon (portal hypertensive colopathy). These lesions can cause a lower GI bleed, that is red blood per rectum, often in the absence of hemodynamic instability. Other locations where portosystemic collaterals may form include the umbilicus (caput medusae; low spontaneous bleeding risk) and the retroperitoneum (e.g. spontaneous splenorenal shunt; low spontaneous bleeding risk but high rate of portosystemic encephalopathy). In patients with an intestinal stoma, the area around the stoma (stomal varices) has a high spontaneous bleeding risk and is very difficult to manage, therefore do not advise this surgery in a cirrhotic.

It goes without saying that hematemesis and melena are by no means pathognomonic for liver disease nor for portal hypertension as they may occur secondary to a variety of lesions, including severe gastroesophageal reflux disease and Mallory–Weiss tears, gastric and duodenal ulcers, and colonic cancer, to name just a few. Of note, gastric and duodenal ulcers are more common in cirrhotic patients than in the normal population. Thus, even in the presence of known portal hypertension, any hematemesis or melena requires expedited endoscopic diagnosis of the bleeding source (and, if necessary, appropriate endoscopic therapy).

As is the case with fluid retention, portal hypertensive bleeding does not typically occur in acute liver disease. In chronic liver disease, a portal hypertensive GI bleed (hematemesis or melena) does not allow one to draw conclusions as to the etiology of the underlying cause of portal hypertension. Having said that, the presence of gastric, in the absence of esophageal, varices must raise the differential of isolated splenic vein thrombosis with left-sided portal hypertension (formation of collaterals via the short gastric veins).

Cognitive dysfunction (hepatic encephalopathy)
Patients with liver disease (or their family members) may complain about subtle cognitive dysfunction, such as difficulties in concentrating and impaired short-term memory. These and a reversal of the day–night cycle, that is

Table 1.1 Hepatic encephalopathy	
Grade	**Symptoms/signs**
Minimal*	Subtle cognitive impairment (difficulties concentrating, impaired short-term memory); reversal of the day/night cycle
I	Lethargy (slowly thinking/speaking), asterixis† possible
II	Confusion (disorientation to time, location and/or person); asterixis† typical
III	Stupor, asterixis† often absent
IV	Deep coma, no asterixis†

*Sometimes also termed "subclinical" or "stage 0" hepatic encephalopathy.
†Asterixis or flapping tremor is the characteristic five to six times per minute tremor observed in patients with hepatic encephalopathy who are asked to hold their hands in a fixed position (with wrists pulled back, fingers spread out, and eyes closed).

day-time fatigue and night-time insomnia, are subtle symptoms of what is called minimal (stage 0) hepatic encephalopathy. Hepatic encephalopathy is a neuropsychiatric disorder of varying severity associated with liver disease and typically classified into stages 0 to IV (Table 1.1). Hepatic encephalopathy is thought to result from an imbalance of excitatory and inhibitory neurotransmitter activities in the brain. While the exact mechanism(s) remain debated, it is generally thought that gut-derived central nervous system inhibitory substances become systemically available secondary to portosystemic shunting and/or an impaired metabolic capacity of the liver (hepatic encephalopathy does not occur in those whose only cause for portal hypertension is a portal vein thrombosis). While arterial ammonia levels are typically elevated in hepatic encephalopathy, the extent of this elevation correlates poorly with the clinical picture and abnormalities in many neurotransmitters systems have been described. Hepatic encephalopathy is a diagnostic hallmark of fulminant hepatic failure. Early in the course of the disease it is often mild (stage 0–II) but often progresses rapidly to coma. The presence/absence of hepatic encephalopathy does not allow any conclusion as to the etiology of the underlying liver disease.

Other, less frequent symptoms and signs
The following symptoms and signs (described in random order) may be associated with liver disease but are less commonly reported by patients with liver disease.

Some patients with liver disease complain of non-specific, dull **abdominal discomfort**. Except for its capsule, the liver has no innervation and sharp pain is not a typical symptom/sign of liver disease. Dull right upper quadrant discomfort/low-intensity pain can be observed in acute hepatitis and is thought to be caused by an acute enlargement of the liver, distending its capsule. Right upper quadrant discomfort is also a common complaint of patients with chronic biliary disease, for example primary biliary cirrhosis and primary sclerosing cholangitis even in the absence of gall stones. Many patients with ascites, especially when new in onset or increasing in volume, complain of bilateral discomfort/low-intensity pain in the lower abdomen; this is probably caused by distension of the abdominal wall. Patients with a massively enlarged spleen secondary to portal hypertension my rarely develop splenic infarcts, which can cause sharp left-sided abdominal pain.

Other gastrointestinal symptoms, such as **a poor appetite** (anorexia) with or without **vomiting**, are not infrequently reported by patients with liver disease (generally with acute liver disease), while **dysgeusia** (altered taste) is a rarer complaint. These symptoms are non-specific, occur in acute and chronic liver disease, and do not offer etiologic clues. Early morning nausea/vomiting (vomitus matutinus) relieved by alcohol (eye opener) is a sign of alcohol dependence.

Pruritus with or without visible scratch marks, but without a visible causative skin lesion, can be a leading presenting symptom of liver diseases, particularly in chronic cholestatic liver disorders such as primary biliary cirrhosis (PBC). Pruritus is, however, not pathognomonic for liver diseases and can be observed in many other conditions, including uremia and many skin disorders. Hepatic pruritus is not specific for PBC and is also observed with other intra- and extrahepatic causes of cholestasis. Rarely, it may even accompany viral hepatitis (particularly in a young woman taking the oral contraceptive pill). Hepatic pruritus is said to be aggravated by warmth, and many report it worsens when going to bed. The mechanism(s) for hepatic pruritus remain(s) debated. It is generally thought that endogenous substances (possibly endorphin-like) normally excreted into bile are retained in cholestasis and act on the central nervous system to cause pruritus.

Primary biliary cirrhosis may be associated with the **sicca syndrome** and/or **Raynaud phenomenon**. These patients may complain of a dry mouth and/or dry eyes, with or without frequent conjunctivitis. Additionally, they may notice that in the cold their fingers turn purple or white ("dead fingers").

Since advanced stages of acute and chronic liver diseases are often associated with decreased synthesis of coagulation factors (increased INR) and a low platelet count, complaints about easy skin **bruising**, gum **bleeding** when brushing their teeth, and/or spontaneous nose bleeds are common. As is the case for most symptoms/signs associated with liver disease, they are non-specific for the presence/etiology of liver disease.

Muscle cramps are a frequent complaint of patients with liver diseases, especially when on diuretic therapy, and are thought to be caused by electrolyte imbalance.

Most patients with liver disease, especially those with severe chronic disease, experience **impaired sexual function** with decreased libido, irregular menstrual cycles up to complete amenorrhea, and erectile dysfunction up to frank impotence. This is thought to be a result of an androgen/estrogen imbalance.

Dyspnea and/or dry **cough** are non-specific symptoms, but may be caused by hepatic hydrothorax, that is a (typically right-sided) pleural effusion associated with portal hypertension. Hepatic hydrothorax is thought to result from ascites being sucked up through preformed anatomical connections in the diaphragm. Fluid is driven into the pleural cavity by the negative pressure generated during inspiration. Hepatic hydrothorax is typically, but not necessarily, accompanied by clinically detectable ascites. In the context of liver disease, dyspnea may also be a symptom of the hepatopulmonary syndrome, that is a functional right–left shunt potentially forming in the lung circulation of patients with portal hypertension, and characterized by orthodeoxia, that is a drop in peripheral O_2 saturation in the upright position that is improved by laying down. Portopulmonary hypertension, that is pulmonary artery hypertension associated with portal hypertension, is another potential cause of, typically, exertional dyspnea in the patient with liver disease.

Apart from bacterial cholangitis associated with primary sclerosing cholangitis (PSC) and other rare conditions that cause biliary strictures (secondary sclerosing cholangitis), **fever and rigors** are not commonly observed with acute and chronic liver diseases.

Many patients with chronic liver disease complain about **feeling cold** all the time. This is thought to be related to heat loss through the skin secondary to liver-disease-related chronic vasodilatation.

Past medical history, review of systems, and family history

Many patients with liver disease will not spontaneously report the symptoms/signs described above, they may only be revealed during a thorough review of systems. A thorough past medical history and family history may also yield valuable clues in the patient with liver disease. Thus, asking for a history of **autoimmune disorders** frequently associated with autoimmune liver diseases, such as hypothyroidism secondary to autoimmune thyroiditis (Hashimoto disease) may suggest an autoimmune etiology to their liver disease. A history/presence of rheumatoid-type **joint pain** may be associated with PBC; degenerative joint pain and/or diabetes may be a hint towards hemochromatosis. A history/presence of the **metabolic syndrome, obesity**, and/or overt **diabetes** predisposes to the development of non-alcoholic fatty liver disease, which may progress to cirrhosis. Hereditary liver diseases, such as genetic hemochromatosis, α_1-antitrypsin deficiency and Wilson disease may be accompanied by a history of **liver disease/liver-related mortality in first-degree relatives**. In all individuals who test positive for hepatitis B, a detailed family history may reveal family members who have died of liver cancer.

Risk factors for liver disease

An *essential* part of the history in all patients with suspected liver disease is a detailed medication history. Many prescribed and over-the-counter medications are able to cause acute or chronic liver disease, either in a dose-dependent or a dose-independent (idiosyncratic) manner. Medications include prescription and non-prescription drugs, as well as herbal and other over-the-counter, alternative medicines.

Taking a history of elements predisposing to liver disease (risk factors for liver disease) is mandatory in all patients with suspected liver issues; these factors are summarized in Table 1.2.

Physical examination

The conduct of the physical examination in a patient with possible liver disease should not be different from a routine physical in anyone. The following highlights some specific aspects to be looked for in a patient with suspected liver disease.

General condition and vital signs. Many, but by no means all, patients with advanced chronic liver disease are **malnourished** and exhibit profound **muscle wasting** and poor dentition. Patients with cirrhosis typically have a hyperdynamic circulation, characterized by a low peripheral vascular resistance (vasodilatation) and a compensatory high cardiac output. Consequently, cirrhotic patients often have blood pressures that are below and heart rates that are above those of an age-matched, normal population.

Nervous system. Look for signs of **hepatic encephalopathy** (Table 1.2) and test for **asterixis**. Patients with alcoholic liver disease may present with signs of organic brain disease such as **Korsakow** or **alcoholic dementia**, as well as **alcohol-induced peripheral polyneuropathy**. **Wilson disease** may affect the central nervous system, its presentation ranging from **slurred speech** (dysarthria) to a **Parkinson-like syndrome** and even to frank **psychosis**.

Head and neck. Special attention is directed to the eyes for detection of a potential **scleral icterus** (see above). A **sicca syndrome** is often only detectable by quantitating tear production using a commercially available filter paper (Schirmer test). A **Kayser–Fleischer ring**, visualized as a circular copper deposit in the rim of the iris, in the context of liver disease is pathognomonic for Wilson disease. Confirmation of its presence/absence usually requires a slit lamp examination by an ophthalmologist. A **hypertrophy of the parotid**, characterized by a bilateral painless palpable enlargement of the gland, may be observed in patients with liver disease thought to be attributable to heavy alcohol consumption.

Table 1.2 Risk factors for liver disease

Risk factor	Comments
Ethnicity or geographic area of origin	Coming from high prevalence areas such as Asia/Pacific for HBV and Egypt or Pakistan for HCV predisposes to the respective chronic viral hepatitis
Sexual preference and behavior	HBV is sexually transmitted; men who have sex with men and individuals with promiscuous life styles are at increased risk of acquiring HBV infection in addition to HIV
History of incarceration or other institutionalization	Incarceration and other institutionalization is associated with a increased risk of acquiring HBV and HCV infection
Illicit drug use	A history or current use of illicit drugs by the i.v. route (or by snorting with a straw) carries an increased risk of acquiring not only HCV, but also HBV and HAV infection
Piercings and tattoos	Non-professionally performed piercings and tattoos carry the risk of HBV and HCV transmission
Transfusions (blood and blood products)	A history of transfusion of blood and blood products prior to introduction of routine HCV testing in the early 1990s is a risk factor for acquiring HCV
Alcohol consumption	Regular consumption of alcohol increases the risk for developing alcoholic liver disease; while individual susceptibility varies and there is no clear dose threshold for harmful drinking, consumption of $\geq$40–60 g of alcohol a day for women and $\geq$60–80 g of alcohol a day for men is generally thought to convey an increased risk for alcoholic liver disease About 10–20% of individuals drinking these or larger amounts of alcohol over a 10-year period develop alcoholic liver cirrhosis Small amounts may be responsible for elevated liver biochemistries
Travel history	Travel into regions of the world where HAV and HBV are prevalent combined with respective sexual or dietary risk behavior predisposes to HBV, HAV, and HEV infection, respectively

HAV, hepatitis A virus, HBV, hepatitis B virus; HCV, hepatitis C virus; HEV, hepatitis E virus.

Abdomen. Bulging flanks with shifting dullness indicate the presence of **ascites**. Ascites predisposes to the development of umbilical and inguinal **hernias**. Patients with portal hypertension often have **prominent abdominal wall veins**, which connect to the umbilical vein as part of portosystemic shunts and typically fill rapidly from caudal, less so from cranial, when effaced. This is similar to the fully developed **caput medusae**, periumbilical shunts between umbilical and abdominal wall veins (rarely observed).

Percussion of the liver in the midclavicular line allows a rough estimate of its size, which is confirmed by palpation of the liver's lower edge. The latter also gives an impression of its consistency and tenderness. In acute liver disease, the liver is often enlarged and tender. In chronic liver disease the liver is typically firm, sometimes with a palpable nodular edge. The liver may be normal in size or even enlarged, depending on the etiology of the chronic liver disease. The liver may become small and shrunken when disease is in an advanced stage. Chronic cholestatic liver diseases (e.g. primary biliary cirrhosis and primary sclerosing cholangitis) may be associated with an enlarged liver even very late into the disease evolution. An extremely firm ("hard as a rock"), indolent, and massively enlarged liver must raise the suspicion of **hepatic amyloidosis**. A hard, enlarged, grossly nodular, sometimes tender liver is suspicious for widespread **metastatic disease** or **extensive primary liver cancer**.

With large hepatocellular cancers an arterial **bruit** may be heard on auscultation over the liver. This is attributable to a high flow into the feeding artery, hepatocellular carcinomas being primarily perfused via branches of the hepatic artery. A bruit may also be heard in other situations where large arteriovenous shunts may form in the liver, such as after a liver trauma or in the rare hereditary hemorrhagic telangiectasia (Osler–Weber–Rendue disease).

In the context of liver disease, an **enlarged palpable spleen** is a sign of portal hypertensions. These sometimes extremely large spleens may reach down to the right side of the pelvis and may be missed if palpation is not started in the left lower abdomen. Portal hypertensive splenomegaly is firm and non-tender.

Chest. Examination of the chest may reveal gynecomastia, that is a mammary gland in a male patient that palpably extends beyond the area of the nipple. Gynecomastia may or may not be tender and is thought to reflect a estrogen/ androgen imbalance secondary to advanced chronic liver disease. Enlarged pectoral fat pads (without enlargement of the mammary gland) is not infrequently observed in male patients with cirrhosis, especially when caused by alcoholic or non-alcoholic fatty liver disease.

In patients with massive ascites, bilaterally decreased air entry into and dullness on percussion over the basal lung fields likely reflects an **elevated diaphragm secondary to ascites**. It may, however, also indicate the presence of pleural effusions, that is **hepatic hydrothorax**. The latter may be present in the absence of clinically detectable ascites and typically, but not necessarily, is right sided or right side dominant, rather than left sided.

Apart from the signs of a **hyperdynamic circulation** (see above), which may also be associated with a functional systolic ejection murmur, examination of the heart is usually unremarkable in patients with liver disease. However, acute and chronic right and left heart failure may cause acute and chronic liver dysfunction, respectively, presenting as "shock liver" (caused by a low flow state due to acute right or left heart failure) or cardiac cirrhosis. It is therefore important to *exclude* by appropriate cardiac examination that the liver disease is not a consequence of heart disease.

Skin and nails. Spider nevi are arteriovenous shunts in the skin formed by a small central artery from which venous collaterals radiate. Upon emptying the spider nevus by applying pressure with a fingertip, the venous collaterals fill from the central small artery once pressure is removed. "Spiders" are suggestive, but not pathognomonic, for liver disease; they may occur in other states associated with a hyperdynamic circulation such as pregnancy. However, numerous spiders (more than three in women, more than two in men) are not typically seen in the absence of liver disease. They are most frequent on chest, neck, and hands, but may occur anywhere. The highest numbers are said to be found in florid alcoholic liver disease and autoimmune hepatitis. **Palmar erythema** is a blotchy, purplish-red discoloration of the thenar and hypothenar eminences and is frequently, but not exclusively, observed in chronic liver disease (it also occurs in rheumatoid arthritis). **Petechial hemorrhage** and **bruising** are consequences of thrombocytopenia, with or without a coagulopathy, commonly associated with liver disease and portal hypertension. **Scratch marks** are a reflection of severe pruritus and may be found in cholestatic liver diseases. **Vitiligo** may be associated with other autoimmune diseases, including autoimmune hepatitis. A **feminine pattern of body hair distribution** is common in men with cirrhosis and is attributed to a estrogen/androgen dysbalance. **Clubbing**, an abnormal shape of the finger nail characterized by an emergent angle of the nail of more than 180° and extreme nail convexity, sometimes forming so-called "drum stick" fingers, may, in the context of cirrhosis, be associated with the hepatopulmonary syndrome or portopulmonary hypertension. "**Terry's nails**" are a whitish discoloration of the nails to within 1–2 mm of the end. They may be observed in cirrhosis, but also in other conditions including congestive heart failure, rheumatoid arthritis, and the nephrotic syndrome.

Miscellaneous. Dupytren's contracture of a palmar tendon is not infrequently observed in individuals with alcoholic liver disease, but also occurs in the absence of alcohol misuse and liver disease, for example traumatic injury. **Testicular atrophy** occurs in men with cirrhosis and is thought to be a result of cirrhosis-related estrogen/androgen dysbalance.

Fever with or without shaking chills may be a result from biliary sepsis, for example PSC or infected ascites (spontaneous bacterial peritonitis) or a liver abscess.

Case study 1.1

A 42-year-old male construction worker, who was laid off 6 months ago, presents with anorexia, increasing abdominal girth, swollen ankles, and jaundice. His symptoms started about 4 weeks ago and have increased. Since the death of a friend in a motor vehicle accident 3 months ago, the patient reported adding three to four whiskeys to his daily alcohol consumption (six beers daily since age 16). Upon direct questioning, he admits to regular vomiting in the morning when brushing his teeth. A month ago he started to drink a shot of whiskey immediately after getting out of bed as this prevented the early morning vomiting.

Physical examination revealed profound jaundice and moderate muscle wasting. The patient was oriented three times and had no asterixis. Examination of the abdomen showed moderate ascites and hepatomegaly (measuring 18 cm in the midclavicular line). The liver was firm, and the spleen palpable to about 4 cm below the costal margin. Moderate "pitting edema" on both lower extremities was present to the knees. He had multiple, large spider nevi on the chest, marked palmar erythema, and bilateral Dupuytren's contractures.

A presumed diagnosis of acute alcoholic hepatitis superimposed on alcoholic cirrhosis was made, later confirmed with appropriate lab tests, an ultrasound, and a transjugular liver biopsy (see Chapter 8).

Multiple choice questions

1. Which of the following symptoms/signs is NOT causally related to liver disease?
   A. Fluid retention
   B. Reversal of the day/night cycle
   C. Circular lipid disposition in the rim of the cornea (arcus senilis)
   D. Dyspnea
   E. Fatigue
   F. Muscle wasting
   G. None of the above
   H. All of the above

2. Which of the following statements is correct?
   A. Risk factors for chronic liver disease include ALL of the following: history of recreational i.v. drug use, blood transfusions, cannabis smoking, piercings and/or tattoos, time spent in countries of the developing world.
   B. Tender hepatomegaly can be observed in early stages of fulminant hepatic failure.
   C. Splenomegaly is typically observed in acute liver disease, because enlargement of the spleen is associated with portal hypertension.

D. Spider nevi never occur in the absence of liver disease.

E. A family history of autoimmune disorders is typically observed in patients with hereditary liver diseases.

F. Many symptoms and signs of liver diseases allow precise conclusions as to the underlying etiology.

G. None of the above

H. All of the above

Answers

1. C
2. B

Further reading

Bellentani S, Tiribelli C. The spectrum of liver disease in the general population: lesson from the Dionysos study. J Hepatol 2001; 35: 531–7.

Duseja A, Chawla YK, Dhiman RK, et al. Non-hepatic insults are common acute precipitants in patients with acute on chronic liver failure (ACLF). Dig Dis Sci 2010; 55: 3188–92.

Polat M, Oztas P, Ilhan MN, et al. Generalized pruritus: a prospective study concerning etiology. Am J Clin Dermatol 2008; 9: 39–44.

Reisman Y, Gips CH, Lavelle SM, et al. Clinical presentation of (subclinical) jaundice—the Euricterus project in the Netherlands. United Dutch Hospitals and Euricterus Project Management Group. Hepatogastroenterology 1996; 43: 1190–5.

Initial diagnosis, workup, and assessment of severity of liver disease in adults

CHAPTER 2

Scott K. Fung

Division of Gastroenterology, Department of Medicine, University of Toronto, Toronto, Ontario, Canada

Key points

- The initial diagnosis of liver disease begins with a complete history, physical examination, and simple liver biochemical blood tests.
- Liver biochemistry determines the pattern of liver enzyme elevation—hepatocellular versus cholestatic liver disease.
- An accurate assessment of severity of liver disease is important to determine prognosis and management.
- The degree of liver dysfunction is determined primarily by blood work, such as total bilirubin and INR.
- Liver biopsy may be used to make an accurate diagnosis and remains the gold standard to stage the degree of hepatic fibrosis in those with chronic liver disease.
- Child–Turcotte–Pugh score and the Model for End-stage Liver Disease score offer the best estimate of survival for patients with cirrhosis (see Chapter 4).
- Abdominal ultrasound is best used to identify space-occupying lesions and evaluate venous supply and drainage—but is not reliable to diagnose cirrhosis.
- Non-invasive laboratory testing, including FibroTest and FibroScan, may reduce the need for biopsy to confirm cirrhosis, but neither have been validated for all etiologies of liver disease.

Introduction

The initial diagnosis and workup of liver disease begins with a complete patient history (including thorough review of prescribed and non-prescribed drug use), physical examination, and simple liver biochemical blood tests. Accurate assessment of disease severity depends, in part, on the possible cause

Hepatology: Diagnosis and Clinical Management, First Edition. Edited by E. Jenny Heathcote.
© 2012 John Wiley & Sons, Ltd. Published 2012 by John Wiley & Sons, Ltd.

of liver disease. For example, the prognosis of chronic viral hepatitis and alcoholic liver disease depend on the degree of fibrosis and inflammation on liver biopsy, whereas biliary disease severity can be determined by simple blood tests.

The severity of the underlying liver disease indicates prognosis and determines the timing for treatment. Patients with cirrhosis require prompt attention and intervention, if a treatment is indeed available. A general approach to assessment of liver disease is illustrated in Fig. 2.1.

History

Clues as to the presence of liver disease and its etiology may be found in a patient's complete medical history:
- the ethnicity and country of birth (which may be risk factors for viral hepatitis);
- risk factors for viral liver disease such as blood transfusion, injection drug use, sexual promiscuity, or exposure to improperly sterilized needles (e.g. tattoos);
- a family history of viral hepatitis, cirrhosis, and liver cancer is important;
- genetic risks for liver disease, such as Wilson disease and hereditary hemochromatosis;
- alcohol consumption—total daily amount and the pattern of drinking as determined by the CAGE questionnaire are helpful features in distinguishing alcoholic liver disease from non-alcoholic fatty liver disease;
- a careful medication history, including all prescription, over-the-counter, and herbal medications, is key to the diagnosis of drug-induced liver injury (DILI);
- medical comorbidities, including diabetes mellitus, hypertension, and dyslipidemia, are associated with non-alcoholic fatty liver disease with or without cirrhosis;
- a personal or family history of autoimmune disease, such as rheumatoid arthritis, thyroiditis, and inflammatory bowel disease, may raise suspicion for autoimmune hepatitis, primary biliary cirrhosis (PBC), and primary sclerosing cholangitis (PSC);
- history of pruritus—typical in those with cholestatic liver disease;
- onset of symptoms—jaundice, dark urine, increasing abdominal girth, leg swelling, fever, or acute confusion are all worrisome features both in those with acute liver disease as well as for those with known chronic liver disease:
  - dark urine implies conjugated hyperbilirubinemia and indicates some degree of hepatic or biliary disease
  - worsening of jaundice and dark urine/pale stools suggests complete biliary obstruction;
- melena and/or hematemesis caused by gastroesophageal varices indicates a poor prognosis, since upper gastrointestinal bleeding is associated with high mortality;

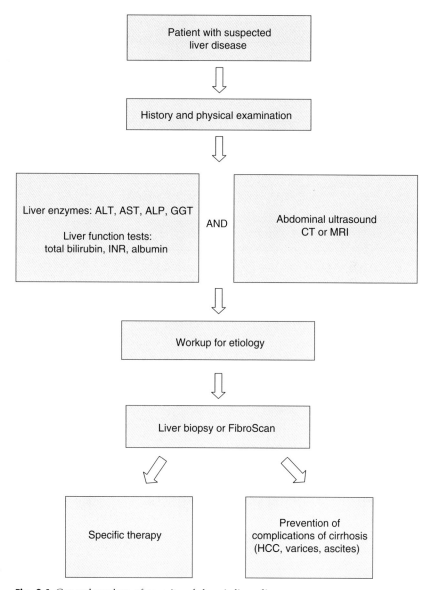

Fig. 2.1 General workup of severity of chronic liver disease.

- right upper quadrant abdominal pain may be present in biliary diseases such as acute cholecystitis but also may be present in patients with chronic liver disease (e.g. PSC).

  Clues from the history that may indicate the cause of liver disease are summarized in Table 2.1.

Table 2.1 Clues to diagnosis of liver disease on history

Disease	Clues in patient history/symptoms
Hepatitis B	Born in an endemic area (SE Asia, sub-Saharan Africa, Eastern Europe) Family history of hepatitis B, cirrhosis, or liver cancer Traumatic sexual activity
Hepatitis C	Previous or current injection drug use/tattoos Born in area where exposure to non-sterile procedures common Receipt of an i.v. blood product (date needed)
Hepatitis A/E	Travel to endemic area (Asia, Indian subcontinent, Latin America) Exposure to contaminated food, water, raw shellfish
Alcohol-related liver disease	Long-term alcohol consumption or binge drinking: women >2 drinks/day; men >4 drinks/day Positive CAGE questionnaire* (>1 positive response in men)
Non-alcoholic fatty liver disease	Diabetes mellitus/hypertension/dyslipidemia Obesity/sedentary lifestyle/poor dietary habits
Drug-induced liver injury (DILI)	New medication exposure within last 12 weeks No known pre-existing liver disease
Autoimmune hepatitis	Personal or family history of autoimmune disease
Hereditary hemochromatosis	Family history of diabetes mellitus/arthralgias/cardiomyopathy
Wilson disease	Family history of cirrhosis, hepatitis, liver failure Personal or family history of psychiatric disease
Primary biliary cirrhosis	Fatigue/pruritus/hypercholesterolemia Personal or family history of autoimmune disease
Primary sclerosing cholangitis	Jaundice and/or pruritus/right upper quadrant pain Recurrent episodes of "cholangitis"

*CAGE questionnaire: Has anyone asked you to **C**ut down on drinking alcohol?; Do you feel **A**nnoyed when asked to cut down?; Do you feel **G**uilty about your drinking?; Do you need an **E**ye-opener?

Physical examination in patients with suspected liver disease

Physical examination in patients with suspected liver disease is as follows.
Skin:
- Scleral icterus is only visible when total bilirubin levels rise above two to three times the upper limit of normal.
- Needle track marks indicate prior injection drug use, which is a risk factor for viral hepatitis.
- Porphyria cutanea tarda, lichen planus, and cutaneous vasculitis represent extrahepatic manifestations of hepatitis C.
- Spider nevi (confined to upper body) and/or easy bruising are signs of chronic liver disease.

Cardiac:
- Signs of congestive heart failure and an enlarged, pulsatile liver suggest a congestive hepatopathy.

Abdomen:
- General inspection of the abdomen may reveal central obesity, abdominal masses, striae, abdominal wall collateral vessels, umbilical hernia, and ascites.
- When palpating the abdomen, particular attention should be paid to the liver span and consistency of the liver edge.
  - Common causes of hepatomegaly include fatty liver and other infiltrative disorders. A normal liver edge is soft and smooth; a hard, liver edge may be palpated in cirrhosis, amyloidosis or liver metastases.
- Splenomegaly is commonly detected in patients with portal hypertension due to cirrhosis or portal vein thrombosis.
- Auscultation may reveal peritoneal friction rubs or bruits over the liver in patients with alcoholic hepatitis, liver metastases, or hepatocellular carcinoma.
- The presence of ascites—bulging flanks, shifting dullness, or a positive fluid wave test—is an indicator of severe portal hypertension. Ascites can be confirmed with a bedside abdominal ultrasound.

Central nervous system:
- Flapping tremor.
- Orientation and level of consciousness (LOC): patients with overt hepatic encephalopathy and who have decreased LOC may require monitoring in the ICU setting. Of note, encephalopathic patients in acute liver failure who also develop jaundice are unlikely to survive without a liver transplant.
- Peripheral neuropathy: alcoholic and/or diabetic.

Key findings of chronic liver disease on physical examination are found in Fig. 2.2, while Fig. 2.3 illustrates clues to the etiology of liver disease based on the physical examination.

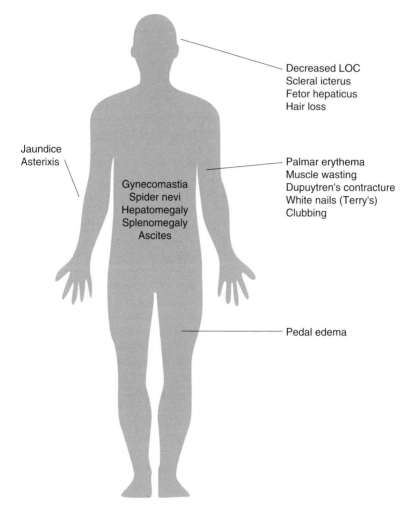

Decreased LOC
Scleral icterus
Fetor hepaticus
Hair loss

Jaundice
Asterixis

Gynecomastia
Spider nevi
Hepatomegaly
Splenomegaly
Ascites

Palmar erythema
Muscle wasting
Dupuytren's contracture
White nails (Terry's)
Clubbing

Pedal edema

Fig. 2.2 Physical examination for signs of chronic liver disease. LOC, level of consciousness.

Laboratory tests

Measurement of liver enzymes is relatively sensitive but not entirely specific for liver disease. For example, elevated aminotransferases may be found in cardiac or musculoskeletal disease. However, entirely normal aspartate aminotransferase (AST) and alanine aminotransferase (ALT) values may be present in patient with well-documented cirrhosis. The degree of liver enzyme elevation is generally not predictive of disease severity, whereas abnormalities in the markers of liver synthetic function, such as albumin, total bilirubin, and the international normalized ratio (INR), do indicate the severity of liver dysfunction.

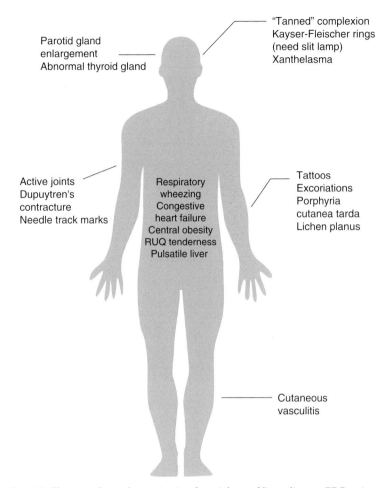

Fig. 2.3 Clues on physical examination for etiology of liver disease. PBC, primary biliary cirrhosis; NASH, non-alcoholic steatohepatitis.

AST, ALT, ALP (alkaline phosphatase), and GGT (γ-glutamine transaminase)

Elevated aminotransferases/transaminases are a sensitive indicator of hepatocellular damage. They are important in monitoring liver disease activity and response to treatment (e.g. autoimmune hepatitis). However, a one-time elevation in ALT in patients with chronic hepatitis B or C is unreliable and cannot be used to determine need for antiviral therapy. The *trend* in ALT levels is much more useful in ascertaining which patients with chronic hepatitis (B or C) may require therapy. It has been recommended that the upper limit of normal for ALT be reduced from 40 IU/L to 30 IU/L in men and 19 IU/L in women.

The pattern of liver enzyme elevation is typically classified as hepatocellular (AST and ALT elevation > alkaline phosphatase (ALP) elevation) or cholestatic

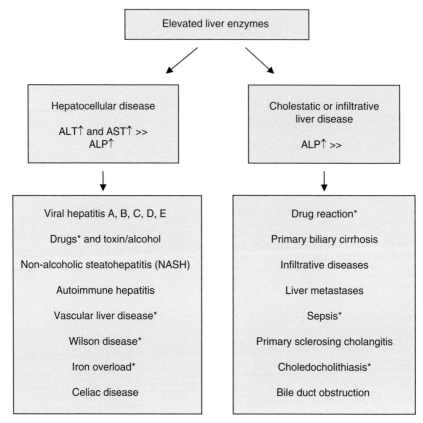

Fig. 2.4 Patterns of liver enzyme elevation. *Can be associated with both hepatocellular and cholestatic features (mixed).

(ALP elevation > AST or ALT elevation), as illustrated in Fig. 2.4. Elevation of GGT is really too non-specific to be of clinical help in formulating a diagnosis. GGT is rarely a helpful test as it may be elevated in all forms of liver disease or as a result of drug induction (e.g. antiepileptics).

Pattern of liver test abnormalities: differential diagnosis
- Hepatocellular disease includes various forms of viral hepatitis, drug induced liver disease, alcoholic hepatitis, non-alcoholic steatohepatitis, and autoimmune hepatitis.
- Cholestatic liver disease can be intra- or extrahepatic in origin. Intrahepatic causes include PBC, drugs and toxins, total parenteral nutrition (TPN) cholestasis, and infiltrative conditions such as metastases, sarcoidosis, and amyloidosis. Extrahepatic causes encompass hepatobiliary obstruction by gallstones, tumors such as cholangiocarcinoma and strictures, for example postoperative, PSC, and parasitic infections.

- Unconjugated hyperbilirubinemia may be due to increased bilirubin production due to ineffective erythropoiesis, hemolytic anemias, or reduced bilirubin uptake or conjugation (Gilbert syndrome) in the liver.
- Isolated conjugated hyperbilirubinemia, in which all other liver enzymes are normal, points to rare inherited disorders such as Dubin–Johnston or Rotor syndrome.
- A mixed liver enzyme profile (both ALT and ALP levels are elevated) occurs commonly with drug-induced liver injury and sepsis, even a liver abscess. Illustrative cases are discussed in Case studies 2.1 and 2.2.
- Liver biochemistry may be nearly normal in those with quiescent liver disease, for example Wilson disease, hereditary hemochromatosis, and chronic viral hepatitis.

There is a short differential diagnosis for very high ALT (>1000 IU/L). The usual suspects include acute viral hepatitis, autoimmune hepatitis, drug- or toxin-induced liver injury and ischemic hepatitis (e.g. due to cocaine use), and common bile duct stones and acute fatty liver (in poorly controlled diabetes). Although these blood tests can be alarmingly high, they do not necessarily predict a poor outcome. Depending on the degree of liver function (INR) impairment, such patients may be managed in the out-patient clinic. Serum transaminase values tend to change rapidly throughout the course of liver disease. In ischemic hepatitis, ALT can rise above 10 000 IU/L but this dramatic elevation does not predict outcome whereas in acetaminophen overdose, ALT may begin to fall or normalize just before INR and total bilirubin rise in the clinical course of fulminant liver failure.

Laboratory testing to evaluate liver disease severity
Total bilirubin
Hyperbilirubinemia occurs in the setting of increased supply of bilirubin (hemolysis), or decreased removal from the serum (hepatic dysfunction or bile duct obstruction), although all three conditions may be present simultaneously. Elevated total bilirubin is not specific for hepatic dysfunction and fractionation is necessary. Normally, hepatocytes are very efficient at removal of bilirubin bound to serum albumin even in severe cirrhosis. Thus, hyperbilirubinemia is a late feature in the course of chronic liver disease, and occasionally in acute liver disease.

In drug-induced liver injury, development of jaundice portends a poor prognosis: Hy's law predicts a mortality of 10–50% in patients who develop jaundice due to drug exposure. In addition, bilirubin is critical component of the Maddrey Discriminant Function in alcoholic hepatitis and in the King's College criteria for acetaminophen toxicity. Jaundice in patients with cirrhosis of any etiology tends to occur late in the course of disease and, once detected, also carries a poor prognosis.

INR
The prothrombin time (PT/INR) is a sensitive marker of liver synthetic function, but it can also be found in states of vitamin K depletion, such as severe

Table 2.2 Child–Turcotte–Pugh score for patients with cirrhosis

	Score		
	1	2	3
Serum bilirubin (μmol)	<34	34–51	>51
Serum albumin (g/L)	>35	28–35	<28
INR	<1.7	1.7–2.3	>2.3
Ascites	None	Easily controlled	Poorly controlled
Hepatic encephalopathy	None	Stages 1–2	Stages 3–4

Class A, 5–6 points; Class B, 7–9 points; Class C, >10 points.

celiac disease. In compensated cirrhosis, PT/INR remains normal but both are elevated with decompensated cirrhosis and acute fulminant liver failure—even after the administration of vitamin K. INR should be monitored on a daily basis in patients hospitalized for acute or chronic liver failure. A rapidly increasing INR in the absence of anticoagulants prompts urgent listing for liver transplantation. As expected, improvement in INR generally accompanies resolution of liver dysfunction.

Albumin
Albumin is made in the liver but the low levels of albumin in serum which may be present in those with chronic liver disease (rarely with acute liver disease) is most often secondary to hemodilution. Loss of albumin, for example in protein-losing enteropathy and nephrotic syndrome, are two other causes of low levels of serum albumin. In certain parts of the world protein malnutrition may be so severe that hypoalbuminemia is found. Albumin, INR, total bilirubin, the presence of ascites, and encephalopathy comprise the Child–Pugh–Turcotte score, which predicts survival of cirrhotic patients (see Table 2.2).

Assessment of severity of chronic liver disease
See Chapter 4.

Assessment of severity of acute liver failure
Acute (fulminant) liver failure (ALF) refers to sudden loss of liver synthetic function in a patient without pre-existing liver disease. ALF represents a syndrome rather than a specific disease and is manifested by coagulopathy (INR >1.5) and any degree of hepatic encephalopathy in a non-cirrhotic patient. It is rare (1 in 50000–100000). The course of disease is unpredictable. The etiology of ALF is variable and the prognosis depends on the underlying etiology. In the Western world, the major cause is drug-induced liver injury caused by

acetaminophen. Other commonly offending drugs include isoniazid (INH), antibiotics, anticonvulsants, and herbal medications. Less commonly, acute viral hepatitis (hepatitis A, B, D, and E) is a cause of ALF.

The severity of ALF is determined by simple biochemical tests. Elevated INR and conjugated bilirubin more than ten times the upper limit of normal imply severe disease. In patients with acetaminophen-induced liver failure, the King's College criteria are predictive of the severity of liver disease and the need for liver transplantation. In cases of non-acetaminophen-induced liver failure, a similar predictive model incorporating other factors, such as patient age and specific etiology of acute liver disease, is used. The best prognosis in ALF has been reported in cases of DILI (drug-induced liver injury) and acute HAV infection. A general approach to management of acute liver disease is shown in Fig. 2.5.

Alcoholic hepatitis is a severe complication of alcoholic liver disease. Patients present with nausea, vomiting, jaundice, and possibly fever, precipitated by a recent change in alcohol consumption. The short-term mortality is high (over 40% at 1 month).

Abdominal imaging

Ultrasound of the liver is an essential baseline test for the workup of liver disease. The test is quick, in many places readily accessible, and does not expose patients to radiation. However, the technique, and thus the results, are very operator dependent. Although there are no contraindications for ultrasound, obesity and massive ascites prevent optimal visualization of the liver. The sensitivity of ultrasound for detection of cirrhosis ranges from 40 to 90%, with a specificity of approximately 80%. The sensitivity for detection of fatty liver by ultrasound is high, but the test is unable to distinguish simple hepatic steatosis from active steatohepatitis. Ultrasound is indispensable for the detection of hepatocellular carcinoma (HCC). Please refer to Chapter 7 for further information on the imaging modalities to evaluate HCC.

Computed tomography (CT) is not recommended as a screening test for liver disease because it involves radiation and there is a risk of contrast-induced nephropathy. Magnetic resonance imaging (MRI) is another modality but it requires longer scan times and is not suitable for claustrophobic patients, those with metal implants, or those who cannot tolerate breath-holding. In patients with hereditary hemochromatosis, MRI may have a specific role in quantifying hepatic iron content and appears to be useful in monitoring response to chelation therapy.

Liver biopsy

Liver biopsy is the single most important test to evaluate of underlying etiology and severity of hepatic fibrosis. Liver biopsy remains a relatively safe diagnostic test if performed by experienced (trained) personnel. Although etiology of

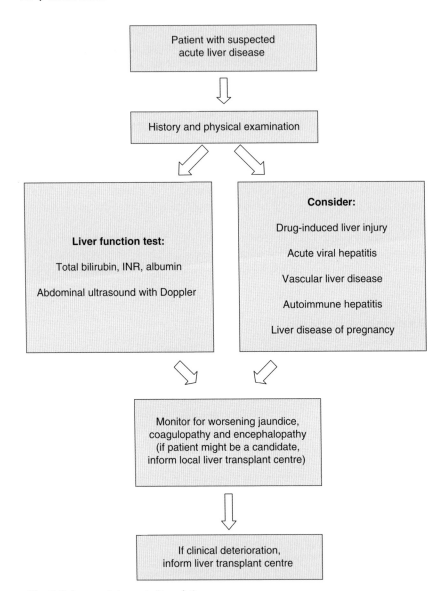

Fig. 2.5 Approach to acute liver failure.

the liver disease may often be ascertained by less invasive tests, an adequately sized (>2.5 cm on the slide from 15 gauge needle) biopsy interpreted by a hepatopathologist gives the most reliable diagnosis. Valuable information is obtained from the necroinflammatory score and grade of hepatic fibrosis (Table 2.3). Additionally, evaluation of the portal tracts documenting type of inflammatory cells and notation of abnormal deposits e.g. copper, amyloid, leukemia/lymphoma.

Table 2.3 METAVIR stage/grade for liver biopsy	
METAVIR grade/stage	**Description**
A1	Mild chronic hepatitis
A2	Moderate chronic hepatitis
A3	Severe chronic hepatitis
F1	Mild portal fibrosis
F2	Periportal fibrosis
F3	Severe bridging fibrosis
F4	Cirrhosis

Box 2.1 Requirements for out-patient liver biopsy

Co-operative and reliable adult patient

Adult accompaniment on day and night of biopsy

Dedicated nursing unit with experienced staff

Onsite blood bank facility in case of need for transfusion

Access to interventional radiology and hepatobiliary surgery for complications, if necessary

Access to in-patient bed for overnight monitoring if necessary

The major indications for liver biopsy include the following:
- to confidently establish etiology (sometimes more than one disease can be present);
- to establish liver disease severity (in terms of fibrosis) in those with no clinical evidence of liver failure;
- to guide the need for initiation or need to continue therapy in autoimmune hepatitis (AIH);
- to confirm the diagnosis of space-occupying lesion by guided biopsy;
- to exclude rejection in the postliver transplant patient.

There are several requirements for liver biopsy (Box 2.1). A dedicated nursing unit is optimal to monitor patients for at least 4 hours post procedure. Patients must be reliable, cooperative, and preferably to have eaten recently (then the gallbladder is empty). Ideally, patients should live within 1 hour (by car) of the hospital, and they must return if any symptoms related to bleeding develop, for example fainting, pain or overt bleeding from the site. Although there is a recent trend for interventional radiologists to perform an ultrasound-guided liver biopsy, studies do not convincingly show lower rates of complications following a guided biopsy. A 15-gauge Jamshidi aspiration needle is recommended to acquire a core of tissue at least 2.5 cm in length (11–15 portal tracts), which allows for accurate staging of fibrosis (Table 2.3). Underestimation of

Table 2.4 Comparison of non-invasive testing for detection HCV liver fibrosis

Test	Components	AUROC (F2–F4 vs. F0–F1)	Sensitivity (%)	Specificity (%)
APRI	AST, platelets	0.88	91	47
FibroTest	α-2 macroglobulin, haptoglobin, GGT, bilirubin, apolipoprotein	0.84	51	94
FibroMeter	α-2 macroglobulin, hyaluronic acid, AST, platelets, PT, urea	0.85	80	76
FibroScan	Tissue elastography	0.90	87	91

AST, aspartate aminotransferase; GGT, γ glutamine transaminase; PT, prothrombin time.

fibrosis occurs in at least 30% of patients when short and/or narrow (if an 18-gauge needle used) cores of liver tissue are obtained (as occurs with an ultrasound-guided needle).

The transjugular approach to the liver allows a liver biopsy to be conducted in those with ascites and/or significant coagulopathy. Liver tissue is obtained using a special needle that is passed into the right or left hepatic vein. This technique is also preferred if measurement of the hepatic venous pressure gradient (HVPG, wedged minus free hepatic venous pressure) is required. Clinically significant portal hypertension occurs when HVPG exceeds 12 mmHg. Cores of liver tissue obtained transjugularly are typically smaller and more fragmented, making accurate staging of fibrosis more difficult. The risk of hemorrhage is minimal but other complications such as cardiac arrhythmias, hepatic capsule perforation (needle track should routinely be plugged with gel or a foam plug at the end of the procedure if the capsule is perforated), and biliary–portal fistulae may occur (1–3%).

Contraindications and complications to percutaneous liver biopsy
There are only a few major contraindications to percutaneous liver biopsy (Box 2.2). Antiplatelet therapy, NSAIDs, and anticoagulants (prescribed such as warfarin and non-prescribed such as garlic or ginseng) should be discontinued 1 week prior to the procedure and resumed 2–3 days post biopsy. Pain or discomfort over the site of the biopsy or in the right shoulder occurs in 20% of patients. The risk of major bleeding—subcapsular or intrahepatic—requiring blood transfusion or surgery is 1 in 1000 to 5000 patients. The risk of mortality following a liver biopsy is very low (1 in 10 000–20 000). Several novel non-invasive tests have been developed for hepatitis C patients and may eventually reduce the need for liver biopsy (Table 2.4).

Box 2.2 Contraindications to percutaneous liver biopsy

Unco-operative patient

Ascites

INR >1.3 (due to any cause, e.g. anticoagulants)

Platelets <70 000/mm^3

Focal lesion lying in the path of the needle tract

Case study 2.1

A 53-year-old female of Greek descent is referred to the Liver Clinic for an isolated elevation of serum alkaline phosphatase (ALP) 195 IU/L. She complains of moderate fatigue and generalized pruritus over the last 6 months. She is otherwise healthy and on no medications. She is a non-smoker and consumes minimal amounts of alcohol. The family history was significant for diabetes mellitus in her mother and rheumatoid arthritis in a maternal aunt. Abdominal examination revealed a palpable spleen but no ascites or other masses.

The following blood tests were provided by her primary care physician:

Test	Value (normal)
ALT	48 IU/L (<30 IU/L)
AST	32 IU/L (<30 IU/L)
ALP	195 IU/L
Total bilirubin	11 μmol
INR	0.9
Albumin	40 g/L
Hemoglobin	121 g/L
WBC	4.5 billion/L
Platelets	127 billion/L

Abdominal ultrasound showed a slightly coarse liver with no focal liver lesions. There was mild splenomegaly but no ascites and extrahepatic bile ducts appeared normal.

Further workup revealed a positive antimitochondrial antibody, negative antinuclear antibody, and negative smooth muscle antibody. IgG and IgA levels were normal, but IgM level was elevated at 6.8 g/L. A diagnosis of primary biliary cirrhosis (PBC) was made. Staging of her disease was achieved via a liver biopsy. Classic features of primary biliary cirrhosis were seen and stage 4 fibrosis, that is cirrhosis, was confirmed histologically (predicted by her low platelet count). As osteoporosis complicates all chronic cholestatic liver disease and because she has biopsy-proven cirrhosis, bone mineral density testing and screening upper endoscopy were arranged. Treatment with ursodeoxycholic acid was initiated with a good response.

Case study 2.2

A 42-year-old male Caucasian financial planner was found to have abnormal liver enzymes on routine testing when he applied for life insurance. He was entirely asymptomatic aside from mild fatigue (overweight) particularly after working long hours. He was taking multivitamins on a daily basis and drank approximately 10 alcoholic drinks weekly. He admitted to injection drug use from the age of 19 to 23. There was a significant family history of cirrhosis in a paternal uncle who was known to be a heavy drinker. On examination, he had a small forearm tattoo. The abdominal exam showed mild hepatomegaly but no other stigmata of chronic liver disease.

The following blood tests were provided by his primary care physician:

Test	Value
ALT	76 IU/L
AST	58 IU/L
ALP	80 IU/L
Total bilirubin	9 μmol
INR	1.1
Albumin	42 g/L
Hemoglobin	150 g/L
WBC	5.1 billion/L
Platelets	200 billion/L

An abdominal ultrasound showed an enlarged fatty liver with no focal liver lesions. There was no splenomegaly or ascites and bile ducts appeared normal.

Further serologic workup revealed a positive hepatitis C antibody, and HCV RNA detectable at a level of 1.5×10^6 IU/mL, genotype 1a infection. Testing for HBsAg and HIV antibody was negative. A diagnosis of hepatitis C was made. FibroScan revealed a liver stiffness measurement of 19.6 kPa, suggesting cirrhosis. No esophageal or gastric varices were visualized on screening endoscopy. The patient undewent triple combination antiviral therapy and achieved a sustained virologic response.

Multiple choice questions

1. According to blood work below, which of the following patients has the poorest liver synthetic function?

	ALT (IU/L)	AST (IU/L)	INR	Total bilirubin (μmol)
A.	2500	3540	1.1	16
B.	58	64	0.9	12
C.	352	412	1.6	52
D.	98	75	0.5	26
E.	157	214	2.2	107

2. Cirrhosis secondary to chronic hepatitis C infection can be most accurately diagnosed by all of the following methods except:
   A. AST : platelet ratio
   B. Abdominal ultrasound
   C. FibroScan
   D. Liver biopsy
   E. FibroTest

3. Which of the following parameters is least helpful in determining the prognosis of a patient with cirrhosis?
   A. Hepatic encephalopathy
   B. Renal function
   C. INR
   D. ALP
   E. Ascites

4. A young male patient with ulcerative colitis is found to have an isolated elevated alkaline phosphatase level during routine blood work. What is the most likely diagnosis?
   A. Non-alcoholic fatty liver disease
   B. Hepatitis C
   C. Primary sclerosing cholangitis
   D. Hepatic amyloidosis
   E. Wilson disease

Answers

1. E
2. A
3. D
4. C

Further reading

Bedossa P and the METAVIR cooperative study group. An algorithm for the grading of activity in chronic hepatitis. Hepatology 1996; 24: 289–93.

Bravo AA, Sheth SG, Chopra S. Liver biopsy. N Engl J Med 2001; 344: 495–500.

Castera L, Forns X, Alberti A. Non-invasive evaluation of liver fibrosis using transient elastography. J Hepatol 2008; 48: 835–47.

Castera L, Vergniol J, Foucher J, et al. Prospective comparison of transient elastography, FibroTest, APRI and liver biopsy for the assessment of fibrosis in chronic hepatitis C. Gastroenterology 2005; 128: 343–50.

Child III CG, Turcotte JG. Surgery and portal hypertension. In: Child III CG, ed. The Liver and Portal Hypertension. Philadelphia: Saunders, 1964, pp. 50–64.

Ghent CN. Percutaneous liver biopsy: reflections and refinements. Can J Gastroenterol 2006; 20: 75–9.

Kamath PS, Wiesner RH, Malinchoc M, et al. A model to predict survival in patients with end-stage liver disease. Hepatology 2001; 33: 464–70.

Kim HC, Nam CM, Jee SH, et al. Normal serum aminotransferase concentration and risk of mortality from liver diseases: prospective cohort study. BJM 2004: 328: 986–6C.

Poynard T, McHutchison J, Manns M, et al. Biochemical surrogate markers of liver fibrosis and activity in a randomized trial of peginterferon alfa-2b and ribavirin. Hepatology 2003; 38: 481–92.

Prati D, Taioli E, Zanella A, et al. Updated definitions of healthy ranges for serum alanine aminotransferase levels. Ann Intern Med 2002; 137: 1–9.

Rockey D, Caldwell S, Goodman Z, et al. Liver biopsy. Hepatology 2009; 49: 1017–44.

Wai CT, Greenson JK, Fontana RJ, et al. A simple non-invasive index can predict cirrhosis in patients with chronic hepatitis C. Hepatology 2003; 38: 518–26.

Pediatric liver disease: an approach to diagnosis and assessment of severity

CHAPTER 3

Binita M. Kamath and Vicky L. Ng

University of Toronto, and Division of Gastroenterology, Hepatology and Nutrition, The Hospital for Sick Children, Toronto, Ontario, Canada

Key points

- The rapid growth of pediatric hepatology as a specific and focused field of interest is attributable to the importance of the dramatic physiologic variables occurring in the maturing liver, as well as recognition of the unique nature of the liver diseases that affect infants and children.
- As with adults, the assessment of liver disease in children requires a careful history and physical examination; however, further investigations are directed by likely diagnoses, which differ significantly by age. Infants and young children, in particular, require careful assessment for congenital and inherited metabolic diseases.
- The assessment of liver disease in children involves directed laboratory investigations, radiologic investigations, and often a liver biopsy. The interpretation of these data requires the input of pediatric subspecialists.

Introduction

As in adults, the adequate evaluation of an infant, child, or adolescent with suspected liver disease involves an appropriate and accurate history, a carefully performed physical examination, and skillful interpretation of signs and symptoms. Further evaluation is aided by judicious selection of diagnostic tests, and in pediatrics special consideration is given to the selection and timing of invasive investigations. The initial approach for the health-care provider first encountering a child with suspected liver disease may address some of the following issues, including: (1) is liver disease present and, if so, what is the nature of the liver disease; (2) what is the severity; and (3) is there specific

Hepatology: Diagnosis and Clinical Management, First Edition. Edited by E. Jenny Heathcote.
© 2012 John Wiley & Sons, Ltd. Published 2012 by John Wiley & Sons, Ltd.

treatment available. Subsequent considerations may include: (4) how to monitor the response to treatment; and (5) the prognosis of the liver disease.

Clinical presentations and common diagnoses

Asymptomatic elevation of liver transaminase levels

With routine laboratory testing now automated and so easily available, physicians often encounter the child with asymptomatic elevation of serum liver transaminase levels. Serum aminotransferase levels are sensitive indicators of liver cell injury and are helpful in recognizing hepatocellular diseases such as those caused by viral, drug-induced or autoimmune hepatitis, non-alcoholic fatty liver disease, or certain chronic liver diseases associated with metabolic conditions previously undiagnosed in the child. It is noteworthy to mention that the normal range for serum aminotransferase levels varies widely among laboratories, along with the recent realization that upper limits of normal may be too high for pediatric patients. This may result in missed opportunities to diagnose liver disease in children. If the results of repeated tests are abnormal, further evaluation is indicated to assess potential etiologic conditions (Box 3.1).

Box 3.1 Causes of asymptomatic elevation of serum aminotransferase levels in children

Hepatic causes
- Chronic viral hepatitis (hepatitis B, hepatitis C, hepatitis D)
- Medication (drug-induced hepatitis)
- Non-alcoholic fatty liver disease (NAFLD)
- Autoimmune hepatitis
- Alcohol
- Other autoimmune disorders such as systemic lupus erythematosus
- Metabolic disorders associated with chronic liver disease (in order of prevalence)
  - α_1-antitrypsin deficiency
  - Wilson disease
  - Tyrosinemia
  - Glycogen storage disease
  - Galactosemia

Non-hepatic causes
- Celiac disease
- Inherited disorders of muscle metabolism
- Acquired muscle diseases
- Cardiomyopathy (serum AST levels >> serum ALT levels)

Other
- Cystic fibrosis
- Other rare metabolic conditions: Niemann–Pick disease

A reliable body of literature to enable unequivocal recommendations for the diagnostic evaluation of children with abnormal liver chemistry tests is lacking.

Jaundice

Jaundice, when it affects children, most commonly presents in the first few months of life. The most common cause of jaundice in the neonate is physiologic and is manifested by predominantly unconjugated hyperbilirubinemia. Any infant jaundiced beyond 14 days of life warrants a fractionated serum bilirubin. Conjugated hyperbilirubinemia (>20% of total bilirubin) is always pathologic and requires assessment by a pediatric hepatologist. A discussion of unconjugated hyperbilirubinemia is beyond the scope of discussion here. Generally, in the assessment of conjugated hyperbilirubinemia, historical clues are unhelpful in the diagnosis, except to elucidate if the infant has recently been systemically unwell. There are a multitude of diagnoses that can cause jaundice before the age of 1 year, which typically present with conjugated hyperbilirubinemia (Box 3.2). Some of these diseases require a prompt diagnosis, for

---

Box 3.2 Diseases in infants and children commonly presenting with jaundice

Children <1 year of age
- Biliary atresia
- Choledochal cyst
- Alagille syndrome
- α_1-antitrypsin deficiency
- Progressive intrahepatic cholestasis (PFIC)
- Tyrosinemia
- Galactosemia
- Hypopituitarism/hypothyroidism
- Bacterial sepsis, particularly urosepsis
- Viral infections: cytomegalovirus, enterovirus
- Congenital infections: syphilis, rubella
- Hepatitis A in day care centers

Children aged 1–18 years
- Hepatitis A infection
- Autoimmune hepatitis
- Primary sclerosing cholangitis
- Choledochal cyst
- Obstructive gallstones (common bile duct stones, i.e. may never have been in gall bladder e.g. MDR3 mutation)
- Wilson disease
- Benign recurrent intrahepatic cholestasis (BRIC)
- Drug-induced: estrogens, erythromycin, acetaminophen

example biliary atresia, treatable metabolic disease, and it is therefore important to rule out these diagnoses without delay. In particular, it is optimal for a baby with biliary atresia to undergo corrective surgery before 60 days of age to maximize the likelihood of successful long-term survival with native liver. Infants with biliary atresia or a choledochal cyst may be jaundiced but look quite well clinically. Stool color is a key part of the history as both of these diagnoses lead to obstructive jaundice, which can cause a pale or acholic stool. Infants with Alagille syndrome may have evidence of cardiac involvement in association with jaundice. Infants with the metabolic diseases tyrosinemia, galactosemia, or hypopituitarism are likely to present early with jaundice and will often look unwell—there is a classic association of *Escherichia coli* sepsis in association with galactosemia. However, any bacterial infection can manifest with jaundice in the neonatal period. Urinary tract infections commonly present within the first 2 months of life with jaundice, lethargy, or poor feeding but rarely with fever. Children with progressive familial intrahepatic cholestasis (PFIC) present later (under 6 months) and have severe pruritus that is disproportionate to the degree of jaundice. The child will also often have evidence of failure to thrive.

Older children presenting with jaundice generally appear well. Children with hepatitis A infection may have a history of travel abroad or eating contaminated food. Children with obstructing gallstones may have a history of acute recurrent abdominal pain. Obstructing stones or a choledochal cyst often manifest with the classic triad of jaundice, pale stools, and dark urine. Primary sclerosing cholangitis and autoimmune hepatitis may present with non-specific symptoms of malaise and fatigue. There may be a positive family history of other autoimmune diseases. Children with inflammatory bowel disease in association with primary sclerosing cholangitis may report, when asked, altered bowel habits. A child with Wilson disease may have a history of neurologic symptoms or deterioration in school performance. Finally, patients with benign recurrent intrahepatic cholestasis (BRIC) reveal a history of intermittent jaundice, often with very severe pruritus. These episodes are followed by asymptomatic intervals and they never develop progressive liver disease.

Hepatomegaly, splenomegaly, and hepatosplenomegaly
Enlargement of the liver and/or spleen commonly occurs with many of the aforementioned causes of jaundice, as well as with any disease causing portal hypertension. This section will focus on etiologic conditions in which organomegaly rather than jaundice is the primary presenting feature. This is a large group of conditions, which may be primarily hepatic or extrahepatic (Box 3.3).

Storage disorders are important causes of pediatric liver disease. Glycogen storage diseases usually present with hepatomegaly and hypoglycemia. Gaucher disease is the most common lysosomal storage disease; the majority of cases are discovered because of hepatomegaly. Associated neurologic findings are only seen in a minority of cases. Niemann–Pick C is a disorder of lipid trafficking and is usually associated with symptomatic, progressive

---

Box 3.3 Disorders associated with liver and/or spleen enlargement in children

- Storage disorders
  - Glycogen storage diseases
  - Lysosomal disorders: Gaucher disease, Niemann–Pick C
- Portal vein thrombosis with cavernous transformation
- Metabolic liver diseases: α_1-antitrypsin deficiency
- Cirrhosis of any cause, e.g. fatty liver disease
- Congenital hepatic fibrosis
- Infection: chronic viral hepatitis, EBV infection
- Malignancy
  - Acute lymphoblastic leukemia
  - Hepatoblastoma
- Rheumatologic diseases, e.g. juvenile rheumatoid arthritis
- Hematologic disorders, e.g. sickle cell disease, hereditary spherocytosis

---

neurocognitive dysfunction such as clumsiness and poor school performance. Physical examination reveals splenomegaly and/or hepatomegaly in most instances.

Cavernous transformation of the portal vein following thrombosis is a relatively common cause of splenomegaly, with or without an initial presentation of gastrointestinal bleeding. This is described in more detail in Chapter 5. Congenital hepatic fibrosis is a fibrocystic disease of the liver, often related to autosomal recessive kidney disease but it can also be associated with other syndromes. This condition may also present with splenomegaly and/or gastrointestinal bleeding.

Fulminant liver failure

All health-care providers must be aware that children in acute liver failure may not fulfill the expected altered mental status criteria of hepatic encephalopathy required for the classic definition of fulminant liver failure in adults. In a pediatric patient with no known liver disease, who has an uncorrectable coagulopathy with clinical and/or biochemical evidence of acute liver injury, prompt admission is critical. Immediate initiation of appropriate supportive therapy focused on preventing or treating complications, and arranging for early referral to a pediatric transplant center, may be life saving.

A number of difficulties exist with applying the classic definition of "fulminant liver failure" in pediatric patients. Herein, "pediatric acute liver failure (PALF)" will be used interchangeably with fulminant liver failure. Firstly, hepatic encephalopathy is often difficult to recognize and diagnose in infants and small children, particularly in the early stages of illness, such that PALF may be present without clinical evidence of encephalopathy. Secondly, the presence of uncorrectable coagulopathy is an important (overt bruising may occur), consistent and reliable finding in children with PALF, even in the absence of hepatic encephalopathy. Thirdly, PALF can present in infants less than 8 weeks of age, and even during the first days of postnatal life. For these and other reasons, a consensus working definition for the clinical condition of acute liver failure in children was derived and currently being applied by the NIH funded Pediatric Acute Liver Failure (PALF) Study Group:

1 evidence of acute liver injury with no known prior evidence of chronic liver disease

   and

2 biochemical and/or clinical evidence of severe liver dysfunction as follows:

   (i) hepatic-based uncorrectable coagulopathy defined as an international normalized ratio (INR) of ≥1.5, despite the use of vitamin K (approximately a prothrombin time [PT] of 15s), in the presence of encephalopathy

   or

   (ii) INR >2.0 despite the use of vitamin K (approximately a PT >20s) even without encephalopathy.

Box 3.4 highlights important questions to ask in the history-taking assessment of a child presenting in acute liver failure. There are many possible etiologies of acute liver failure in children and these are best considered by age (Table 3.1). This then leads to a rationalization of the important diagnostic investigations (Box 3.5).

In conclusion, PALF is a serious and potentially devastating, although fortunately an infrequent, clinical condition. Prompt identification of treatable underlying causes and the institution of appropriate supportive and

---

Box 3.4 Important questions to ask in the assessment of a child presenting with acute liver failure

General history: timing of jaundice, fevers, rashes, behavioral/personality changes, tachypnea, recent weight gain (ascites), abdominal pain, sick contacts, history of international travel

Ingestions: over the counter drugs (including specific dosing, concentration and timing of all medications, especially acetaminophen), other herbs, mushrooms, naturopathic/homeopathic medications or vitamins. Be sure to ask ALL care providers of the child

Birth history: complications of pregnancy, neonatal sepsis with previous child, history of spontaneous abortions, early infantile death, siblings with metabolic conditions, parental consanguinity

Past medical history: bleeding or clotting tendencies, seizure disorder, developmental delays

Family history: liver diseases or metabolic syndromes, autoimmune conditions, malignancies, bleeding or clotting tendencies

Table 3.1 Conditions associated with acute liver failure at different ages

Etiology	Neonate	Infant	Child	Adolescent
	Patient age			
Drugs/toxins	Unusual	Acetaminophen, valproate, TMP/SMX	Acetaminophen, valproate, antibiotics (e.g. TMP/SMX, rifampin), lisinopril, mushrooms	Acetaminophen, valproate, TMP/SMX, rifampin, lisinopril, mushrooms
Metabolic syndromes	Galactosemia, tyrosinemia, HFI, urea cycle defects, neonatal hemochromatosis, mitochondrial disorders, bile acid synthesis defects, Niemann–Pick type C	HFI, fatty acid oxidation defects, bile acid synthesis defects, mitochondrial disorders, perinatal hemochromatosis, Niemann–Pick type C	Wilson disease, mitochondrial disorders, α_1-antitrypsin deficiency, Reye syndrome, Niemann–Pick type C	Wilson disease, fatty liver of pregnancy, Niemann–Pick type C
Infections	HSV, adenovirus, echovirus, Coxsackie virus, HBV, parvovirus B19, VZV, CMV, EBV, measles	HAV, HBV, NANB, adenovirus, EBV, echovirus, Coxsackie virus	Adenovirus, VZV, other herpes viruses (CMV, EBV), paramyxovirus, influenza virus, HAV, HBV, NANB	Adenovirus, VZV, other herpes viruses, paramyxovirus, influenza virus, HAV, HBV, HEV, NANB
Vascular/ischemic	Severe asphyxia, congenital heart disease, cardiac surgery	Myocarditis, severe asphyxia, cardiac surgery, congenital heart disease	Budd–Chiari syndrome, myocarditis, postoperatively, cardiomyopathy	Budd–Chiari syndrome, myocarditis, postoperatively, cardiomyopathy
Autoimmunity	N/A	N/A	Autoimmune hepatitis	Autoimmune hepatitis
Malignancy	Neonatal leukemia, hemophagocytic lymphohistiocytosis	Hemophagocytic lymphohistiocytosis	Hemophagocytic lymphohistiocytosis	Hemophagocytic lymphohistiocytosis

EBV, Epstein–Barr virus; HFI, hereditary fructose intolerance; HAV, hepatitis A virus; HBV, hepatitis B virus; HEV, hepatitis E virus; NANB, non-A, non-B hepatitis virus; VZV, varicella zoster virus; TMP/SMX, trimethoprim/sulfamethoxazole; PALF, pediatric acute liver failure.

> **Box 3.5 Important diagnostic investigations**
>
> Blood
> - Liver synthetic function tests: INR, glucose, albumin, ammonia, conjugated bilirubin
> - Tests of liver injury: ALT, AST, LDH, ALP, GGT
> - ABG/serum amino acids
> - Na, K, chloride, CO_2, Ca, Mg, phosphate, urea, creatinine
> - CBC with differential, blood type and screen, Coombs
> - Blood culture
> - Viral hepatitis serologies (anti-HAV IgM, HBsAg, anti-HBc IgM, anti-HEV and anti-HCV)
> - Autoimmune markers (ANA, ASMA, anti-LKM, immunoglobulin levels)
> - Ceruloplasmin level
> - Acetaminophen level and toxin screen
> - HIV serology
>
> Urine
> - Urine toxicology screen
> - Urine culture
> - Urine organic acids
> - 24-h urine collection for copper
> - Urine β-HCG
>
> Imaging
> - Abdominal ultrasound with Doppler
>
> Consults required
> - Pediatric ICU
> - Pediatric GI
> - Transplant center
> - Ophthalmology (Wilson disease)
> - Toxicology
>
> AP, alkaline phosphatase; ABG, arterial blood gas; β-HCG, β human chorionic gonadotropin; HIV, human immunodeficiency virus.

therapeutic measures are essential for optimization of the clinical management of PALF patients. Intensive support and liver transplant hold the greatest potential for survival.

Biochemical investigations

Common laboratory tests used to confirm or screen for liver disease include serum aminotransferase levels, alkaline phosphatase activity, and γ-glutamyl transpeptidase (GGT) levels. Often, the prothrombin time, albumin levels, and serum bilirubin levels are simultaneously determined. These tests are complementary and provide an estimation of hepatic synthetic and excretory functions. They may be helpful to guide the stratification of the disturbance. Hence, the sensitivity and specificity of screening laboratory tests in the detection of liver disease may be increased when used as a battery. When more than one test within a battery is serially abnormal the probability of liver disease increases. When all test results within the battery are normal, the probability of missing occult liver disease is lowered. Ultimately, the clinical significance of any liver chemistry test abnormality in a child must be interpreted in the context of the clinical setting.

Acute liver cell injury (parenchymal disease) in viral hepatitis, drug- or toxin-induced liver disease, shock, hypoxemia, or metabolic disease is best reflected in marked increases in serum aminotransferase activities. Even in situations where blunt abdominal trauma is a possible etiology, elevations in activity of these enzymes may provide an early clue to hepatic injury. Cholestasis (obstructive disease) involves regurgitation of bile components into serum; accordingly, the serum levels of total and conjugated bilirubin and serum bile acids will be elevated. Elevations in serum alkaline phosphatase and GGT are also sensitive indicators of obstructive processes or of inflammation of the biliary tract, including biliary atresia, cholelithiasis, and cholangitis, among others.

A predominant elevation in the conjugated fraction provides a relatively sensitive index of hepatocellular disease or hepatic excretory dysfunction. Hepatic synthetic function is reflected in prothrombin times and serum protein levels.

A markedly elevated level of in α-fetoprotein in the serum may suggest hepatoblastoma. Hypoalbuminemia caused by depressed synthesis may complicate severe liver disease and serve as a prognostic factor.

The severity of the liver disease may be reflected in:

1 clinical signs: worsening jaundice, onset of ascites, variceal hemorrhage, occurrence of hepatic encephalopathy (less common in children than in adults), apparent shrinkage of liver mass owing to massive necrosis or

2 biochemical alterations: persistent or worsening cholestasis/conjugated hyperbilirubinemia, marked hypoalbuminemia, prolonged prothrombin times or INR values unresponsive to parenteral administration of vitamin K, hypoglycemia, hyperammonemia, electrolyte imbalance.

Deficiencies of factor V and of the vitamin K-dependent factors (II, VII, IX, and X) may occur in patients with severe liver disease or acute liver failure (see previous section). If the prothrombin time is prolonged as a result of intestinal malabsorption of vitamin K (resulting from cholestasis) or decreased nutritional intake of vitamin K, then parenteral 2–10 mg administration of vitamin K should correct the coagulopathy leading to normalization within 12 h. Unresponsiveness to vitamin K suggests hepatic disease. Persistently low levels of factor VII are evidence of a poor prognosis in pediatric acute liver failure. Interpretation of serum ammonia values must be carried out cautiously because of variability in their physiologic determinants and the inherent difficulty in laboratory measurement (it must be an arterial blood sample, measured immediately).

Interpretation of biochemical tests of hepatic structure and function must be made in the context of age-related changes. For example, the activity of alkaline phosphatase varies considerably with age, reflecting predominantly the activity of the isoenzyme that originates in bone. An isolated increase in alkaline phosphatase particularly in children may *not* indicate hepatic or biliary disease, if other liver function tests results are normal, as levels of alkaline phosphatase from bone are normally elevated until the epiphyses are closed.

Radiologic investigations

Ultrasound
Diagnosis. An ultrasound with Doppler is an essential investigation in any child suspected of liver disease. This can be diagnostic (e.g. a choledochal cyst, cavernous transformation of the portal vein, or Budd–Chiari syndrome) or in other cases it may be suggestive of a diagnosis, such as the absence of a gallbladder and polysplenia, as seen in some cases of biliary atresia. Ultrasound cannot generally differentiate among conditions with homogenous enlargement of the liver; even the appearance of fat may be due to multiple underlying diagnoses. A mass can be readily identified on ultrasound, and in a few cases a particular diagnosis can be made, for example central scar in focal nodular hyperplasia.

Assessment of disease severity. Ultrasound also has a clear role in the assessment of liver disease severity. Certainly, in any progressive liver disease, an ultrasound is helpful to identify reversal in portal blood flow, increasing spleen size, and the presence of ascites. In severe liver disease, evolving cirrhosis of the liver and gastroesophageal varices may also be detected on ultrasound. Ultrasound also has a role in cancer screening in children with chronic liver disease, such as HBV.

Radionuclide scan (hepatoiminodiacetic acid [HIDA] or di-isopropyl iminodiacetic acid [DISIDA])
Diagnosis. This test relies on the uptake of a radioisotope by the liver and subsequent excretion into the bile. When this test is normal, extrahepatic biliary patency is established and biliary atresia is excluded. Therefore, this investigation is performed in infants with conjugated hyperbilirubinemia. Traditionally, this test has been performed after 5 days of oral administration of phenobarbital, though this is not mandatory and can lead to unnecessary delay in the work-up of a cholestatic infant.

Current pediatric guidelines suggest that radionucleotide scans are of limited value in the evaluation of cholestatic infant. A hepatitis from any cause can result in poor uptake of the tracer, making subsequent assessment of biliary excretion impossible. In the majority of infants with conjugated hyperbilirubinemia, a liver biopsy is more useful.

Assessment of disease severity. A radionuclide scan generally does not have any value in the assessment of liver disease severity.

Magnetic resonance cholangiopancreatography (MRCP)

Diagnosis. MRCP has a useful adjunct role in the diagnosis of some pediatric biliary disorders. It is not widely used in infants, as sensitivity is limited due to their small size. In older children who can remain still (if asked) for a prolonged period, MRCP can be helpful to delineate the anatomy of a choledochal cyst and to identify the extent of biliary involvement in primary sclerosing cholangitis. In congenital hepatic fibrosis an MRCP is a useful tool in evaluating the nature of biliary involvement—cystic dilatation of the intrahepatic tree in addition to congenital hepatic fibrosis is diagnostic of Caroli syndrome.

Assessment of disease severity. An MRCP generally does not have any value in the assessment of liver disease severity.

Invasive investigations

Liver biopsy

Diagnosis. Liver biopsy is the most sensitive and specific investigation in the diagnosis of pediatric liver disease. In many centers, liver biopsy is now performed under ultrasound guidance by interventional radiologists, rather than by the blind percutaneous approach by trained hepatologists. In experienced hands, the risk of bleeding and other complications is very low, even in small infants. A single pass is usually required to yield sufficient tissue for both light and electron microscopy (need to be put in two bottles as different preservatives required). Appropriate evaluation of the tissue by an experienced pediatric pathologist is vital. Obviously, it is necessary to make sure to correct any coagulopathy prior to the procedure.

Assessment of disease severity. Liver biopsies are not routinely performed to assess liver disease severity in pediatrics, for example chronic viral hepatitis.

Endoscopy

Diagnosis. Upper endoscopy is not a useful diagnostic tool in the evaluation of pediatric liver disease, other than in the event of a gastrointestinal bleed, in which case it is both a therapeutic and diagnostic tool. Colonoscopy is recommended in children with primary sclerosing cholangitis to identify subclinical inflammatory bowel disease even in the absence of overt gastrointestinal symptoms.

Assessment of disease severity. Children with liver disease do not routinely undergo upper endoscopy to identify esophageal varices and assess liver disease severity. Primary prophylaxis of variceal bleeding is not performed in children, thus upper endoscopy is only useful in select cases.

Intraoperative cholangiogram

This is the gold standard investigation in the evaluation biliary tree patency in an infant with conjugated hyperbilirubinemia and a suspected diagnosis of biliary atresia. This is the only role for this test.

Endoscopic retrograde cholangiopancreatography (ERCP)

ERCP has been described in infants in a few expert centers, but in general babies undergo a percutaneous transhepatic cholangiogram (PTC) or an intraoperative cholangiogram. In larger children, ERCP has value as both a diagnostic and therapeutic tool. In particular, it is useful in the management of primary sclerosing cholangitis, in the event of a dominant biliary stricture, stent placement can re-establish biliary drainage and reduce the progression of biliary fibrosis.

FibroScan

FibroScan is not routinely performed in children on a clinical basis.

Conclusions

The approach to pediatric liver disease rests on the same principles of history, physical examination, and appropriate investigations, as in adult medicine. However, in order to streamline the investigative approach appropriately, it is important to have an understanding of the different likely etiologies of a presentation by age, since these vary considerably. Furthermore, it should be appreciated that children usually manifest subtle clinical features of their disease, often until the process is quite advanced. Therefore careful attention must be applied to nuances in the history, such as poor feeding and lethargy in an infant or deteriorating school performance in an adolescent, and appropriate investigations arranged rapidly. This appreciation of subtleties is the cornerstone of success in the approach to pediatric liver disease.

Case study 3.1

A 6-week-old baby presents to an emergency room with persistent jaundice. She is the product of an unremarkable pregnancy and delivery and has been jaundiced since the first few days of life. She has no fever and is breast feeding and gaining weight well. Her stools are beige in color but there is some variability and sometimes they appear light yellow. The parents have been told by their family doctor that this is likely to be physiologic jaundice of the newborn and no laboratory investigations have been performed. On physical examination, she is icteric, with no dysmorphic features. She has no murmur and her abdomen is soft with 3 cm of hepatomegaly palpable below the xiphoid (no palpable splenomegaly).

Comment. This is the typical presenting scenario for biliary atresia. These infants look remarkably well and there is a temptation to reassure the parents and discharge them without further intervention. Since it is well established that the outcomes from Kasai portoenterostomy are best if surgery is performed before 60 days, it is imperative to perform baseline investigations in a child such as this. Laboratory tests did indeed reveal conjugated bilirubin 118 μmol/L, unconjugated bilirubin 48 μmol/L, ALT 109 IU/L, GGT 853 IU/L, INR 1.1. An abdominal ultrasound demonstrated polysplenia and the absence of a gallbladder, all very suggestive of biliary atresia. At this point, consultation with a pediatric hepatologist is essential and arrangements for a liver biopsy would be appropriate. It should also be noted that the variation in stool color is not unusual in infants with biliary atresia and lightly pigmented stools may also signify biliary tract disease.

Case study 3.2

A 10-year-old girl with no previous known medical conditions presents to her general pediatrician with a chief complaint of periumbilical abdominal pain for the past several months. History is notable for absence of vomiting, diarrhea, hematochezia, weight loss, or fever, with no prodromal illness. She has always been an excellent straight A student. Physical examination is notable for a palpable liver edge 2 cm below the right costal margin. Screening blood tests are ordered, and she is referred to the Liver Clinic for further investigations of a serum AST level 160 IU/L and ALT level of 148 IU/L. Further liver chemistry test results include alkaline phosphatase 454 IU/L, GGT 50 IU/L, serum albumin 46 g/L, conjugated bilirubin 0 μmol/L, unconjugated bilirubin 11 μmol/L, INR 1.2. All her hepatitis serology was negative, serum immunoglobulin levels normal, and serum autoantibodies negative. Serum ceruloplasmin level 109 (normal 264–473) mg/L, serum copper 7.7 (normal 13.2–21.4) μmol/L. The basal 24-h urinary copper excretion is 2.87 (reference normal is <0.6) μmol/24 h. Ultrasound shows coarse hepatomegaly and mild splenomegaly.

Comment. The spectrum of liver disease encountered in patients with Wilson disease can be highly variable, ranging from asymptomatic biochemical abnormalities to acute liver failure (see Chapter 23). As in this case, children may be entirely asymptomatic, with hepatic enlargement or abnormal serum aminotransferase levels found only incidentally. The degree of elevation of aminotransferase activity may be mild and does not reflect the severity of the liver disease. Modestly subnormal serum ceruloplasmin levels suggest further evaluation for Wilson disease is necessary. Basal 24-h urinary excretion of copper should be obtained in all patients in whom the diagnosis of Wilson disease is suspected. A slit-lamp examination by an experienced observer is required to identify Kayser–Fleischer rings in most patients, but these are not entirely specific for Wilson disease, being present in only 44–62% of patients with mainly hepatic disease at the time of diagnosis. Arrangement for a liver biopsy with quantification of hepatic parenchymal copper concentration is appropriate, in order to confirm a diagnosis of Wilson disease in this patient.

Multiple choice questions

1. Which of the following causes of neonatal cholestasis are the most important to identify and suspect on the FIRST patient encounter?
   A. Hypothyroidism
   B. Bacterial sepsis
   C. Galactosemia
   D. Biliary atresia
   E. All of the above

2. All of the following investigations are commonly used in the assessment of liver disease in children, except:
   A. Liver biopsy
   B. Radionuclide scan (HIDA/DISIDA)
   C. FibroScan
   D. Ultrasound
   E. MRCP

Answers

1. E
2. C

Further reading

Dhawan A. Etiology and prognosis of acute liver failure in children. Liver Transpl 2008; 14: S80–S84.

Mouzaki M, Ng VL. Acute liver failure in children. Clin Pediat Emerg Med 2010; 11: 198–206.

Moyer V, Freese DK, Whitington PF, et al. Guideline for the evaluation of cholestatic jaundice in infants: recommendations of the North American Society for Pediatric Gastroenterology, Hepatology and Nutrition. J Pediatr Gastroenterol Nutr 2004; 39: 115–28.

Schwimmer JB, Dunn W, Norman GJ, et al. SAFETY study: alanine aminotransferase cutoff values are set too high for reliable detection of pediatric chronic liver disease. Gastroenterology 2010; 138: 1357–64, 64 e1–2.

Natural history of the cirrhotic patient

CHAPTER 4

Jordan J. Feld

University of Toronto, and Division of Gastroenterology, Toronto Western Hospital, University Health Network, Toronto, Ontario, Canada

Key points

- Cirrhosis may be entirely asymptomatic with no clinical signs.
- Routine laboratory tests that may suggest underlying cirrhosis include: thrombocytopenia, hyperbilirubinemia, and hypoalbuminemia.
- Non-invasive tests (serum panels and transient elastography) are valuable to rule in or rule out cirrhosis.
- Decompensation of cirrhosis is often precipitated by infection, medications, and medical procedures (especially surgery).
- Child–Pugh–Turcotte Score and MELD score are used to assess prognosis in cirrhotic patients regardless of etiology.
- All patients with cirrhosis require screening for esophageal varices and ultrasound surveillance for hepatoma.
- Control of the underlying cause of liver disease may lead to fibrosis regression with "resolution" of cirrhosis; however, risk of hepatocellular carcinoma (HCC) persists.

Introduction

The diagnosis of cirrhosis is often first made when a patient develops overt signs of portal hypertension or liver failure; however, cirrhosis will usually have been present in an asymptomatic form for many years prior to the onset of clinical manifestations. Patients with well-compensated cirrhosis may have entirely normal liver synthetic function and no history of complications. Nevertheless, the presence of cirrhosis, even if clinically silent, has important prognostic implications and may significantly affect the course and management of other diseases. Thus a high index of suspicion is needed to recognize cirrhosis.

Hepatology: Diagnosis and Clinical Management, First Edition. Edited by E. Jenny Heathcote.
© 2012 John Wiley & Sons, Ltd. Published 2012 by John Wiley & Sons, Ltd.

The gold standard for the diagnosis remains liver biopsy with demonstration of discrete nodules surrounded by fibrous tissue. However, clinical and laboratory parameters can also be very suggestive of cirrhosis, as can radiological imaging. Recently, non-invasive assessments of hepatic fibrosis using panels of serum tests and transient elastography have been developed. Both correlate fairly well with liver biopsy, particularly in ruling in or ruling out cirrhosis. The advantages and disadvantages of the different diagnostic modalities will be discussed, followed by a description of the natural history of patients with cirrhosis, both with and without treatment of the underlying liver disease.

Diagnosis

History and physical examination in someone suspected of having cirrhosis

In patients with decompensated cirrhosis, the diagnosis is usually clinically obvious with the presence of ascites/edema, hepatic encephalopathy, and/or jaundice, whereas in well-compensated cirrhosis many patients have no symptoms or signs and therefore a high index of suspicion is necessary to recognize cirrhosis.

Even in patients with previous episodes of hepatic decompensation, the diagnosis may not be clear if neither the patient nor their physician relate their past symptoms to the liver. As a result, all patients with possible liver disease should be asked specifically about past or present:
- ascites
- ankle edema
- jaundice
- GI bleeding (melena, hematemesis)
- encephalopathy
- pruritus
- dyspnea
- non-specific symptoms (fatigue, unexplained weight loss/gain).

Patients may have difficulty distinguishing "abdominal bloating" from **ascites**. Increasing belt/pant size associated with increasing weight, persistence of the "abdominal swelling," and **ankle edema** are suggestive that the abdominal swelling is due to ascites. Patients and even family members may also not recognize **jaundice**, particularly when it develops slowly over time. However, the onset of darkening of the urine (± staining of underwear) is typically noticed. This is a useful clue to the first appearance of jaundice, which may help clarify if a specific incident occurred that may have precipitated worsening of the clinical condition. **Hepatic encephalopathy** may also be difficult to appreciate in its early stages. A reversal of the day/night sleep pattern with insomnia at night and daytime somnolence is often the first sign. Subtle impairments in memory and/or executive function should be corroborated by friends or family members. Focal neurological deficits are uncommon with encephalopathy but can occur and reverse with treatment. Persistence of the deficits despite improvement in cognition suggests other etiologies, such as a cerebrovascular event. **Pruritus** in patients with cirrhosis is most common in biliary diseases but may develop in patients with cirrhosis (or even acute hepatitis). Liver-related pruritus is generalized with no associated rash (although skin markings from excessive scratching may develop) and may be very severe. Pruritus may be exacerbated by certain medications, particularly estrogens and any other medications associated with cholestasis. **Dyspnea** is not a common symptom of cirrhosis but its presence may have important implications. Patients with ascites who develop shortness of breath may have progressed to **hepatic hydrothorax** due to defects in the diaphragm with resultant translocation of fluid from the abdomen to the thorax due to the lower intrathoracic pressure. Dyspnea may also signify the presence of **hepatopulmonary syndrome**[1] with intrathoracic right to left shunts. Classically in this setting, patients describe improvement in shortness of breath with lying down, so-called platypnea, thought to be due to a predominance of shunts in the lower lung fields. Dyspnea may also occur in **portopulmonary hypertension**, a condition in which pulmonary hypertension develops due to primary portal hypertension. Dyspnea may also be unrelated to cirrhosis. Patients may also complain of non-specific symptoms such as fatigue.

Physical examination should include a full examination with a particular focus on signs of chronic liver disease:

- hands: clubbing, Terry's nails (hypoalbuminemia), palmar erythema, muscle wasting, Dupuytren's contracture
- head and neck: scleral icterus (best seen in natural sunlight), parotid enlargement, temporal muscle wasting, hepatic fetor
- chest: spider nevi, pleural effusion (hydrothorax usually right-sided)
- cardiac: non-specific findings (low JVP, tachycardia, relative hypotension)
- abdomen: ascites (bulging flanks sensitive test, fluid wave specific test, other tests including shifting dullness), caput medusa (dilated superficial periumbilical veins), liver size (may be large or small), splenomegaly (by percussion using Castell's test or by palpation), hepatic bruit (may indicate HCC)
- neurological: asterixis, focal deficits
- extremities: pitting edema.

When evaluating patients who have signs of cirrhosis, it is important to consider the context in choosing the tests to perform. If the clinical suspicion for cirrhosis is low, the goal should be to use sensitive tests to rule out cirrhosis, with a move to more specific tests as the diagnosis seems more likely. This is best illustrated with tests for ascites and splenomegaly. Almost all patients with ascites have bulging flanks and thus this test has a high sensitivity, but many patients with bulging flanks are just obese without ascites and therefore this sign is not very specific. In contrast, only patients with fairly tense ascites have a positive fluid wave test meaning that it is not very sensitive, but this finding is present only in patients with peritoneal fluid and therefore is very specific. If a patient does not have bulging flanks, the examination for ascites can stop there, as this is the most sensitive test for the condition. There is no need to assess for shifting dullness or a fluid wave, both of which are more specific but less sensitive. In a patient with a protuberant abdomen, the fluid wave test is very helpful for confirming the presence of ascites. If available, a bedside ultrasound done by an experienced operator is both sensitive and specific. Similarly, Castell's sign (dullness to percussion in the last intercostal space in the midaxillary line upon inspiration) has a high sensitivity for splenomegaly but modest specificity, while palpation of the spleen is very specific but only possible with significant splenic enlargement and therefore is not very sensitive. Therefore if Castell's sign, the sensitive test, is negative, there is no need to try to palpate the spleen.

Liver biopsy

Biopsy remains the gold standard for assessing hepatic fibrosis and diagnosing cirrhosis. Biopsy may also provide information on the etiology of the underlying liver disease. Because of the small size of the sample, liver biopsy specimens are subject to sampling error. Biopsies of at least 2cm in length (after fixation, i.e. 3–4cm of fresh tissue) are required for accurate diagnosis. Although very significant fibrosis may be seen on the H&E stain, fibrosis is best appreciated on the Masson trichrome stain, which stains collagen green. The pattern of fibrosis differs by etiology of liver disease, but once cirrhosis is established the patterns may look very similar. Occasionally, if a biopsy is performed in the middle of a large macronodule, it may be difficult to appreciate the degree of fibrosis and cirrhosis may be missed; however, an experienced pathologist should recognize the histologic asymmetry. Alternatively, a superficial biopsy involving mostly liver capsule may overestimate the degree of fibrosis.

Liver biopsy may be performed percutaneously, with or without ultrasound guidance, or via the transjugular route. Transjugular biopsy allows liver tissue to be obtained in patients with impaired coagulation or thrombocytopenia because the biopsy site is within the liver and thus any bleeding will be tamponaded by the surrounding liver. With a percutaneous approach, a tract is made from the liver to the skin and thus if bleeding occurs, it may be very severe. The disadvantages of the transjugular approach are the use of smaller-gauge needles and the need to pass the catheter via the heart, increasing the risk of other complications. A major utility of the transjugular approach is the ability to measure **free and wedged hepatic vein pressures** to estimate portal pressure. The wedged hepatic vein pressure is an estimate of the transmitted portal vein pressure, similar to the concept of a pulmonary artery pressure approximating the left atrial pressure with a Swan–Ganz catheter. The difference in free and wedged hepatic vein pressure is referred to as the **hepatic venous pressure gradient** (HVPG). HVPG greater than 5mmHg indicates the presence of **sinusoidal portal hypertension**, the most common cause of which is cirrhosis. HVPG also correlates with the risk of complications. HVPG of greater than10mmHg is associated with development of ascites and increased likelihood of the presence of esophageal varices. Variceal hemorrhage does not occur with HVPG less than 12mmHg in the setting of cirrhosis. HVPG may underestimate the degree of portal hypertension in patients with cirrhosis if they also have a cause for **presinusoidal portal hypertension**, such as portal vein thrombosis or granulomatous liver disease (e.g. primary biliary cirrhosis or sarcoidosis). This is because the HVPG focuses only on the gradient across the liver. If the portal pressure is elevated before it reaches the liver (e.g. portal vein thrombosis), the gradient across the liver will still be normal despite the presence of presinusoidal portal hypertension. Similarly, patients with **postsinusoidal portal hypertension** (e.g. IVC web, heart failure, constrictive pericarditis, pulmonary hypertension) will have elevated free and wedged pressures but a normal gradient (HVPG) across the liver.

Imaging

Cirrhosis may be suggested by the contour and appearance of the liver on abdominal imaging; however, in early cirrhosis, the liver may look entirely normal on all types of imaging. Although fairly specific, imaging is quite insensitive for the diagnosis of cirrhosis. The diagnostic accuracy of imaging is improved if other factors are also taken into account. The presence of signs of portal hypertension suggesting cirrhosis include: splenomegaly, increased portal vein diameter, intra-abdominal varices, and patent umbilical vein.

Non-invasive testing

Serum tests

Numerous panels of serum tests have been developed to predict the presence of cirrhosis. Some rely on readily available laboratory tests, while others require specialized testing (see Table 4.1 and Chapter 2).

Most panels have good sensitivity and specificity for diagnosing or excluding cirrhosis but are less predictive for intermediate stages of fibrosis. The tests have been best validated in viral hepatitis (particularly HCV infection) and may not be as accurate in other causes of liver disease. Beyond the panels of tests, routine laboratory parameters can also be helpful in diagnosing cirrhosis. Progressive thrombocytopenia develops in the setting of cirrhosis and portal hypertension due to splenic sequestration and reduced hepatic thrombopoeitin production in advanced disease.[2] Patients with cirrhosis also develop a polyclonal hypergammaglobulinemia due to high titer antibodies to gut bacteria, which is secondary to portosystemic shunting. In most causes of chronic liver disease, the alanine aminotransferase (ALT) is elevated more than the aspartate aminotransferase (AST); however, as fibrosis progresses, the ratio ALT:AST changes. If the AST is greater than ALT, this is suggestive of advanced fibrosis or cirrhosis.

Transient elastography (TE)

TE uses modified ultrasound to evaluate the speed of propagation of a sound wave through the liver to estimate liver stiffness, which correlates with hepatic fibrosis. TE samples a greater area of the liver than liver biopsy and can be

Table 4.1 Serum tests to diagnose cirrhosis

Test	Components	Thresholds	AUROC	Sensitivity (%)	Specificity (%)
Fibrotest	α2-macroglobulin apo-lipoprotein A2 haptoglobin GGT Bilirubin Age Sex	>0.6 = F3 <0.3 = <F2	0.87	47 90	90 Not reported
APRI	AST Platelet count	>1.0 = F4 <0.5 = <F3	0.82	86 81	71 50
FIB-4	Age AST Platelet count ALT	>3.6 = F4	0.93	30	98
Forns	Platelet count GGT Cholesterol Age	>5.2 = F4	0.70	99	26

AST, aspartate aminotransferase; ALT, alanine aminotransferase; GGT, γ glutamyl transpeptidase.
FibroTest: proprietary
APRI: (aspartate aminotransferase to platelet ratio index) = ([AST/ULN]/platelet [10^9/L]) × 100
FIB-4: (age [years] × AST [IU/L])/(platelet [10^9/L] × ALT [IU/L]$^{1/2}$)
Forns: 7.811 − 1.131 × ln(platelet count) + 0.781 × ln(GGT) + 3.467 × ln(age) − 0.014 × (cholesterol)

easily performed in the out-patient setting, with immediate results. Liver stiffness continues to increase once cirrhosis is established and may provide prognostic information about the risk of developing complications. TE is inaccurate in the setting of ascites and may be difficult to perform in overweight patients. TE may also be falsely elevated in patients with acute hepatitis.

Natural history

Compensated cirrhosis refers to cirrhosis with preserved liver synthetic function (bilirubin, albumin, and INR) and no portal hypertension (no splenomegaly, varices, ascites) or other complications. Once complications develop, either acutely or chronically, **decompensated** cirrhosis is diagnosed and this has important prognostic implications. The likelihood of progressing from compensated to decompensated cirrhosis depends on the underlying etiology of liver disease but is also influenced by many other, sometimes external, factors. Patients with well-compensated, stable cirrhosis may develop acute decompensation with systemic insults, particularly infections, surgery/ anesthesia, sudden hemorrhage or any cause of profound hypotension (see below), and use of specific medications.

Cirrhosis used to be viewed as an irreversible state; however, recent evidence clearly shows that hepatic fibrosis regresses over time and even cirrhosis can be reversed with removal of the chronic liver insult (e.g. cure of hepatitis C infection, long-term suppression of hepatitis B, abstinence from alcohol, etc.). Regression of fibrosis reduces but does not eliminate the risk of development of complications, such as the risk of hepatocellular carcinoma (HCC).

Prognosis

The prognosis of cirrhosis is highly variable, depending on the etiology of liver disease, presence of complications, and comorbid diseases. Predictive models have been developed to help estimate the survival of patients with cirrhosis.

Child–Turcotte–Pugh score

The Child–Turcotte score was originally designed to predict outcome in patients undergoing portocaval shunting in the presence of cirrhosis and included: albumin, bilirubin, ascites, encephalopathy, and nutritional status. The score was modified for patients undergoing non-shunt surgery (Child–Pugh; Table 4.2). Nutritional status was removed as a parameter and the prothrombin time/ INR was added. The score only applies to patients with cirrhosis. The minimum score is 5 (i.e. 1 point for each factor assessed).
- Grade A (well compensated): score of 5–6
- Grade B (significant functional compromise): score of 7–9
- Grade C (decompensated disease): score of 10–15.

Table 4.2 Child–Pugh score

Factor	1 point	2 points	3 points
Albumin (g/L)	>35	28–35	<28
PT (>control, seconds)	<4	4–6	>6
INR	<1.7	1.7–2.3	>2.3
Bilirubin (μmol/L)	<17	17–34	>34
Ascites	Absent	Slight	Moderate
Encephalopathy	None	Grade 1–2	Grade 3–4

The Child–Pugh grade is predictive of 1- and 2-year survival:
- Grade A: 100% 1-year, 85% 2-year survival
- Grade B: 80% 1-year, 60% 2-year survival
- Grade C: 45% 1-year, 35% 2-year survival.

The Child–Pugh score is also predictive of mortality with abdominal surgery: Grade A 10%, Grade B 30%, and Grade C 82%.

Model for end-stage liver disease (MELD)

The MELD score was developed using regression modeling based on the 3-month survival of patients post-TIPS (transjugular intrahepatic portosystemic shunting) insertion. MELD score includes bilirubin, INR, and creatinine in the following formula:

$$\text{MELD score} = 3.8[\text{Ln serum bilirubin (mg/dL)}] + 11.2[\text{Ln INR}]$$
$$+ 9.6[\text{Ln serum creatinine (mg/dL)}]$$

The original version of the MELD score included points for the etiology of liver disease; however, this factor has now been removed. MELD is designed to have a minimum value of 3. Because logarithms are used, values below 1.0 are not permitted to avoid negative numbers. Hence the minimum values to be included are bilirubin 1 mg/dL, INR 1.0, and creatinine 1 mg/dL. This is often relevant for patients with early decompensation as creatinine values may be below 1.0 mg/dL because of low muscle mass. In such cases, MELD scores should be calculated using a creatinine of 1 mg/dL.

MELD has proven to be of prognostic utility in many circumstances and for most chronic liver diseases. It is now used for organ allocation on the liver transplant waiting list in the USA. Minimal MELD score for transplant is usually around 15. This is based on the fact that at a MELD of 15, the 1-year survival probabilities with and without a transplant become equivalent (80 vs. 81%). With lower MELD scores survival without a transplant is greater than with a transplant and for higher MELD scores transplantation improves survival.

Modifications to MELD. Modifications have been proposed including: inclusion of serum sodium concentration, serum albumin concentration, and different weighting of the bilirubin, INR, and creatinine. These modifications may ultimately be adopted for organ allocation. The MELD score is modified if HCC is present because patients may have poor survival based on the presence of HCC despite relatively preserved liver synthetic function, and thus low MELD scores. Very early tumors are not given extra MELD points. Tumors of 2–5 cm or two to three lesions of less than 3 cm are assigned a MELD score of 24 (15% mortality at 3 months) and the score increases every 3 months equivalent to an increase of 10% risk of mortality. The number of MELD points at each interval differs based on the severity of disease at the time of evaluation because the

MELD score is not linear, with small absolute differences in MELD score predicting greater changes in mortality rate at higher baseline MELD scores (e.g. a change of MELD from 9 to 11 is of less significance than from 24 to 26).

MELD has also been validated as a predictor of survival in the following conditions:
- alcoholic hepatitis
- hepatorenal syndrome (MELD >20 predicts worse survival)
- acute variceal hemorrhage in cirrhotic patients
- sepsis in cirrhotic patients as long as unrelated to spontaneous bacterial peritonitis
- abdominal, orthopedic, and cardiac surgery in known cirrhotic patients.

Clinical stages of cirrhosis: prognosis

The Baveno classification system categorizes patients with cirrhosis based on clinical factors only, which have proven to be useful for prognostication at the population level.[3]

Stage 1: uncomplicated cirrhosis (no varices/ascites)

Stage 2: cirrhosis with varices (no ascites or bleeding)

Stage 3: cirrhosis with ascites with or without varices

Stage 4: cirrhosis with GI bleeding with or without ascites.

Stages 1 and 2 are compensated while Stages 3 and 4 have signs of decompensation.

Registry studies suggest that the risk for decompensation is greatest in the first year after diagnosis of cirrhosis. This is likely due to bias with early decompensation leading to the initial diagnosis. However, based on these data, after adjusting for age and gender, 31% (95% CI 29–33%) of patients decompensate in the first year after diagnosis. Rates of decompensation are higher for alcohol-related cirrhosis (38%) than non-alcohol-related cirrhosis (25%) in the first year after diagnosis.

Beyond the first year after diagnosis, rates of decompensation are much lower with rates of 7.3% per year reported for those with alcohol-related cirrhosis and 5.5% per year for those with cirrhosis from other etiologies. Patients in Stages 1 or 2 have an approximately 7% chance of death within 1 year, without first progressing to decompensated disease (Stages 3/4) (i.e. predominantly non-liver-related mortality). In contrast, patients in Stages 3 or 4 have an 18–20% chance of death within 1 year.

Patients in Stages 1 or 2 progress to Stages 3 or 4 at a rate of 17–20% within 1 year. Over longer follow-up, patients in Stages 1 and 2 have a 13–15% chance of death without first progressing to decompensation (predominantly non-liver-related mortality). This suggests that these patients truly have compensated cirrhosis and means that they are likely dying of causes not directly related to their liver disease. These data are largely derived from patients with alcohol and viral hepatitis-related liver disease. Patients with autoimmune liver disease have a much slower rate of progression and these data likely do not apply.

Practical considerations for patients with cirrhosis

Patients with cirrhosis may remain stable for many years if they can avoid insults that acutely worsen their condition. Avoiding specific insults is often as important to prevent decompensation of liver disease as treating the underlying conditions. It is critical to explain to patients with cirrhosis that they must take precautions to prevent their liver disease from getting worse. This is particularly true for patients with well-compensated disease who are likely entirely asymptomatic.

Patients should be advised to inform all doctors and dentists with whom they interact that they have cirrhosis, as this information may affect many aspects of their clinical care. Patients with cirrhosis should be advised of the following (providing patients with a card to give to all relevant practitioners is often useful):

1 Complete abstinence from alcohol is required.
2 If pain or fever medications are required, acetaminophen is the preferred agent. Up to 2 g of acetaminophen (four extra-strength tablets) per 24 hours are safe but it is important for all cirrhotic patients to read labels because some people will be given multiple, different medications that contain acetaminophen. The total dose per day cannot exceed 2 g.
   Explanation: Acetaminophen is safe in patients with liver disease. Confusion often arises by the fact that overdoses of acetaminophen cause liver failure; however, standard doses (up to 2 g per day) are well tolerated. A common cause for acetaminophen overdose is inadvertent consumption of multiple acetaminophen-containing agents.
3 Non-steroidal anti-inflammatory agents, such as ibuprophen, naproxen, and aspirin, *should be avoided*, particularly in patients with ascites.
   Explanation: Renal perfusion in patients is very dependent on prostaglandin-mediated vasodilation. Prostaglandin inhibition due to NSAID use can precipitate renal failure, particularly in patients with ascites. GI bleeding is a secondary but less important concern.
4 Aminoglycoside antibiotics should be avoided.
   Explanation: Aminoglycosides may precipitate renal failure in patients with cirrhosis, particularly those with ascites.
5 *If surgery is required*, patients must inform surgeons or dentists that they have cirrhosis and advise them to contact the primary liver doctor prior to the procedure (see Boxes 4.1 and 4.2).
   Explanation: As discussed below, surgery may precipitate hepatic decompensation. Care must be taken to avoid hypotension during induction of anesthesia. Alternatives to general anesthesia are preferred if feasible. Ascites may develop postoperatively in patients with cirrhosis due to fluid shifts and excessive use of both colloid and/or crystalloid replacements. Electrolyte imbalances, particularly hypokalemia and alkalosis, postoperative ileus, and the use of opioids may precipitate hepatic encephalopathy. The risk of postoperative infection is increased. Patients with advanced disease, that is

Box 4.1 Practice points: optimizing medical therapy for cirrhotic patients going for surgery

Any operation in a cirrhotic patient carries an increased risk of mortality: Child's C > B > A, mostly as a consequence of hypotension.

Medical optimization:

- Avoid any surgery in patients with acute severe hepatitis or Child's C cirrhosis.
- Replace fluid loss with colloids (blood/albumin), minimal normal saline should be given as this will immediately lead to the formation of ascites.
- Avoid benzodiazepines, aminoglycosides, and NSAIDs (use acetaminophen). Proton pump inhibitors should only be used if necessary because of the associated increased risk of infection in this population.
- All patients need treatment of any infection as soon as it is suspected.
- Electrolyte abnormalities, particularly hypokalemia and metabolic alkalosis, should be corrected to reduce the chance of cardiac arrhythmias and hepatic encephalopathy.
- Reduce chance of hepatic encephalopathy by preventing constipation and carefully monitoring the use of opioids.
- Evaluate and monitor renal function throughout hospital stay; i.v. furosemide should be avoided.

Box 4.2 Memo for individuals known to have cirrhosis

You have cirrhosis, so you *must remember*

1 Do not drink alcohol
2 Do not take aspirin or arthritis pills
   Note: for pain or fever it is safe to take Tylenol (acetaminophen) in prescribed doses
3 Do not take sleeping pills/sedatives/or cough syrups that contain codeine or medications that contain narcotics—example: Percocet, Tylenol with codeine (Tylenol 1, 2, 3)
4 Do not add salt to your food or eat salty food (see Table 6.1)
5 Avoid antibiotics called aminoglycosides (example: gentamycin or tobramycin)
6 If you need surgery, discuss with your liver doctor first
7 If you have varices, do not use Viagra or other similar medications
8 Call your doctor if you have black stools
9 Make sure an ultrasound appointment is booked every 6 months
10 Arrange to get your Hep A and B vaccinations
11 Any infection must be treated immediately
12 Wear a medic alert bracelet indicating cirrhosis

those with thrombocytopenia and an elevated INR, may have an increased risk of perioperative bleeding. Patients with cirrhosis should receive standard deep vein thrombosis prophylaxis irrespective of the platelet count and INR as there is an increased rate of deep vein thrombosis in cirrhotic patients, likely due to a reduction in endogenous anticoagulants such as protein C and S.

6 Acid-suppressing medications should not be taken unless clearly necessary.

Explanation: Proton-pump inhibitors have been associated with an increased risk of spontaneous bacterial peritonitis in patients with ascites. If indicated, proton pump inhibitors can be safely used; however, it is important to consider the indication and consider alternatives if available (e.g. prokinetics for reflux disease). H_2-blockers should also be avoided unless necessary.

7 Patients with cirrhosis are at much higher risk for bacterial sepsis and tolerate infections very poorly. Jaundice with or without other signs of decompensation may be the first sign of sepsis. Patients may have relatively few signs and symptoms. Notably, white blood cell (WBC) results in the "normal range" may be elevated in patients with cirrhosis because of baseline low WBC levels due to splenomegaly. Treating physicians should have a low threshold for antibiotic therapy in patients with possible sepsis, even if cultures are negative.

Explanation: The liver plays a major role in clearing pathogens, particularly enteric bacteria which may enter the portal blood stream. Bacterial translocation increases with portal hypertension. Sepsis may exacerbate existing hemodynamic abnormalities present in cirrhosis, which may precipitate renal failure and other complications.

Required screening tests in patients with cirrhosis

Hepatocellular carcinoma (HCC) surveillance

HCC screening should be performed with ultrasound every 6 months (more frequent screening is of no benefit). There is no evidence that screening with computed tomography (CT) or magnetic resonance imaging (MRI) adds significant benefit to screening and in addition to the increased cost, CT also adds a significant exposure to radiation and i.v. contrast. These tests should only be done to investigate lesions first seen on ultrasound. Because ultrasound is very operator dependent, it is preferable to use the same ultrasound facility for all screening, ideally in a center with an interest in liver disease. α-Fetoprotein (AFP) may also be used for HCC screening; however, it has poor sensitivity and specificity and recent guidelines do not recommend its use as a screening test. Many HCCs do not produce AFP, and AFP is often elevated in patients with active hepatitis (especially viral hepatitis), and therefore mild elevations are particularly non-specific. If a mass is identified on ultrasound, a significantly elevated AFP (e.g. >200 ng/mL) supports the diagnosis of HCC. Ultrasound screening also allows for detection of mild ascites before it is clinically detectable.

Esophageal variceal screening

Initial variceal screening with gastroscopy should be done in all patients with cirrhosis, particularly those with platelet counts less than 200 000/μL. If no varices are seen, the test should be repeated every 2 to 3 years. Once varices are detected, the test should be repeated annually to assess for an increase in the size of varices and the need for prophylaxis with non-selective beta-blockers. The latter should be started for Grade 3 varices or varices with any high-risk features (red marks).[4] Once patients are on beta-blockers, provided the heart rate is less than 60 bpm and patients are compliant, there is no need for further variceal screening in the absence of bleeding. For patients intolerant of beta-blockers or those with very large varices with high-risk features, primary prophylaxis with variceal band ligation should be considered. Although band ligation is at least as effective as beta-blocker therapy, there is a small but finite risk of complications with the endoscopic procedure and therefore beta-blockers are still used as first-line therapy. Patients with granulomatous liver diseases (sarcoid, primary biliary cirrhosis) may have portal hypertension out of keeping with their degree of fibrosis due to a presinusoidal component to the elevated portal pressure and rarely may develop varices prior to the development of cirrhosis.

Laboratory testing

Parameters of liver synthetic function and renal function must be monitored: bilirubin, INR, albumin, creatinine, and electrolytes (in patients with ascites). These tests should be done in patients with cirrhosis on at least an annual basis to allow for calculation of MELD score to predict prognosis and timing of liver transplantation.

Diagnostic paracentesis to exclude spontaneous bacterial peritonitis

Any patients with cirrhotic ascites presenting to an unscheduled medical visit should have an immediate diagnostic paracentesis to exclude spontaneous bacterial peritonitis because up to 50% of patients are entirely asymptomatic (Table 4.3).

Management of patients with cirrhosis after successful treatment

Liver diseases with effective treatments that can be given to patients with cirrhosis include hepatitis C, hepatitis B, and alcohol and autoimmune liver disease. The natural history of cirrhosis is markedly different after resolution of the underlying liver disease.

Table 4.3 Routine monitoring required in patients with cirrhosis

Screening indication	Test	Frequency	Notes
HCC	Ultrasound AFP	Every 6 months Only if mass seen on ultrasound; unreliable as screening test	
Varices	Gastroscopy	Every 2 years Increase to annual once varices detected	Patients treated with non-selective beta-blockers do not require ongoing variceal surveillance
Liver function	INR, bilirubin, albumin, creatinine	At least annually for assessment of MELD and prognosis	
Spontaneous bacterial peritonitis	Ascitic fluid for cell count	Every unscheduled medical visit in patients with ascites	Up to 50% entirely asymptomatic

AFP, α-fetoprotein; MELD, Model for End-stage Liver Disease.

Hepatitis C post sustained virological response (SVR)

Patients who have achieved sustained viral eradication with antiviral therapy must continue to be followed if they had underlying cirrhosis prior to therapy. Post SVR, the outcome of cirrhosis is much improved.[5] There is no progression of portal hypertension or synthetic dysfunction (in the absence of other hepatic insults, e.g. alcohol). Therefore, if varices were not present prior to therapy, they do not develop post-SVR and screening is unnecessary. The only major concern post SVR is the persistent, albeit lower, risk of HCC. Patients with cirrhosis (and arguably with F3 fibrosis) prior to therapy may develop HCC after SVR. Consequently, these patients require continued HCC surveillance with ultrasound every 6 months. Whether patients can eventually stop surveillance, particularly if regression of fibrosis occurs, is unknown.

Hepatitis B with HBsAg clearance

Patients with HBsAg clearance prior to age 50 (whether treatment induced or spontaneous) have a very good long-term prognosis. Following HBsAg clearance, complications of cirrhosis do not occur unless either HBsAg reappears (with immunosuppression) or another hepatic insult occurs (fatty liver/ alcohol). Notably, however, even with suppression of HBV DNA to undetectable levels without clearance of HBsAg, complications of cirrhosis, particularly HCC, may develop.

Hepatic fibrosis may regress over time in patients with inactive disease (either spontaneous or treatment induced). Repeat biopsy may no longer show cirrhosis; however, even with regression of fibrosis, the risk of HCC still exists. The risk of HCC is likely lower after HBsAg clearance but surveillance ultrasound is still required because cirrhosis is present.

Abstinence from alcohol

In addition to minimizing further hepatic injury, abstinence may result in improvements in liver synthetic function, portal hypertension, and even hepatic fibrosis. In patients with decompensated alcoholic cirrhosis, complete abstinence may lead to a significant reduction in portal pressure. Portal pressure is often increased in alcoholic cirrhosis more than in other kinds of cirrhosis because the inflammation of acute on chronic alcohol injury can worsen portal hypertension due to edema and sinusoidal compression.

With the reduction in portal pressure, ascites, encephalopathy, and esophageal varices may all improve. Improvements in liver function plateau by 6 months in most patients. If patients remain decompensated despite abstinence, liver transplantation should be considered. In stable patients with alcohol-related cirrhosis who have remained abstinent, ongoing HCC and variceal surveillance is recommended.

Treated autoimmune hepatitis (AIH)

Even patients with severe AIH and cirrhosis usually show dramatic improvements with steroid therapy. Once the disease is quiescent, it may remain stable for years. Some evidence suggests that fibrosis may regress in treated patients with cirrhosis.

Flares of disease may occur with medication withdrawal or non-compliance, or during pregnancy or shortly following delivery, which can lead to decompensation in patients with cirrhosis. The risk of HCC with AIH is much lower than with viral or alcohol-related cirrhosis.

Complications of cirrhosis

See Chapter 5.

Case study 4.1

A 47-year-old man with hepatitis C infection genotype 3 was treated successfully with peginterferon and ribavirin and achieved a sustained virological response (SVR). Prior to therapy, laboratory investigations revealed an elevated ALT (74 IU/L) and AST (123 IU/L), with a bilirubin of 12 μmol/dL, albumin of 36 g/L, and INR of 1.2. Renal function was normal (CrCl 65 mL/min) and CBC was notable only for a

(Continued)

platelet count of 105000/μL. Following treatment, his ALT and AST normalized to 19 IU/L and 24 IU/L, respectively. Ultrasound imaging of the abdomen was reported as normal.

Comment: Although this patient has achieved an SVR, effectively a viral cure of HCV infection, he likely had cirrhosis (judged by his low platelet count) prior to treatment and therefore needs ongoing follow-up. His risk of hepatic decompensation is negligible (unless for some reason he has a secondary insult) but he is still at increased risk of development of HCC and therefore requires ongoing screening with 6-monthly ultrasound examinations. He does not need variceal screening as varices do not develop or enlarge after SVR in the absence of another source of liver injury.

As treatment response rates continue to improve with new therapies for HCV, pretreatment liver biopsies are likely to be performed less frequently. Consequently, a high index of suspicion will be required to identify patients with compensated cirrhosis. The low platelet count and AST greater than ALT are suggestive of advanced fibrosis in this case. Ultrasound is insensitive and cannot be relied upon to identify early cirrhosis. Non-invasive assessments of fibrosis such as transient elastography (FibroScan) or serum panels (FibroTest, APRI, FibroSure, etc.) will be helpful additions. Hopefully, recognition of factors that increase the risk of HCC post-SVR will help identify patients at highest risk to ensure that ongoing HCC screening is done in a cost-effective manner.

Case study 4.2

A 53-year-old man develops marked confusion, low-grade fever, and anasarca 2 days after a routine right hemicolectomy for an early-stage colon cancer. The patient was not known to have any significant past medical history aside from mild hypertension and obesity. He had no known history of liver disease or cognitive impairment. He took hydrochlorothiazide and simvastatin but was on no other regular medications. According to the surgical record, there were no intraoperative complications and no overt signs of portal hypertension were recorded. He is febrile at 38.2°C but the surgical wound looks clean. He has gross ascites and peripheral edema and is disoriented to time and place. Laboratory tests before surgery were notable only for a platelet count of 107000/μL with mildly elevated ALT (48 IU/L) and AST (58 IU/L) but normal bilirubin and creatinine. Repeat investigations reveal an ALT of 52 IU/L, AST of 68 IU/L, ALP of 110 IU/L, bilirubin of 78 μmol/dL, albumin of 32 g/L, and INR of 1.46 with a creatinine of 183 μmol/L (baseline 74 μmol/L).

Comment: This patient has developed acute hepatic decompensation following a routine abdominal surgery. Patients with cirrhosis are at high risk of decompensation with even relatively routine surgeries, particularly intra-abdominal procedures. This patient had only subtle laboratory abnormalities to suggest cirrhosis prior to surgery and was clearly well compensated. Even patients with Child's A cirrhosis with normal synthetic function and no portal hypertension have an approximately 10%

risk of perioperative mortality. This risk increases to 40% for patients with Child's B cirrhosis and may be as high as 70–80% for those with marked decompensation (Child's C) preoperatively. The MELD score can also be used to predict risk. Factors that increase the risk of perioperative decompensation include hypotension at the time of induction of anesthesia or anytime during surgery, fluid overload, particularly with saline postoperatively, and perioperative infections. This patient has developed ascites and needs to have a diagnostic paracentesis to exclude spontaneous or secondary bacterial peritonitis. Even if cultures are negative, he should be treated for presumed sepsis. The cause for cirrhosis should be investigated as well, likely nonalcoholic steatohepatitis (NASH) in this man with metabolic risk factors but no other known risks for chronic liver disease.

Multiple choice questions

1. After successful eradication of HCV (sustained virological response) in patients with underlying cirrhosis, patients:
   A. Do not require any further follow-up
   B. Should continue with variceal surveillance
   C. Are at continued risk of HCC and require ongoing ultrasound surveillance
   D. Will always have cirrhosis because fibrosis is irreversible

2. Common precipitants for hepatic decompensation include all of the following except:
   A. Laparoscopic cholecystectomy
   B. Urinary tract infection
   C. Acetaminophen 2 g per day for back pain
   D. Ibuprophen 800 mg p.o. t.i.d. for back pain
   E. Variceal hemorrhage

Answers

1. C
2. C

References

1. Umeda N, Kamath PS. Hepatopulmonary syndrome and portopulmonary hypertension. Hepatol Res 2009; 39: 1020–2.
2. Qamar AA, Grace ND, Groszmann RJ, et al. Incidence, prevalence, and clinical significance of abnormal hematologic indices in compensated cirrhosis. Clin Gastroenterol Hepatol 2009; 7: 689–95.

3. Fleming KM, Aithal GP, Card TR, et al. The rate of decompensation and clinical progression of disease in people with cirrhosis: a cohort study. Aliment Pharmacol Ther 2010; 32: 1343–50.
4. Garcia-Tsao G, Bosch J. Management of varices and variceal hemorrhage in cirrhosis. N Engl J Med 2010; 362: 823–32.
5. Veldt BJ, Heathcote EJ, Wedemeyer H, et al. Sustained virologic response and clinical outcomes in patients with chronic hepatitis C and advanced fibrosis. Ann Intern Med 2007; 147: 677–84.

Management of complications of portal hypertension in adults and children: variceal hemorrhage

CHAPTER 5

E. Jenny Heathcote,[1] Simon Ling,[2] and Binita M. Kamath[2]

[1] Division of Gastroenterology, Toronto Western Hospital, University Health Network, University of Toronto, Toronto, Ontario, Canada
[2] University of Toronto, and Division of Gastroenterology, Hepatology and Nutrition, The Hospital for Sick Children, Toronto, Ontario, Canada

Key points

- All adult patients known or suspected to have cirrhosis require esophagogastroduodenoscopy (EGD) to check for the presence of varices.
- All adult cirrhotic patients with medium or large varices, and even those with small varices with red spots or red wale marks, should be prescribed long-term prophylactic treatment with a non-selective beta-blocker to reduce the risk of a variceal bleed. Patients with contraindications to or adverse effects of beta-blockers should be treated with prophylactic endoscopic variceal ligation (EVL).
- Application of screening endoscopy and primary prophylactic therapy for children with portal hypertension should only be undertaken in consultation with a specialist pediatric hepatologist, because relevant studies in children have not yet been undertaken.
- Management of presumed variceal hemorrhage in adults and children requires careful volume replacement and treatment with a vasoactive drug (e.g. octreotide or terlipressin), intravenous third-generation cephalosporins, and a proton pump inhibitor. Urgent upper pan endoscopy is required and optimally if the patient is bleeding at the time of the procedure the patient should be intubated prior to EVL.
- Prevention of repeat variceal bleeding episodes is most successful with a combination of non-selective beta-blocker therapy and follow-up endoscopy with EVL until varices are completely eradicated. Thereafter, non-selective beta-blocker therapy needs to be maintained long term (proven value in adults only).

(Continued)

Hepatology: Diagnosis and Clinical Management, First Edition. Edited by E. Jenny Heathcote.
© 2012 John Wiley & Sons, Ltd. Published 2012 by John Wiley & Sons, Ltd.

- Definitive treatment of the cause of portal hypertension should be considered in selected patients (e.g. portosystemic shunt surgery or liver transplantation for those with cirrhosis and in children with portal vein thrombosis, meso-left portal vein bypass surgery should be considered).
- A poor outcome can be predicted in adults by their age older than 60 years, their MELD score more than 18, presence of encephalopathy, or an hepatic venous pressure gradient (HVPG) more than 20 mmHg.

Box 5.1 Other causes of upper gastrointestinal bleed in a cirrhotic

- Esophagitis (often in an immune compromised individual)—may or may not suffer heartburn; esophagitis itself is not a cause of variceal rupture
- Peptic ulcer disease (stomach or duodenum) is not unusual in cirrhotic patients
- Any other cause of upper gastrointestinal bleeding

Introduction

Portal hypertension with variceal bleeding is an important cause of morbidity and mortality in both children and adults with liver disease. In children with liver disease due to biliary tract disease, portal hypertension usually manifests early in their clinical course, prior to the onset of hepatic insufficiency. In adults, the predominant cause of portal hypertension is cirrhosis—the etiology being very closely related to geographic region, for example alcohol liver disease, non-alcoholic fatty liver (NAFL), and hepatitis C in the West and chronic viral hepatitis B or C in the East. As in children, in adults with chronic biliary disease (e.g. primary biliary cirrhosis and primary sclerosing cholangitis) variceal hemorrhage may take place prior to there being overt cirrhosis. It is not unusual for a patient who is bleeding from esophageal and/or gastric varices to have a second pathology, which could also present as hematemesis. Hence the need to fully establish the cause of gastrointestinal bleeding (Box 5.1).

Pathogenesis of portal hypertension (Fig. 5.1, Box 5.2)

Non-cirrhotic portal hypertension: prehepatic, presinusoidal

This results from an obstruction of the portal venous flow to the liver, most often secondary to a thrombosis in the portal and/or splenic vein. Portal vein thrombosis may also complicate advanced cirrhosis, which may cause retrograde flow and turbulence and thus progressive thrombosis in the portal vein. In children, portal vein thrombosis may occur following umbilical vein catheterization in a sick newborn infant, in whom the clinical presentation is

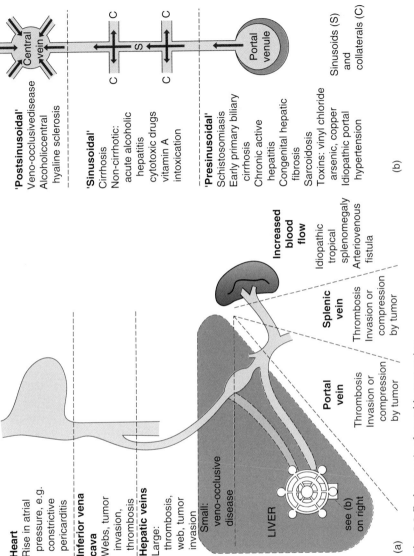

'Postsinusoidal'
Veno-occlusivedisease
Alcoholiccentral
hyaline sclerosis

'Sinusoidal'
Cirrhosis
Non-cirrhotic:
  acute alcoholic
    hepatitis
  cytotoxic drugs
  vitamin A
    intoxication

'Presinusoidal'
Schistosomiasis
Early primary biliary
  cirrhosis
Chronic active
  hepatitis
Congenital hepatic
  fibrosis
Sarcoidosis
Toxins: vinyl chloride
  arsenic, copper
Idiopathic portal
  hypertension

Sinusoids (S)
and
collaterals (C)

(b)

Heart
Rise in atrial
pressure, e.g.
constrictive
pericarditis
**Inferior vena
cava**
Webs, tumor
invasion,
thrombosis
Hepatic veins
Large:
thrombosis,
web, tumor
invasion
Small:
veno-occlusive
disease

LIVER

see (b)
on right

**Increased
blood
flow**
Idiopathic
tropical
splenomegaly
Arteriovenous
fistula

**Splenic
vein**
Thrombosis
Invasion or
compression
by tumor

**Portal
vein**
Thrombosis
Invasion or
compression
by tumor

(a)

Fig. 5.1 Pathogenesis of portal hypertension.

Box 5.2 Pathogenesis of portal hypertension

Prehepatic (presinusoidal): adults and children
- Portal vein thrombosis
- Splenic vein thrombosis
- Splanchnic arteriovenous fistula
- Compression of portal vein by neighboring tumor
- Arteriovenous fistula (Osler–Weber–Rendu syndrome)

Intrahepatic sinusoidal: children
Biliary
- Biliary atresia
- Cystic fibrosis
- Primary sclerosing cholangitis
- Alagille syndrome
- Congenital hepatic fibrosis

Hepatocellular (may all progress to cirrhosis)
- Autoimmune hepatitis
- Chronic hepatitis B and C
- Wilson disease
- α_1-antitrypsin deficiency

Intrahepatic sinusoidal: adults
- Nodular regenerative hyperplasia (commonly mistaken for cirrhosis)
- Portal sclerosis
- Schistosomiasis
- Congenital hepatic fibrosis (e.g. Caroli disease associated with autosomal recessive polycystic kidney disease)
- Primary biliary cirrhosis (but without cirrhosis)
- Primary and secondary sclerosing cholangitis (without cirrhosis)
- Myeloproliferative disease/Hodgkin disease

Hepatocellular
- As for children

Posthepatic (postsinusoidal): adults and children
- Congenital cardiac disease, inherited hypercoagulable states
- IVC obstruction
- Budd–Chiari syndrome
- Congestive cardiac failure
- Veno-occlusive disease

usually with splenomegaly or variceal hemorrhage later in childhood. Prehepatic portal hypertension could also be caused by tumor compression or invasion (e.g. hypernephroma) of the portal vein. An arteriovenous fistula in an individual with Osler–Weber–Rendu syndrome is a rare cause of prehepatic portal hypertension.

Non-cirrhotic portal hypertension very rarely causes catastrophic variceal hemorrhage. If this occurs, liver failure is unusual as there is little actual disease of the liver.

Non-cirrhotic portal hypertension: intrahepatic, sinusoidal

There are several disease of the liver that predominantly affect the portal tracts, which may cause portal hypertension in the absence of cirrhosis. Most often the damage is secondary to inflammation around the hepatic arteries (e.g. PAN) complicated by thrombosis of the veins within the portal triad. This pathologic process causes nodular regenerative hyperplasia (NRH). There are many diseases that promote the development of NRH, that is obliteration of the venules in the portal tracts, for example primary biliary cirrhosis, sarcoidosis, schistosomiasis, and certain toxins such as excess vitamin A. Congenital hepatic fibrosis is often misdiagnosed as cirrhosis if the liver biopsy is poorly interpreted, and is caused by obliteration of the terminal branches of the portal vein. Other diseases may damage the entire portal tract, for example myeloproliferative disease and Hodgkin's disease.

Non-cirrhotic portal hypertension: posthepatic

Any condition that prevents free flow of venous blood from the liver back to the heart gives rise to posthepatic portal hypertension, as occurs with acute thrombosis of the portal venous radicals (e.g. Budd–Chiari syndrome) for which there are several precipitants, the most common being a congenital disease affecting coagulation. Other slower, even transient, causes are congestive cardiac failure or inferior vena cava obstruction.

Although portal hypertension due to outflow tract obstruction (e.g. Budd–Chiari syndrome) most often presents with marked hepatomegaly, splenomegaly, and ascites, it may, albeit rarely, present with variceal hemorrhage and inactive cirrhosis.

Portal hypertension due to cirrhosis of any cause

Chronic intrahepatic/sinusoidal disease of any cause may progress to cirrhosis. Under normal conditions, all of the portal venous blood can be recovered from the hepatic veins but in cirrhosis as little as 10% may be recovered; the remainder leaves the liver via collaterals to:

1 esophagus and stomach (via anastomoses between the portal system and intercostals, the esophageal and the azygous veins of the caval system);
2 falciform ligament through para umbilical veins;
3 at sites where abdominal organs are in contact with the peritoneum, particularly at sites of previous abdominal surgery;
4 via the left renal vein from the splenic vein (splenorenal shunt).

Acute and chronic effects of portal hypertension due to cirrhosis

Hemorrhage

Hemorrhage from esophageal and/or gastric varices may present as the following.

1 An upper gastrointestinal bleed usually accompanied by melena is most often precipitated by spontaneous bacteremia.

2 Portal gastropathy causes either acute bleeding presenting as hematemesis and/or melena, or low-grade chronic bleeding, which presents as iron-deficiency anemia.

3 Sudden variceal hemorrhage may be the initial presentation of invasion of the portal vein by hepatocellular carcinoma, less likely a thrombosis of the portal vein.

Palpable splenomegaly is usual in all patients with a variceal hemorrhage.

Central nervous system

Effects of portal hypertension on the central nervous system include the following.

1 Prolonged shunting of portal venous blood away from the liver may be associated with low-grade hepatic encephalopathy, affecting many aspects of cerebral function. Precipitants of overt encephalopathy include sepsis, electrolytic imbalance, and a high protein meal, for example UGI bleed.

2 A spontaneous splenorenal shunt in a patient with otherwise "silent cirrhosis" may present with other, more permanent neurologic disorders, for example a parkinsonian like illness or paraplegia.

Clinical features: rupture of esophageal/gastric varices

Sudden hematemesis results in bright red blood per os and/or melena per rectum (if massive bleed, blood remains bright red). The patient may have no known history of liver disease so there is a need to look for the following.

- Skin stigmata of cirrhosis (spider nevi, palmar erythema, jaundice)—may be present;
- Abdominal examination—abdominal collaterals radiating away from umbilicus;
- Venous hum heard between xiphoid process to umbilicus (Cruveilhier–Baumgarten syndrome)—this is rare;
- Splenomegaly—this is almost universal;
- Liver may be small or large—depending on the etiology of liver disease;
- Liver edge—hard, cirrhosis; soft, suspect extra hepatic portal venous obstruction;
- Ascites—if absent prior to hemorrhage, often develops rapidly following fluid resuscitation if the patient is cirrhotic.

The course of investigation and treatment of possible ruptured esophageal varices (Box 5.3)

The following steps should be carried out in the investigation and treatment of possible ruptured esophageal varices (Fig. 5.2).

- Assess airway, ventilation, and circulation, and provide general resuscitative support as appropriate.
- Transfuse with blood to maintain hemoglobin at 80–100 g/L. More generous transfusion will increase the likelihood of ongoing bleeding.
- Pantoprazole 80 mg i.v. bolus followed by 8 mg/h i.v. infusion to adults until the source of bleeding is defined. Pantoprazole 2 mg/kg i.v. bolus followed by 0.2 mg/h i.v. infusion to children until the source of bleeding is defined.
- If possible, children with a presumed variceal hemorrhage should be transferred to the nearest center with tertiary pediatric hepatology services as soon as they are stable for transport.

Box 5.3 Management of bleeding esophageal varices

- Appropriate attention to airway, ventilation, and circulation
- Blood transfusion aiming to maintain hemoglobin at 80–100 g/L (no higher)
- i.v. vasoactive drug
  Adult: i.v. terlipressin 2 mg 6 hourly for 48 h OR i.v. octreotide 50 μg bolus and then 50 μg/h for 48 h to 5 days
  Child: octreotide 1–5 μg/kg i.v. bolus followed by 1–5 μg/kg per h i.v. infusion
- i.v. third-generation cephalosporin for 5 days
  plus
- i.v. proton pump inhibitors, followed by oral, at least until all varices eradicated
- When patient stable perform EGD with EVL (aim for within 12 h of presentation) (If patient remains unstable with ongoing hemorrhage need intubation and ventilation, i.e. call anesthesia)
- Continuously monitor renal function, cognition, and liver function

Success	Failure (≥2 attempts banding)
Introduce oral non-selective beta-blocker after hemodynamically stable for 5 days	Refer to tertiary center if experience with occlusion tubes is not available
Repeat EGD at monthly intervals with EVL until varices eradicated	Evaluate for suitability for TIPS procedure or portosystemic shunt and Consult liver transplant center
Repeat EGD every 1–2 years	

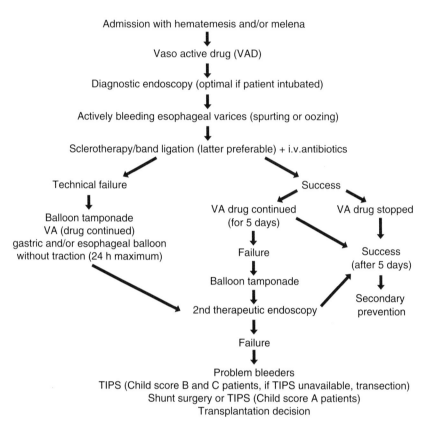

Fig. 5.2 Admission with hematemesis and/or melena.

- Commence intravenous infusion of vasoactive drug doses (see Box 5.3).
- Commence intravenous broad-spectrum antibiotic (e.g. third-generation cephalosporin) to treat associated sepsis (often asymptomatic) this maneuver reduces the risk of rebleeding and improves survival.
- An i.v. proton pump inhibitor will facilitate healing of post banding/sclerosis esophageal/gastric ulceration.
- Arrange for urgent EGD once the patient is hemodynamically stabilized (usual target is within 12h of admission). Procedure should be performed by an endoscopist trained in variceal ligation and interventional endoscopy for management of acute GI bleeding.
- To optimize visibility it is best to perform gastric lavage prior to introduction of the endoscope. If available, introduce a large-bore endoscope with well-functioning suction in place as this optimally demonstrates the site and the source of bleeding.
- If esophageal and/or gastric varices are thought to be the source of bleeding (may be very difficult to determine if patient is hypotensive), banding of the varices at the time of first endoscopy should be performed. Injection

sclerotherapy may be considered in adults and older children (typically >15 kg) if banding is not available, but sclerotherapy is associated with more frequent adverse effects. Injection sclerotherapy is the endoscopic management of choice in infants and small children less than 15 kg.

- If rebleeding occurs, a repeat attempt to band or sclerosis should be made, in the meanwhile arrangement for alternate therapy should be sought.
- Adult patients should be admitted to a tertiary referral center if control of variceal bleeding cannot be achieved. Such patients are most often those with advanced cirrhosis (Child's C). Active management of hypotension will minimize the risk of renal impairment secondary to renal hypoperfusion; particularly in patients with cirrhosis, and regularly monitor renal function. It should however be remembered that over-transfusion many promote further gastrointestinal bleeding, that is keep Hb less than 10 g/L.
- If despite banding or sclerotherapy variceal hemorrhage continues, control of bleeding in the adult patient is most likely to be secured by insertion of a TIPS (transjugular intrahepatic portosystemic shunt) (Fig. 5.3, Plate 5.1), which allows immediate decompression of the portal venous system by the creation of a wide connection between the hepatic vein and a branch of the portal vein but if the radiologist is inexperienced this procedure may be fraught with complications (Box 5.4). Thus TIPS should not be performed unless a trained physician is available.
- When a TIPS is not immediately available, occlusion tubes may be considered for maintenance of hemodynamic stability but only in the short term while planning for further intervention such as TIPS in patients with refractory bleeding. Such tubes include the Linton tube (single gastric balloon), Minnesota or Sengstaken–Blakemore tubes (esophageal and gastric balloons) Fig. 5.4. Their use is associated with significant risk, including esophageal or gastric wall necrosis, ulceration, perforation, and aspiration pneumonia. Therefore, placement of such tubes should *only* be performed by trained and experienced personnel. If neither insertion of an occlusion tube or TIPS is available then immediate transfer to a referral center with expertise in endoscopic procedures is necessary (Box 5.5), and optimally to a liver transplant center. When access to interventional radiology is unavailable, referral to a surgeon for consideration for a portosystemic shunt should be considered (Fig. 5.5).

It should be noted that surgical portosystemic shunting has far poorer results in children with decompensated liver disease when secondary to intrahepatic causes. Thus these children are best offered liver transplantation. Surgical shunts should be considered in pediatric patients with compensated intrahepatic disease or extrahepatic portal hypertension so as to be able to delay or even avoid transplantation.

Prevention of variceal hemorrhage in cirrhotic patients

See Chapter 4.

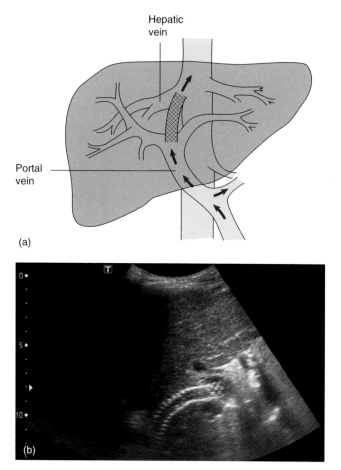

Fig. 5.3 Transjugular intrahepatic portosystemic shunt (TIPS). (a) Diagram of the correct location of a TIPS. (b) Ultrasound image of TIPS.

Box 5.4 Complications of TIPS procedure

Portosystemic hepatic encephalopathy
(reduce size of TIPS by inserting smaller stent)
Frank liver failure (especially if >20% fall in gradient following TIPS)
(NB: TIPS not effective for postbanding ulceration)

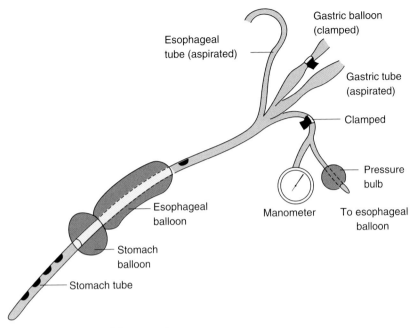

Fig. 5.4 Sengstaken–Blakemore tube.

Box 5.5 Failure to secure hemostasis from variceal hemorrhage

Patient must be intubated
Evaluate MELD score (see Chapter 4)
Insert occlusion tube through mouth and secure with string and 1 liter bottle of i.v. fluid over an "orthopedic" pulley (preferable than via nose)
Physician must be experienced

MELD >18 or age >60 years	MELD <18 and age <60 years
Liver transplant if suitable candidate (TIPS contraindicated)	Evaluate for TIPS (reduce pressure gradient only by 20%)

For children with refractory bleeding, consult pediatric hepatology expert

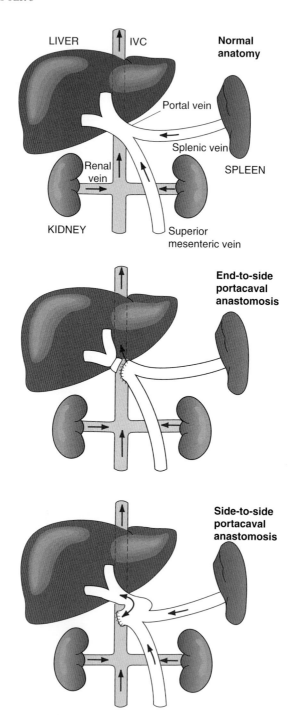

Fig. 5.5 Portosystemic shunts.

Case study 5.1: adult

A 42-year-old man was found lying in the street vomiting bright red blood. Upon arrival at the emergency room he was hypotensive (80/40 mmHg lying) with a pulse of 130 beats/min (regular rhythm). He was observed to have further hematemeses. He was in no obvious pain, gave no history of prior similar episodes, and was fully alert. He had consumed at least 100 g alcohol daily since his early 20s. As a teenager he had used illicit intravenous drugs for several years and as a consequence it was found difficult to access his peripheral veins. He had never been told he had liver disease but rarely sought medical attention.

In view of his continuous hemorrhage and poor venous access, anesthesia was called to potentially intubate the patient and to insert a central line to allow for effective fluid resuscitation. On physical examination:

- He was alert but too unwell to test for an hepatic flap. He was very anxious.
- His sclera were mildly jaundiced (bilirubin 60 μmol/L).
- Multiple spider nevi were visible over his upper chest. His abdomen was flat but he had a large, firm liver (16 cm span) and an easily palpable spleen. No ascites or ankle edema was present.
- Blood work taken at the time of admission showed a hemoglobin of 6 g/dL, WBC 11.6×10^9/L, platelet count 78×10^9/L, and his INR was 1.4.
- He was thought most likely to have cirrhosis due to excess consumption of alcohol, possibly on a background of hepatitis C. However, in view of his near normal INR, minimal jaundice, and lack of fluid retention, his cirrhosis was not thought to be severe.
- Because of his hypotension he was resuscitated initially with normal saline; this was changed to blood once it became available—he was transfused two units, after which his Hb rose to 7 g/L. His pulse rate fell to 100/min and blood pressure rose to 90/60 mmHg. He was maintained on i.v. D5W (note not saline once hemodynamically stable).
- It was assumed that his UGI hemorrhage was variceal secondary to cirrhosis and he was given a bolus of i.v. octreotide (50 μg) and treatment with the same was maintained at a rate of 50 μg/h over the next 24 h.
- As he was fully conscious he was given a small dose of sedation (i.v.) and a Ewald tube was passed and gastric lavage performed. Once no more clots of blood could be removed an upper panendoscopy was performed. Large esophageal varices were visualized with some overlying clot. No lesions in the stomach and duodenum were observed. There was no obvious bleeding and so banding of his varices was performed without difficulty. The patient's recovery was rapid. The sedation given for the procedure did not precipitate an episode of encephalopathy and may have been why he suffered no overt symptoms of acute alcohol withdrawal. He was prescribed a 5-day course of ceftriaxone and a proton pump inhibitor.
- The bleeding stopped following the banding procedure thus there was no need to add any other measures, for example passage of an occlusion tube and/or TIPS.

(Continued)

- He had developed some ascites following admission which responded well to salt restriction and to the diuretic aldactone.
- He underwent further variceal banding (EVL) a few days later and was then discharged. Prior to discharging he was counseled with regard to his alcohol consumption. He was tested for hepatitis B and C and was found to be immune to B but infected with hepatitis C. He was prescribed to take nadolol as a secondary prevention measure.
- Follow-up was arranged for a month when he would undergo repeat endoscopy and further variceal ablation performed if deemed necessary. His lifelong need for daily Nadalol was re-emphasized and the possible need for antiviral therapy for his hepatitis C discussed.

Case study 5.2: child

An 11-year-old boy with a known diagnosis of autosomal recessive polycystic kidney disease and congenital hepatic fibrosis (ARPKD/CHF) experienced a large hematemesis during a baseball game. There was no preceding trauma. He had had no prior episodes of hematemesis. The amount of blood vomited could not be accurately quantified but was described as copious and sufficient to soak the clothes of the child and his baseball coach. On arrival in the emergency room he was pale and clammy to the touch.

Initial examination
- afebrile, HR 160 beats/min, BP 86/40 mmHg lying with 20 mm postural drop;
- conscious but pale, anicteric;
- capillary refill time 5s, weak peripheral pulses;
- respiratory examination unremarkable except for mild tachypnea;
- abdomen distended—marked distention of cutaneous veins, liver palpable 3 cm below the right costal margin and firm, spleen palpable 10 cm below the left costal margin and firm, right kidney palpable, left kidney hard to appreciate due to splenomegaly, minimal ascites, no scrotal edema.

Initial assessment
- Two large-bore cannulae were placed in either arm, basic laboratory tests (hematology, biochemistry, type and cross) were drawn and he was infused rapidly with 20 mL/kg of normal saline.
- A pediatric hepatologist with expertise in therapeutic endoscopy was consulted.
- The patient was closely monitored in the resuscitation room in the emergency room.
- His heart rate fell to 140 after the first fluid bolus, and he received a second bolus.
- He was given an i.v. octreotide bolus 5 μg/kg and started on an infusion at 3 μg/kg per h.

Further history

He was known to have ARPKD/CHF. He had presented antenatally with enlarged echogenic kidneys on ultrasound and was oligouric at birth. He had been closely followed by a nephrologist his whole life and had a slowly rising creatinine and was being considered for renal replacement therapy. He saw a hepatologist once a year and was followed with blood work and ultrasound. He had never had any prior hepatic interventions, such as a liver biopsy or an upper endoscopy. He had experienced no complications, such as cholangitis, ascites, or gastrointestinal bleeding. His parents report that he is known to have a large spleen for which he wore a spleen guard during sports and his platelet count was typically around 60×10^9/L.

Further course

- When his initial laboratory blood work returned, his hemoglobin was 5.5 g/L (baseline 12), his platelets were 58×10^9/L, and his INR was 1.3. His serum transaminases were less than twice the ULN and his conjugated bilirubin was normal.
- In view of ongoing tachycardia and the significant drop in hemoglobin he was taken to the operating room, intubated, and underwent endoscopy where four large varices were successfully banded in the distal esophagus.
- He was monitored in the ICU overnight; the octreotide was continued for 48 h before weaning.
- He was not prescribed antibiotics as he was not cirrhotic.

Comment

This is a typical course for a child with ARPKD/CHF in that he has evolving portal hypertension (as evidenced by the low platelet count). There are no current data to support primary prophylaxis of esophageal varices in children. Children with ARPKD/CHF may remain compensated with their chronic liver disease for many years and are usually managed conservatively without the use of non-selective beta-blockers or prophylactic banding. However, after a presentation such as this, he would now be repeatedly banded on a regular schedule (every 4–6 weeks) until the varices were eradicated and would then continue with surveillance endoscopy. If the varices were refractory to endoscopic ligation and he had continued to have ongoing bleeding, he would have been considered for liver transplantation.

Multiple choice questions

1. A 60-year-old previously healthy man from the Middle East presents to the ER with his first upper gastrointestinal hemorrhage. He had been taking aspirin several times a day for an acute tenosynovitis of his elbow. Examination revealed marked hepatomegaly and a spleen that was just palpable. His blood pressure on arrival was 100/60 mmHg, pulse 110 beats/min, and he had a 15-mm postural drop. Initial hemoglobin was 10 g/L, WBC 6×10^9/L,

platelets $130 \times 10^9/L$, and INR 0.9. Preparation is made for an endoscopic procedure. Which of the following is *incorrect*?

A. His platelet count may be a helpful indicator of an underlying cirrhosis

B. i.v. cephtriaxone was administered and rapidly switched to oral medication to be continued for a further 4 days

C. Esophageal varices seen at endoscopy were banded and once stable the selective beta-blocker metoprolol was prescribed as long-term prophylaxis against further hemorrhage

D. Patient was advised to take acetaminophen and not acetylsalicylic acid for his tenosynovitis or any other pains he may suffer

2. A 9-month-old child with biliary atresia and her native liver presents with hematemesis likely from esophageal varices. What is the appropriate sequence of management?

A. Resuscitation, consult pediatric hepatologist, octreotide, endoscopy with sclerotherapy of varices

B. i.v. octreotide and fluids, consult pediatric hepatologist

C. Octreotide, consult pediatric hepatologist, endoscopy with band ligation of varices

D. Resuscitation, consult pediatric hepatologist, endoscopy, TIPS

E. Resuscitation, consult pediatric hepatologist, octreotide, endoscopy with band ligation of varices

Answers

1. C
2. A

Further reading

Afdhal NH, Curry MP. Early TIPS to improve survival in acute variceal bleeding. N Engl J Med 2010; 362: 2421–2.

Bernard B, Lebrec D, Mathurin P, Opolon P, et al. Propranolol and sclerotherapy in the prevention of gastrointestinal rebleeding in patients with cirrhosis: a meta-analysis. J Hepatol 1997; 26: 312–24.

García-Pagán JC, Caca K, Bureau C, et al; Early TIPS (Transjugular Intrahepatic Porto-systemic Shunt) Cooperative Study Group. Early use of TIPS in patients with cirrhosis and variceal bleeding. N Engl J Med 2010; 362: 2370–9.

Gluud LL, Klingenberg S, Nikolova D, et al. Banding ligation versus beta-blockers as primary prophylaxis in esophageal varices: systematic review of randomized trials. Am J Gastroenterol 2007; 102: 2842–8.

Lebrec D, Poynard T, Hillon P, et al. Propranolol for prevention of recurrent gastrointestinal bleeding in patients with cirrhosis: a controlled study. N Engl J Med 1981; 305: 1371–4.

Lebrec D, Vinel JP, Dupas JL. Complications of portal hypertension in adults: a French consensus. Eur J Gastroenterol Hepatol 2005; 17: 403–10.

Lebrec D, Vinel JP, Dupas JL. Complications of portal hypertension in adults: a French consensus. Eur J Gastroenterol Hepatol 2005; 17: 403–10.

Lo GH, Lai KH, Cheng JS, et al. The additive effect of sclerotherapy to patients receiving repeated endoscopic variceal ligation: a prospective, randomized trial. Hepatology 1998; 28: 391–5.

Pagliaro L, D'Amico G, Sörensen TI, et al. Prevention of first bleeding in cirrhosis. A meta-analysis of randomized trials of nonsurgical treatment. Ann Intern Med 1992; 117: 59–70.

Poddar U, Thapa BR, Singh K. Band ligation plus sclerotherapy versus sclerotherapy alone in children with extrahepatic portal venous obstruction. J Clin Gastroenterol 2005; 39: 626–9.

Qamar AA, Grace ND, Groszmann RJ, et al; Portal Hypertension Collaborative Group. Platelet count is not a predictor of the presence or development of gastroesophageal varices in cirrhosis. Hepatology 2008; 47: 153–9.

Sanyal AJ, Freedman AM, Luketic VA, et al. Transjugular intrahepatic portosystemic shunts for patients with active variceal hemorrhage unresponsive to sclerotherapy. Gastroenterology 1996; 111: 138–46.

Management of ascites

CHAPTER 6

David K.H. Wong

University of Toronto, and Division of Gastroenterology, Toronto Western Hospital, University Health Network, Toronto, Ontario, Canada

Key points

- Ascites in a cirrhotic due to liver failure is a bad prognostic sign. MELD (see Chapters 2 and 4) should be calculated and liver transplantation should be considered. Low albumin states can precipitate ascites in the setting of cirrhosis without liver failure—the MELD is low and so liver transplantation is not the answer.
- Worsening ascites should prompt a search for a cause precipitating the clinical deterioration, such as bacterial infection or renal failure.
- Treating the underlying liver disease to prevent further liver injury can result in resolution of ascites and preventing the need for liver transplantation.

Introduction

It has long been recognized that the development of cirrhotic ascites is associated with a high mortality risk.[1] D'Amico et al. have reported that, in a population where the underlying liver disease was largely untreated, the development of ascites is associated with a 20–26% chance of death over the next 1 year.[2,3] Many liver diseases can now be treated, such as hepatitis B, hepatitis C, Wilson disease, etc. Control of the primary liver disease can lead to fibrosis regression[4] and improvement in liver function to the point where long-term survival without liver transplantation is possible.[5]

Pathogenesis of ascites in cirrhosis

The development of cirrhotic ascites is the end result of physiologic compensatory steps that eventually lead to failure of other body systems.[6] The increased

Hepatology: Diagnosis and Clinical Management, First Edition. Edited by E. Jenny Heathcote.
© 2012 John Wiley & Sons, Ltd. Published 2012 by John Wiley & Sons, Ltd.

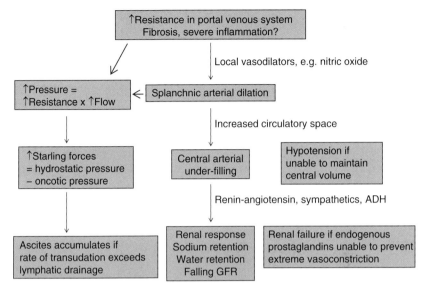

Fig. 6.1 Pathophysiology of portal hypertension: peripheral arteriolar vasodilatation hypothesis. Gradual increase in portal hypertension over years leads to ascites that becomes more difficult to control. ADH, antidiuretic hormone; GFR, glomerular filtration rate.

resistance to blood flow through the cirrhotic liver leads to a progressive, increase in production of vasodilatory substances, such as nitric oxide, in an attempt to minimize resistance (Fig. 6.1). This leads to progressive splanchnic arterial dilation (arterioles arising from the celiac, superior mesenteric, and inferior mesenteric arteries). The combination of increased resistance and increased flow results in increased pressure in the portal venous system, that is portal hypertension. Increased hydrostatic pressure from portal hypertension, in combination with decreased oncotic pressure from reduced liver synthesis of albumin, results in increased Starling forces. This allows increased transudation of albumin-poor plasma from the liver and mesentery into the peritoneal cavity. Ascites accumulates when the rate of transudation into the peritoneal cavity exceeds the rate of lymphatic drainage from the peritoneal cavity.

In addition, simultaneous splanchnic arterial dilation leads to an overall increased vascular space and under-filling of the central arterial compartment. To compensate, the kidneys retain sodium and water, resulting in a larger total plasma volume. As both the cirrhotic process and increase in liver resistance progress with time, there is progressive splanchnic arterial dilation leading to greater stimulation of the renin–angiotensin system, sympathetic nervous system, and release of antidiuretic hormone, causing vasoconstriction in the kidneys and even more sodium retention, further worsening ascites control

Table 6.1 Progression of cirrhosis leads to ascites that becomes more refractory to treatment

Phase	Ascites control	Description
1	Subclinical	Sodium retention is mild and most of dietary sodium intake can be cleared by the kidneys. The mildly increased fluid transudate is cleared by the lymphatics and so clinical ascites does not develop. Severe sodium loading, for example after intravenous fluid resuscitation for a variceal bleed, can lead to transient ascites.
2	Diet control	Sodium retention is moderate but high sodium intake can lead to ascites accumulation whereas a dietary sodium restriction can still lead to resolution of ascites.
3	Diuretics	Renal sodium restriction is much lower (<10 mEq/day) due to increased stimulation of the renin–angiotensin system, the sympathetic nervous system, and production of ADH. Dietary sodium restriction alone will not prevent ascites accumulation. Despite increasing renal vasoconstriction, GFR is maintained due to local production of prostaglandins. Blockage of prostaglandins through NSAIDs can lead to renal failure.
4	HRS-2	Serum creatinine > 1.5 mg/dL or GFR has fallen to <40 mL/min due to renal vasoconstriction and all other causes of renal dysfunction have been excluded, no improvement after at least 2 days of diuretic withdrawal and plasma volume expansion with albumin. Ascites control becomes more difficult despite diuretics. Prognosis for survival is poor: 50% at 5 months and 20% at 1 year.
5	HRS-1	Rapidly progressive renal failure to >2.5 mg/dL (221 μmol/L) within 2 weeks, usually in the setting of pre-existing HRS-2. Frequently precipitated by physiologic stress: major surgery, gastrointestinal bleeding, sepsis such as spontaneous bacterial peritonitis. Prognosis for survival is very poor: 20% at 2 weeks.

Management of ascites: dietary sodium restriction to <2 g/day is effective for up to phase 2. Diuretics are required from phase 3 onwards, with higher doses of diuretics required to phase 4. By phase 4, diuretics may not work adequately and therapeutic paracentesis may be needed. However, survival is not improved by paracentesis—a transplant is needed to improve prospects for long-term survival.

ADH, antidiuretic hormone; GFR, glomerular filtration rate; HRS, hepatorenal syndrome; NSAID, non-steroidal anti-inflammatory drug.

(Table 6.1). These compensatory mechanisms eventually fail, resulting in renal failure from renal ischemia and circulatory failure from under-filling of the central arterial space.

Ascites is best detected by ultrasound during routine ultrasound surveillance for liver cancer in the patient with known cirrhosis. In those with unsuspected cirrhosis, ascites volume must exceed 1.5 L before bulging flanks are evident. Shifting dullness is reported to have 83% sensitivity and 56% specificity for the detection of ascites, but the performance characteristics depend on the volume of ascites, with massive ascites being obvious on clinical exam and small ascites essentially undetectable without ultrasound.[7]

Paracentesis to remove ascites is safe (see below for discussion of what tests should be done of ascites fluid). The complication rate of the procedure is low—approximately 1% for abdominal wall hematomas. Serious complications, such as bowel perforation, are rare, and the rate is estimated at less than 1/1000 procedures. Clotting factors such as plasma are not required prior to paracentesis, even if the INR is elevated to 9. The sites used for paracentesis are the left or right lower quadrant, approximately 3 cm cephalad and 3 cm medial to the anterior superior iliac spine. The right side is less optimal if the cecum is dilated as may occur with chronic lactulose use. Bedside ultrasound guidance is useful, especially if the clinician is not confident of the site for paracentesis.

Diagnostic paracentesis should be done for *all* patients with ascites. A serum to ascites albumin gradient (SAAG) more than 11 g/L is supportive of the diagnosis of cirrhotic ascites (Tables 6.2 and 6.3). The white blood cell (WBC) count and differential must always be evaluated on ascites fluid, where a finding of more than 250 neutrophils/μL (0.25×10^9 neutrophils/L) is supportive of infection. If infection is suspected because of low-grade fever, abdominal pain, or elevated leukocyte count from baseline, ascites fluid should be cultured in blood culture bottles as this increases the yield of a positive culture.

Table 6.2 Routine tests of ascites fluid for uncomplicated ascites

Tests	Interpretation
Albumin	SAAG = serum albumin − ascites albumin SAAG > 11 g/L is consistent with cirrhotic ascites and portal hypertension plus second cause of ascites formation
Cell count and differential	PMN ≥ 250 cells/μL (0.25×10^9/L) supports diagnosis of spontaneous bacterial peritonitis Empiric therapy with a third-generation cephalosporin × 5 days should be started, but can be modified based on results of bacterial culture/sensitivity testing

PMN, polymorphonuclear cells; SAAG, serum ascites albumin gradient.

Table 6.3 Special tests of ascites fluid

Indication	Tests	Interpretation
Suspect infection	Bacterial culture in blood culture bottle	Positive cultures can guide antibiotic therapy; positive in 50%
Intestinal perforation	PMN extremely high Multiple organisms Protein > 10 g/L Glucose < 3.0 mmol/L ALP > 240 IU/L CEA > 5 ng/mL	Search for site of perforation
Peritoneal carcinomatosis, ovarian carcinoma, gastric carcinoma	Cytology	Rarely positive in other cancers such as primary liver cancer
High risk for tuberculous peritonitis: endemic area, HIV	Mycobacterial culture	Sensitivity only ~50%
Chylous (milky) fluid	Triglycerides > 100 mg/dL	Although possible with cirrhotic ascites, rule out lymphatic obstruction or lymphatic disruption

ALP, alkaline phosphatase; CEA, carcinoembryonic antigen; PMN, polymorphonuclear cells.

Antibiotics (third-generation cephalosporin or amoxicillin–clavulanic acid i.v.) should be started if the fluid neutrophil count is elevated—do not wait for results of the culture as they may not be available for 24 hours. Infection is usually caused by Gram-negative bacteria from normal intestinal flora. Although routine culture of ascites fluid is not necessary, it should be done if the ascites WBC is more than 250 neutrophils/μL. Diagnostic paracentesis should be repeated if there is no clinical improvement after 48 hours of antibiotics. If the ascites WBC and neutrophils remain high (<25% fall from baseline), a change in antibiotics, taking into account local antibiotic resistant strains, should be considered. After recovery from an episode of spontaneous bacterial peritonitis, secondary prophylactic antibiotics (norfloxacin 400 mg/day or ofloxacin 400 mg/day, or Septra 750 mg once weekly indefinitely) should be prescribed.

Management of cirrhotic ascites

Given the pathogenesis of cirrhotic ascites, therapy is directed at minimizing sodium intake and diuretics to enhance sodium excretion if necessary (Table

6.1). This strategy will not work for those with SAAG less than 11 (ascites not associated with cirrhosis) and is likely to result in renal insufficiency. Once the diagnosis of cirrhotic ascites is established, the most important long-term management strategy is to treat all treatable underlying liver diseases. Alcohol consumption should be minimized, hepatitis B should be controlled, and so forth. In cases where the underlying cause of liver disease is not yet effectively treatable (e.g. fatty liver), ascites control will become increasingly more difficult and will eventually require liver transplantation.

Sodium restriction

Dietary sodium intake should be restricted to 2000 mg/day (88 mmol/day). Maintenance intravenous fluids should be given with caution as they can be significant sources of sodium intake. For example, 1 liter of normal saline contains 154 mmol sodium, almost 2 days worth of dietary sodium intake. More stringent restriction is not recommended because food becomes less palatable and more difficult to find, making malnutrition a significant risk. As long as the daily urinary excretion of sodium exceeds 88 mmol/day, ascites should decrease and resolve (phase 2). If ascites seemingly cannot be controlled by sodium restriction, urine biochemistry should be performed. If a random urinary sample yields a sodium level greater than potassium or a 24-h urine collection shows very high levels of sodium excretion (>100 mmol/day), then high dietary sodium intake is the likely cause of ascites accumulation. Fluid restriction is usually not necessary as water loss passively follows sodium loss. Chronic hyponatremia correlates with the severity of cirrhosis but on its own is seldom morbid unless the hyponatremia is corrected too rapidly.

Diuretics

Once the daily urinary excretion of sodium falls below 78 mmol/day, ascites will accumulate despite sodium restriction (phase 3). Diuretics can increase urinary sodium excretion. The usual approach is to introduce a combination of oral diuretics, typically furosemide 40 mg and spironolactone 100 mg daily. Diuretics are advised to be taken in the morning—night time dosing will lead to nocturia and disturbed sleep. Weight loss should be limited to no more than 0.5 kg/day if there is no underlying edema. When diuretics are first required, the response is usually dramatic and ascites quickly resolves. Even if ascites resolves, the Model for End-stage Liver Disease (MELD) should be calculated and a referral for liver transplantation assessment be made if MELD is elevated to the criteria of your local transplant center (e.g. MELD ≥15 for Toronto in 2011). If the underlying liver disease is untreated and cirrhosis progresses, urinary sodium excretion continues to fall and higher doses of diuretics are required. Before raising the doses of diuretics, it is worthwhile reviewing dietary sodium restriction. Adequate naturesis can be checked by testing the urine; a random urine sodium/potassium ratio more than 1 or a 24-h urine sodium more than 78 mmol/day suggests adequate diuresis with current doses of diuretics but inadequate dietary sodium restriction. The doses of diuretics

---

Box 6.1 Diagnosis of hepatorenal syndrome

1 Cirrhotic ascites
2 Serum creatinine > 133 μmol/L (1.5 mg/dL)
3 Creatinine remains over 133 μmol/L after at least 2 days of:
   (i)   Diuretic withdrawal
   (ii) Volume expansion with albumin 1 g/kg/day (max 100 g/day)
4 Absence of shock
5 No current or recent exposure to nephrotoxic drugs
6 Absence of primary renal disease:
   (i)   Proteinuria > 500 mg/day
   (ii) Hematuria > 50 red blood cells/high-power field
   (iii) Abnormal renal parenchyma on imaging

---

can be increased, trying to maintain the ratio of furosemide 40 mg to spironolactone 100 mg, in steps of 40 mg and 100 mg, respectively, to a maximum dose of furosemide 160 mg and spironolactone 400 mg once daily in the morning (i.e. not divided doses). As the doses of diuretics required increase, the serum creatinine also increases, and is suggestive of type 2 hepatorenal syndrome when serum creatinine is more than 133 μmol/L (Box 6.1).[8] Spironolactone can cause tender gynecomastia, which can be significant. Amiloride (10–40 mg) can be used to as a substitute for spironolactone but, in general, it is less effective than spironolactone. Careful monitoring of electrolytes and creatinine should be done (at least monthly) after starting diuretics and after each change in dose of diuretics. Diuretics should be held and reassessed if there are unexpected increases in fluid loss (vomiting, diarrhea) or if complications of uncontrolled/recurrent encephalopathy, significant hyponatremia (Na <120 mmol/L) despite fluid restriction, or renal insufficiency (creatinine >133 μmol/L) develops (Box 6.1).

Paracentesis
Therapeutic large-volume paracentesis is useful to relieve tense ascites, which may accumulate despite adequate dietary sodium restriction and maximally tolerated doses of diuretics (phase 4). Refractory ascites is defined as ascites that is unresponsive to sodium restriction and maximal dose diuretics (furosemide 160 mg and spironolactone 400 mg) and recurs rapidly after therapeutic paracentesis. Others may not be able to tolerate maximal doses of diuretics because of the complications listed above. Serial therapeutic large-volume paracenteses may be required.

The role of intravenous albumin replacement after paracentesis remains controversial and data supporting its use are not conclusive. Furthermore, albumin is very expensive. Nevertheless, most centers advocate i.v. albumin with therapeutic paracentesis when over 5 liters ascites has been removed, at a dose of 6–8 g albumin per liter ascites removed above 5 liters. In Toronto, this translates to 25% albumin × 100 mL infused after 5 liters removed, and a second 100 mL after 8–10 liters removed. The insertion of a transjugular intrahepatic portosystemic shunt (TIPS) shunt for refractory ascites remains experimental. Liver transplantation seems to be the only treatment option that can improve the dismal 20% 1-year survival in those with refractory ascites.

Hepatorenal syndrome

Type 1 hepatorenal syndrome is a clinical finding of acute and rapidly progressive renal failure that does not improve despite stopping diuretics and a trial of plasma volume expansion for at least 2 days (Fig. 6.2). Other causes of renal disease should also be excluded (nephrotoxic drugs, parenchymal renal disease as suggested by the finding of proteinuria and/or microscopic hematuria). Nevertheless, hepatorenal syndrome can develop in those with underlying primary renal disease. Type 1 hepatorenal syndrome is typically seen in the setting of those with type 2 hepatorenal syndrome who then go on to experience a significant physiological stress, such as sepsis, gastrointestinal bleeding, exposure to nephrotoxic drugs, etc. (Fig. 6.3). Prognosis is extremely poor, usually with death within 2 weeks. Treatment with albumin 10–20 g/day infusion plus octreotide 200 μg s.c. t.i.d. and midodrine titrated to a maximum dose of 12.5 mg t.i.d. orally, to achieve an increase in mean blood pressure of 15 mmHg, may reverse type 1 hepatorenal syndrome. Terlipressin (unavailable in North America) has also been used to reverse type 1 hepatorenal syndrome. The role of TIPS for type 1 hepatorenal syndrome remains experimental. Even if type 1 hepatorenal syndrome resolves, mortality is still high without liver transplantation.

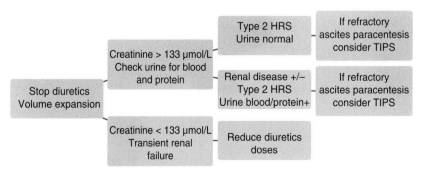

Fig. 6.2 Approach to slowly worsening renal function in those with cirrhotic ascites on diuretic therapy. HRS, hepatorenal syndrome; TIPS, transjugular intrahepatic portosystemic shunt.

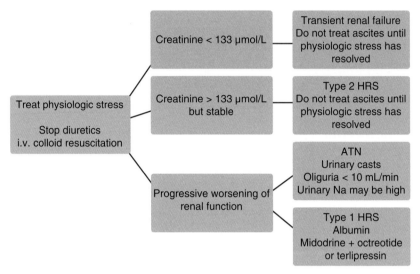

Fig. 6.3 Renal failure in the setting of physiologic stress, such as bacterial infection, gastrointestinal bleed, etc. The physiologic stress should be treated appropriately (band ligation of esophageal varices, antibiotics for spontaneous bacterial peritonitis), plasma volume should be expanded with the appropriate colloid (bleeding may require blood or fresh frozen plasma whereas spontaneous bacterial peritonitis would benefit from albumin). ATN, acute tubular necrosis; HRS, hepatorenal syndrome.

Case study 6.1

A 78-year-old woman with fatty liver (risks: non-insulin dependent diabetes, hyperlipidemia, hypertension, body mass index (BMI) 30) is found to have a liver that appeared cirrhotic during cholecystectomy in 1995. Liver biopsy at the time confirmed fatty liver and cirrhosis. Ascites was first noted in 2007 and was initially controlled with dietary sodium restriction. Diuretics (furosemide 40 mg and spironolactone 100 mg) were introduced in 2008 and the doses of diuretics needed to control the ascites have been gradually increased since 2010. In 2011, she was taking furosemide 120 mg and spironolactone 300 mg with reasonable control; although some ascites persists, it is not uncomfortable. She now presents with a 2-day history of malaise, light headedness, and abdominal tenderness. In the emergency department, she looked comfortable. Vital signs: temperature 37.2°C, HR 88, BP 90/48 supine. Physical examination showed evidence of muscle mass loss and almost tense ascites. Routine lab tests: ALT 62 IU/L, AST 81 IU/L, INR 1.9, albumin 27 g/L, bilirubin 44 μmol/L, Hb 152 g/L, WBC 5.8 × 10^9/L, platelets 58 × 10^9/L, Na 128 mmol/L, K 5.1 mmol/L, creatinine 148 μmol/L. Comparing her labs to those drawn 1 month before, the WBC is higher from her baseline of 2.3 × 10^9/L and creatinine has risen from 130 μmol/L. Ultrasound today shows a cirrhotic liver, massive ascites, and no hepatoma. Diagnostic paracentesis shows WBC 720 cells/µL, neutrophils 82%, consistent with spontaneous bacterial peritonitis.

Comment
This case illustrates the progression of cirrhosis through the various stages of ascites, as described in Fig. 6.1 and Table 6.1, with stage 1 in 1995, stage 2 in 2007, stage 3 in 2008, and stage 4 in 2010. When ascites worsens, a precipitating cause should be sought; a history of increased sodium intake either through diet or intravenously from hospital care, a history of stopping diuretics, acute renal insufficiency precipitated by hypovolemia (over-diuresis, acute intercurrent illness limiting oral intake or increased loss with diarrhea), non-steroidal anti-inflammatory drug (NSAID) use, or infection. This case also illustrates that spontaneous bacterial peritonitis does not always cause fever and so a diagnostic paracentesis is mandatory, both in new-onset ascites and in the setting of worsening ascites. Leukocytosis is only apparent if her baseline values are taken into account. The BMI is not accurate in this setting as a significant proportion of the mass is due to ascites fluid. The MELD score 1 month prior to current presentation was 22 but her advanced age precludes liver transplantation. Current management is to treat the infection with intravenous antibiotics, either a third-generation cephalosporin or a quinolone. She is at high risk for acute renal failure due to the physiological stress of infection, resulting in hepatorenal syndrome type 1 (stage 5) and so i.v. albumin (1 g/kg/day, maximum 100 g/day) should be given and diuretics should be stopped during the acute infection. She is also at risk for esophageal variceal bleed as portal pressures will increase due to increased portal venous flow resulting from a combination of hyperemic reaction during peritonitis and increased plasma volume from fluid resuscitation. Gastroscopy, if not done in the last 12 months, should be performed and large varices should be banded. Beta-blockers are not a realistic option given the low blood pressure associated with advanced cirrhosis. Prophylactic antibiotics (norfloxacin 400 mg/day, or ofloxacin 400 mg/day, or Septra 750 mg once weekly indefinitely) should be given post discharge from hospital. Finally, a frank discussion with the patient and her family to inform them of her prognosis—survival estimated to be 20% over the next year or two—as well as the likely need for increasing medical support for ascites that is increasingly more difficult to manage. Since liver transplantation is not an option, end of life discussions should be held with this patient.

Case study 6.2

A 52-year-old man presents with increased abdominal girth of 2 weeks' duration, otherwise well. He knows that he is a "hepatitis B carrier" but has never been sick in his life and so does not see doctors. He has noted that his energy levels have decreased over the last year but he is still able to work long hours. He drinks three to six standard alcoholic drinks a day with work clients. His weight today is

(Continued)

unchanged from a year ago, BMI 27, but he notes that the muscle mass around his face, upper extremities, and chest has decreased whereas his abdomen is now distended and bloated. Clinical examination shows ascites with shifting dullness. Initial laboratory investigations show ALT 1421 IU/L, AST 1350 IU/L, INR 1.6, albumin 28 g/L, bilirubin 44 μmol/L, Hb 152 g/L, WBC 2.8 × 10⁹/L, platelets 78 × 10⁹/L, creatinine 98 μmol/L. Hepatitis B is active: HBeAg negative, anti-HBe positive, HBV DNA 4.25 × 10⁷ IU/mL. Ultrasound confirms a cirrhotic-looking liver and ascites.

Comment

Liver disease with or without liver cirrhosis is usually asymptomatic until the development of liver failure. Ascites is a sign of liver failure associated with significant liver synthetic failure. This is usually preceded by muscle mass loss (and falling serum albumin levels). The current weight suggests that over the last year, 4–5 kg of muscle mass has been lost and he now has 4–5 liters of ascites fluid. A diagnostic tap should be done to confirm an elevated SAAG in cirrhotic ascites (see Table 6.2). Furosemide 40 mg and spironolactone 100 mg daily can be prescribed and should be very effective in new-onset ascites. Given the INR 1.6, bilirubin 44 μmol/L, creatinine 98 μmol/L, the MELD is 16, which meets criteria for liver transplantation. However, he has two potentially treatable causes of cirrhosis: hepatitis B and alcohol. Of the two, hepatitis B is probably the major cause of injury as the ALT and AST are far too high to attribute to alcohol. With effective hepatitis B antiviral therapy and alcohol cessation, liver inflammation can resolve, allowing liver fibrosis to regress within 6–12 months such that ascites can potentially then resolve, MELD improve to less than 15, and liver transplantation may no longer be necessary. With improving liver function, the doses of diuretics need to be re-assessed and diuretics may no longer be needed within 6–12 months.

Case study 6.3

A 58-year-old man presents with a 6-month history of abdominal discomfort. Ultrasound shows ascites. The liver is enlarged and looks fatty but not obviously cirrhotic. Routine lab. tests are as follows: ALT 22 IU/L, AST 31 IU/L, INR 1.0, albumin 27 g/L, bilirubin 14 μmol/L, Hb 152 g/L, WBC 4.8 × 10⁹/L, platelets 148 × 10⁹/L, creatinine 98 μmol/L. Diagnostic paracentesis confirms uncomplicated cirrhotic ascites. Workup for liver disease uncovers risk factors for fatty liver (BMI 36, diabetes, hyperlipidemia) and hepatitis C infection. The FibroTest (FibroSure) is 0.82, suggesting cirrhosis. FibroScan failed to get a reading, likely because of body shape associated with central obesity (see Chapters 2 and 4). Physical examination shows hypertension with BP 200/110 as well as pitting edema to the ankles, pretibial skin hyperpigmentation, previously thought to be due to chronic venous stasis from diabetes. On further questioning, there is also a history of intermittent red skin lesions affecting the legs for years. Tests for serum cryoglobulins are positive, urinalysis shows both blood and proteins, and 24-h urine collections is positive for protein up to 1.8 g/day.

Comment

This case illustrates that ascites may not be obvious in those with pre-existing central obesity. Furthermore, liver disease can exist even if liver enzymes (ALT and AST) are in the normal range, and that cirrhosis can exist even if the liver does not look cirrhotic on imaging. It should be noted that liver enzymes may have been high in the remote past when he was not being monitored. Although the development of ascites is usually a poor prognostic marker, which should prompt an evaluation for liver transplantation, there is a discrepancy between MELD 7 and Child–Pugh–Turcotte score 8 (grade B) (see Chapter 4). In this case, MELD is a more accurate reflection of liver disease as the liver synthetic function is normal other than the very low albumin level, which results in decreased oncotic pressure and therefore increased Starling forces for fluid transudation and ascites formation. This should prompt an investigation for protein loss. In this case, renal protein loss has been identified. Even if skin biopsy of the intermittent red spots confirms leukocytoclastic vasculitis, it is not possible to distinguish renal disease from hepatitis C-associated symptomatic cryoglobulinemia and membranoproliferative glomerulonephritis (MPGN) from other causes of renal disease, such as diabetic nephropathy, unless a renal biopsy is done. Treatment should be directed at the ongoing proteinuria. If this is hepatitis C-associated cryoglobulinemia and MPGN as opposed to diabetic nephropathy, immune suppression is rarely successful. MPGN can improve with plasma pharesis but the benefit is temporary. Eradication of hepatitis C infection can help as it eliminates the ongoing antigenic stimulation driving the over-active B-cell response, which is the underlying cause of cryoglobulins. Anti-B cell therapy with rituximab (anti-CD20) can theoretically be of benefit as well.

Multiple choice question

1. A 48-year-old woman with alcoholic cirrhosis presents with gradually worsening ascites. Ascites first presented 2 years ago and has been controlled with furosemide 40 mg and spironolactone 100 mg daily. Labs today are: ALT 24 IU/L, AST 48 IU/L, ALP 104 IU/L, Na 138 mmol/L, K 3.8 mmol/L, creatinine 102 μmol/L, Hb 138 g/L, WBC 3.1×10^9 cells/L, platelets 62×10^9/L, INR 1.58, albumin 28 g/L, bilirubin 42 μmol/L. Urinalysis shows no proteins or blood, urine Na 22 mmol/L, K 37 mmol/L. The most appropriate management is:
   A. Repeat counseling about dietary sodium restriction
   B. Increase diuretics to furosemide 80 mg and spironolactone 200 mg daily
   C. Diagnostic paracentesis and empiric antibiotics
   D. Gastroscopy to rule out large varices
   E. Referral for liver transplantation

Answer

1. E. Referral for liver transplantation is the only thing that will improve her prospects for survival given MELD 16. Dietary sodium restriction is unlikely to help given the low urinary sodium : potassium. Increasing doses of diuretics may help but will not affect prospects for survival. A diagnostic paracentesis should be done but empiric antibiotics should only be given if the ascites fluid analysis is suggestive of infection as there are no other clinical features of infection. Gastroscopy to look for large varices should also be done but once again, will not affect long-term survival given MELD 16.

References

1. Gines P, Quintero E, Arroyo V, et al. Compensated cirrhosis: Natural history and prognostic factors. Hepatology 1987; 7: 122–8.
2. D'Amico G, Garcia-Tsao G, Pagliaro L. Natural history and prognostic indicators of survival in cirrhosis: A systematic review of 118 studies. J Hepatol 2006; 44: 217–31.
3. D'Amico G, Villanueva C, Burroughs AK, et al. Clinical stages of cirrhosis: a multicenter cohort study of 1858 patients. AASLD 2010. Hepatology 2010; 52 (Suppl.): A20.
4. Wanless IR, Nakashima E, Sherman M. Regression of human cirrhosis: Morpholic features and genesis of incomplete septal cirrhosis. Arch Path Lab Med 2000; 124: 1599–607.
5. Villeneuve J-P, Condreay LD, Willems B, et al. Lamivudine treatment for decompensated cirrhosis resulting from chronic hepatitis B. Hepatology 2000; 13: 207–10.
6. Arroyo V, Colmenero J. Ascites and hepatorenal syndrome in cirrhosis: pathophysiological basis of therapy and current management. J Hepatolol 2003; 38 (Suppl. 1): S69–S89.
7. Runyon BA. Management of adult patients with ascites due to cirrhosis: An update. Hepatology 2009; 49: 2087–107.
8. Guevara M, Arroyo V. Hepatorenal syndrome. Expert Opin Pharmacother 2011; 12: 1405–17.

Masses in the liver

CHAPTER 7

Morris Sherman

Toronto General Hospital, University Health Network and University of Toronto, Toronto, Ontario, Canada

Key points

- Investigation of masses in the liver is largely radiological and biopsy is only necessary if radiological investigations fail to identify a cause with certainty.
- Hemangiomas are harmless and once diagnosed do not need any further follow-up.
- Hepatocellular carcinoma is no longer the universal death sentence it once was.
  - Regular screening liver ultrasound can identify the majority of cancers at a size that is amenable to cure.
  - Therefore all patients with cirrhosis of any cause should undergo 6-monthly surveillance.
  - Patients with hepatitis B at risk for hepatocellular carcinoma should be identified using published nomograms.

There are many different tumors that may grow in the liver. Apart from metastases from other organs, most are rare and do not merit more than a passing mention. Liver abscesses are not common, but are potentially fatal and so deserve mention. This discussion will therefore be limited to abscesses and to the three most common benign masses or tumor-like lesions, hemangioma, focal nodular hyperplasia, and hepatic adenoma, and the two most common malignant tumors of the liver, hepatocellular carcinoma (HCC) and intrahepatic cholangiocarcinoma (ICC). These five entities account for the vast majority of nodular lesions found on radiological examination of the liver in children and adults.

Hepatology: Diagnosis and Clinical Management, First Edition. Edited by E. Jenny Heathcote.
© 2012 John Wiley & Sons, Ltd. Published 2012 by John Wiley & Sons, Ltd.

Liver abscess

Patients with a liver abscess usually present with fever and pain in the right upper quadrant. They are more frequent in areas of the world where hepatocellular carcinoma (HCC) is also prevalent—a simple clinical test to differentiate the two is to "spring" the lower chest—the individual with an abscess will feel sudden pain whereas this is unlikely if the liver mass is an HCC.

Amoebic liver abscess

Entamoeba histolytica may exist in an environment in a "vegetative" form. When consumed it excysts in the colon to the trophozoite form and may invade the mucosa (possible over several years) causing "flask-shaped" ulcers, which lead to systemic infection, initially via the portal system to the liver but may also be transported to the lungs and brain. The organism produces proteolytic enzymes, which causes the microabscesses to coalesce to a large abscess, generally in the right lobe of the liver.

The patient may present just with fever or just weight loss and/or abdominal pain. Typically, the patient is found to have an elevated serum alkaline phosphatase (ALP) without anemia. Ultrasound shows the presence of an intrahepatic fluid collection. If the edge of the abscess is close to the liver surface rupture is imminent, and treatment needs to be instituted quickly. Diagnosis can be confirmed serologically with antibody tests—EIA and fluorescent antibodies (IgG). But, since this takes time, often treatment has to be instituted before these test results are available. The radiological appearances (ultrasound or CT scan) are often typical and allow rapid diagnosis. Aspiration of the abscess may be necessary for diagnosis if radiology is not typical. It is important to drain all of the red/brown necrotic material ("anchovy paste") because the amoebae are found in or close to the abscess wall, and are often only found in the last samples taken. Treatment with metronidazole 750 mg t.i.d. for 5–10 days is curative and the outcome is excellent. If drainage for diagnosis has not been required, drainage is not standard therapy but may be required in abscesses that are at risk of rupture.

Pyogenic liver abscess

Pyogenic liver abscess is much harder to diagnose as it has an insidious onset and often complicates other intra-abdominal or systemic diseases. The risk factors include:

- recent surgical, endoscopic, or radiologic procedures;
- chronic biliary disease, e.g. primary sclerosing cholangitis, Caroli disease;
- damage to the hepatic artery, e.g. following infusions of chemotherapy to ablate liver tumors;
- neonatal umbilical sepsis;
- portal pyemia/septic embolus, e.g. secondary to gallbladder infection, diverticulitis, or pancreatitis;

- immunocompromised patients—those with organ transplant, leukemia, HIV infection.

The diagnosis is easy to miss as the patient is often already unwell and then further deterioration may be slow. A fall in hemoglobin and/or serum albumin commonly accompanies development of a liver abscess (or abscesses) but may be thought to be secondary to their primary disease. Abdominal pain with or without fever has an insidious onset. Leukocytosis is common, though jaundice is unusual. The diagnosis should be confirmed by ultrasound, CT scan, and/or MRI—sharp borders between normal liver and abscess become obvious. Aspiration under ultrasound guidance is required and cultures for *both* aerobic and anaerobic organisms should be requested.

Treatment

Treatment should be relief of biliary obstruction if present and systemic antibiotics. The prognosis for those with multiple abscesses is poor, whereas that for a single abscess is better.

Hemangioma

Epidemiology

Hemangioma is the most common liver tumor, found in up to 20% of autopsy series. They occur more frequently in women for unknown reasons. They may be single or multiple and may vary in size from a few millimeters to 10 cm or more, although most are smaller than 5 cm in diameter. They consist of vascular channels lined by a single endothelial layer, supported by fibrous tissue. The vascular spaces may contain thrombi, which may calcify.

Hemangioma is a benign lesion, and never develops into malignancy. Whether the lesion is hormone sensitive is controversial. There are case reports of enlargement of hemangiomas with pregnancy or exogenous estrogen administration. However, hemangiomas may enlarge in the absence of these stimuli. Despite this, the vast majority of hemangiomas are clearly not hormone sensitive and do not grow significantly, either spontaneously or under hormonal influences.

Diagnosis

Because the majority of hemangiomas are clinically silent, they most commonly present as an incidental finding on an ultrasound done for unrelated purposes. The diagnosis of hemangioma is radiological.[1] Typically, hemangiomas are described as brightly echogenic on ultrasound. The nature of the lesion can be confirmed by one of several methods. A labeled red blood cell scan shows pooling of the label in the lesion that persists into the delayed phases (late portal phase). However, the sensitivity of this nuclear medicine study is dependent on the size of the lesion. This technique is not highly sensitive or specific, and its use is declining. Hemangiomas that are smaller than about 2 cm may not be detected by labeled red blood cell scanning. All forms of dynamic imaging, that is contrast ultrasound, tri- or four-phase CT scanning or MRI are more sensitive and specific for the detection of hemangioma[2] than red cell scans. The characteristic features are centripetal filling of the lesion with contrast agent, and peripheral nodularity in the venous or late phases.

Clinical features

Hemangiomas of the liver rarely cause symptoms. Thrombosis of very large lesions may present as pain. This can be diagnosed radiologically, using a dynamic contrast-enhanced study. Usually analgesia is the only treatment required, since once the thrombus has formed and is stable the pain will subside. Occasionally giant hemangiomas may bleed, either into the liver or into the peritoneal cavity. Rupture has also been reported associated with enlargement during pregnancy. These are exceptionally rare events, and are the only indications for resection of these lesions.

Large hemangiomas may rarely be associated with thrombocytopenia (Kasabach–Merritt syndrome), particularly in children. Fibrin deposition within the lesion has been reported to cause hypofibrinogenemia.

Practice point. Ultrasound is frequently the only test necessary to confirm hemangioma.

Practice point. Hemangioma virtually never causes symptoms and do not need to be followed at all.

Focal nodular hyperplasia

Focal nodular hyperplasia (FNH) is a tumor-like lesion that consists mainly of normal hepatocytes and fibrous stroma. It has no malignant potential. FNH occurs more frequently in women. The etiology is unknown. Some believe that the FNH is a hypertrophic lesion that grows in response to the development of a spider-like arterial vascular abnormality. The cause of the initial vascular abnormality is unknown. In most instances, the lesion presents as an incidental finding on an imaging study ordered for other reasons. While there are reports of apparent enlargement of FNH in response to estrogen exposure it is difficult to know whether the association is real or due to selective reporting. There are few prospective series that included sufficient subjects to completely exclude the possibility that some FNHs do develop in relation to sex hormone exposure, but the vast majority of FNH are not hormone sensitive[2] and do not enlarge, and the presence of an FNH is not a contraindication to pregnancy.

FNH may vary in size from smaller than 2 cm to many cm in diameter. Very large lesions may infarct or may bleed. External rupture into the peritoneum is rare. Occasionally, FNH may shrink in size or even regress completely.[3]

Pathology

The lesion consists of normal hepatocytes in plates two to three cells thick (compared to the single or double cell plates in normal liver). The arteries drain directly into the sinusoids between adjacent plates. In the center of the lesion there is usually a fibrous stellate scar, carrying the vascular supply (arterial only), which, if present, is characteristic of FNH.

Diagnosis

FNH can usually be diagnosed radiologically without having to resort to biopsy. Perhaps the most sensitive and specific imaging technique is contrast-enhanced ultrasound (CEUS).[3] In this technique microbubbles are injected peripherally and scanned as they flow through the liver. The microbubbles provide multiple surfaces for the incoming sound waves to reflect off, giving a very bright pattern and outlining the blood vessels. CEUS can often clearly demonstrate the feeding artery and the central stellate scar which, if present, is a diagnostic finding. Dynamic MRI and three-phase CT scan can also often show the central scar. However, even in the absence of the scar pattern the enhancement characteristics can distinguish FNH from HCC.

Treatment

Since FNH does not undergo malignant transformation only symptomatic lesions need treatment. Occasionally, very large lesions causing pressure symptoms may need to be resected. Arterial embolization is effective in reducing the size of the lesion, but may not eradicate it completely. Large FNH lesions are at risk for rupture, and may require prophylactic treatment. Lesions that do rupture also require surgical intervention, although embolization has also been used to treat these lesions.

Hepatic adenoma

Epidemiology

This is a rare, benign liver tumor. That adenomas are frequently hormone dependent is now well established.[3] The evidence of a causal association rests on small case series and the temporal relationship between the introduction of the oral contraceptive pill and a sudden significant increase in the number of case reports of hepatic adenoma appearing in the literature. The association was enforced by the finding that hepatic adenoma may enlarge during pregnancy, and may regress after delivery or on withdrawal of the oral contraceptives. Similarly, adenoma associated with androgen use may regress once the androgen therapy is withdrawn. Today's oral contraceptives have much lower estrogen concentrations than those that were in use when the association was first recognized, and some do not even contain the C17-alkyl-substituted estrogens that have been incriminated.

Although development of hepatic adenoma is usually associated with longer-term oral contraceptive use, the development of adenoma has been described after as little as 6 months of use. Hepatic adenomas in men are seen in association with use of anabolic steroids, initially reported with therapeutic use of anabolic steroids for Fanconi anemia or aplastic anemia, and more recently following illicit use of androgens by athletes. Glycogen storage disease type 1A is associated with the development of multiple hepatic adenomas. These are usually multiple, and need to be monitored for malignant conversion. Multiple hepatic adenomatosis is a rare condition, in which the liver may contain 10 or more lesions of various sizes. This may occur in the setting of exogenous hormone administration, although there may be no such history. Hepatic adenomas tend to enlarge over time and have the potential to become malignant. The development of HCC in a pre-existing hepatic adenoma, although well described, is a rare event. Adenomas with malignant potential have a typical staining pattern for β-catenin. Therefore all adenomas should undergo biopsy to look for this staining and the malignant potential that it infers. If this staining is present this may be an indication for resection, particularly if there is no response to estrogen or androgen withdrawal.

Diagnosis

Hepatic adenomas are often incidental findings in patients undergoing radiological imaging, usually ultrasound, for other reasons. Large lesions may cause pressure symptoms, a palpable right upper quadrant mass, or rarely may present with pain due to bleeding into the tumor or rupture into the peritoneum.

Radiological diagnosis is moderately specific. Technetium-labeled liver spleen scans may show a cold area, because the adenoma contains relatively few Kupffer cells. However, this is not a highly sensitive or specific test. The ultrasound appearances are not specific. The lesion may be hyper- or hypoechoic, or of mixed echogenicity. CEUS is useful to exclude the differential diagnoses of HCC and focal nodular hyperplasia, but the appearances are not highly specific for adenoma. CT and MRI may also show rapid arterial enhancement. Other features that may be detected radiologically include the presence of fat in the lesion, abnormal vessels, or intratumoral hemorrhage. Because the radiologic features are not sufficiently specific, needle biopsy of the lesion is always required for a definitive diagnosis.

Pathology

The hallmark of the hepatic adenoma is that it consists solely of hepatocytes, arranged in chords that are seldom more than three cells wide, separated by very narrow sinusoids. The hepatocytes are often larger than normal hepatocytes and may contain fat. Kupffer cells are variably present, although usually in reduced numbers. Bile ducts are absent. Mitoses are rare. The differential diagnosis is primarily with HCC, in which the chords are usually more than three cells wide, and the overall architecture is more disorganized.

Treatment

Hepatic adenomas diagnosed in the setting of exogenous hormone administration often regress when the offending drug is withdrawn, and this constitutes the treatment of choice. Stable lesions can be watched, but growing lesions should be treated, because of the risk of complications related to bleeding or rupture, or to malignant transformation. The usual therapy in the past has been resection, but today local ablation with radiofrequency probes is more commonly used for smaller lesions.

Hepatic adenoma is not a contraindication to pregnancy. Whether treatment of the lesion is required prior to or during pregnancy is controversial. Some advocate ablation or resection of all adenomas prior to pregnancy, or in early pregnancy. This is because of the risk of rupture, which although it is usually associated with larger adenomas, can also occur with smaller lesions. However, an alternative approach would be to monitor the growth of the lesion by frequent ultrasonography and only intervene if the lesion is seen to grow. For those women who are first diagnosed with adenoma during pregnancy the same considerations apply.

Hepatocellular carcinoma

Epidemiology

Hepatocellular carcinoma (HCC) is one of the 10 most common tumors in the world, accounting for more than 300 000 deaths each year.[4] There are close epidemiological links with several diseases that predispose to the development of HCC. The vast majority of HCCs develop on the background of chronic liver disease, usually cirrhosis. HCC arising in a previously normal liver accounts for less than 10% of all HCCs. Worldwide, the most frequent underlying cause of HCC is chronic hepatitis B, followed by hepatitis C. The incidence of HCC is rising in many countries in the West. In some countries, for example Italy, there was a silent epidemic of hepatitis C infection in the period between about 1945 and 1970. In other countries epidemics of hepatitis C occurred as a result of injection drug use, a practice that became widespread during the 1960s and 1970s. Those cohorts have now been infected for up to 40 or more years and are now at risk for the development of HCC. Finally, immigration from parts of the world where hepatitis B and hepatitis C are common is also contributing to the pool of infected individuals in many Western countries, and hence also to the rising incidence of HCC.

Other causes of cirrhosis that predispose to HCC include alcoholic cirrhosis, cirrhosis associated with genetic hemochromatosis, and α_1-antitrypsin deficiency, primary biliary cirrhosis, and more recently it has been recognized that cirrhosis following steatohepatitis is also a risk factor for HCC. Hepatitis B is common in South East Asia and sub-Saharan Africa. In these parts of the world the incidence of HCC is more than 5/100 000 per year, and may be as high as more than 50/100 000 per year in parts of China. In contrast, in parts of the world where chronic viral hepatitis is less common, for example Northern

Europe and North America, the incidence of HCC is closer to 1–5/100000 per year and hepatitis C is the commonest cause.

Practice point. The high prevalence in the West of fatty liver disease and diabetes means that in future these diseases will be the most common causes of HCC.

HCC can also develop in precirrhotic chronic liver injury. This has been well documented in hepatitis B, but also occurs in hepatitis C and non-alcoholic fatty liver disease. The incidence of HCC in these patients is lower than in cirrhosis.

Surveillance for HCC

Surveillance for HCC has become standard of care. This is based on several lines of evidence. A randomized controlled trial in hepatitis B carriers in China that showed that 6-monthly screening with ultrasound and α-fetoprotein resulted in a reduction in mortality of 37%.[5] Several cost–efficacy analyses in various at risk populations have suggested that screening for HCC is cost effective. Patients who undergo surveillance have their HCC diagnosed at an earlier stage.[6] Small HCC can be cured with appreciable frequency (>90%). However, it has become apparent that most of the benefit of surveillance comes from ultrasound, and that the use of serum measurement of α-fetoprotein adds little except cost. Overall, α-fetoprotein screening is insufficiently sensitive and insufficiently specific for general use as a screening test.[7] These results have led to the recommendation by many different groups that patients at risk for HCC should undergo surveillance with ultrasound alone.[8] The screening interval should be 6 months. This is based on the anticipated tumor doubling time, which on average is about 3–5 months. Patients deemed at higher than average risk do not need to be screened more frequently, since the screening interval depends on tumor growth rate, not degree of risk.

With a good ultrasound examination it is possible to detect lesions smaller than 1 cm. With appropriate follow-up and intervention, it is at least theoretically possible to cure the majority of HCC at this size (see below). Thus it is essential to identify patients at risk for HCC, to provide regular surveillance, and to thoroughly investigate lesions discovered on ultrasound to determine whether they are malignant or not.

Practice point. In order to achieve the best outcomes from HCC screening it is important to find the lesions when they are smaller than 2–2.5 cm in diameter, hence 6-monthly screening is better than annual. The cure rate of these lesions is better than 98%.

Diagnosis

Patients whose tumors are diagnosed through screening present with small lesions and are asymptomatic. Unfortunately, even in parts of the world where HCC is common, the majority of patients do not undergo screening, and present with late-stage disease.

HCC can be diagnosed radiologically in the majority of patients, so that biopsy is not necessary. If the typical radiological appearances are present the diagnosis is confirmed. These are that the lesion enhances in the arterial phase of a dynamic contrast study, and is less enhancing than the surrounding liver in the portal venous and late phases of the study. The mechanism is that the tumor is fed exclusively by arterial flow, whereas the liver is fed by arterial and portal venous blood. Thus, in the arterial phase the arterial blood containing contrast is diluted by portal venous blood in the liver but not in the tumor. However, in the venous and delayed phases, the tumor is fed by arterial blood that no longer contains contrast, whereas the portal venous blood in the liver now contains contrast. Lesions that do not match these criteria (and are not clearly FNH, hemangioma, or metastasis) require biopsy.

With improvements in ultrasonography in the recent past we are now able to find lesions that are smaller than 1 cm. However, the smaller the lesion, the more difficult it is to distinguish a benign from malignant nodule, either radiologically or on biopsy. Therefore the algorithm that has been developed to help distinguish these two possibilities has stratified lesions by size, either smaller or larger than 1 cm in diameter. Most lesions smaller than 1 cm are not HCC. The larger the lesion, the more likely it is to be HCC. This algorithm is shown in Figs 7.1 and 7.2.

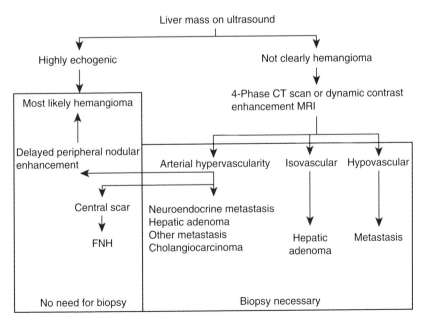

Fig. 7.1 Algorithm for the diagnosis of a liver mass in a patient who does not have any risk factors for hepatocellular carcinoma. FNH, focal nodular hyperplasia.

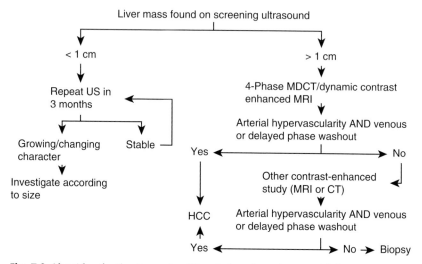

Fig. 7.2 Algorithm for the diagnosis of liver lesions in patients at risk for hepatocellular carcinoma. This algorithm applies only to lesions detected in a cirrhotic liver or in the liver of patients with chronic hepatitis B. In other situations this algorithm is less useful. HCC, hepatocellular carcinoma; MDCT, multidetector computed tomography.

Serum α-fetoprotein concentration has long been used as a diagnostic test for HCC. Given the high specificity of the radiological appearances α-fetoprotein seldom provides additional information.

Pathology

The earliest lesions of HCC consist of well-differentiated cells in plates that may not be more than three cells wide. There may still be portal tracts present, and there may be some arterialization, but portal veins are still present. The cells in these lesions often contain fat, and there is seldom any vascular invasion by tumor cells. These small lesions are often unencapsulated. As the lesion progresses the cellular differentiation changes, more typical nuclear/cytoplasmic ratio changes are seen, and there is nuclear pleiomorphism. These lesions later become encapsulated, and there may be microvascular vessel invasion. More advanced lesions no longer have portal tracts and there are no portal veins. The cells exhibit more features of malignancy, such as altered nucleocytoplasmic ratio, and altered nuclear morphology.

Clinical features

HCC that causes symptoms is late-stage disease, and at that point is seldom curable and often is too far advanced for any form of therapy, including liver transplantation. Late-stage disease usually presents as deterioration in clinical status in a patient known to have liver disease, or as new-onset ascites in

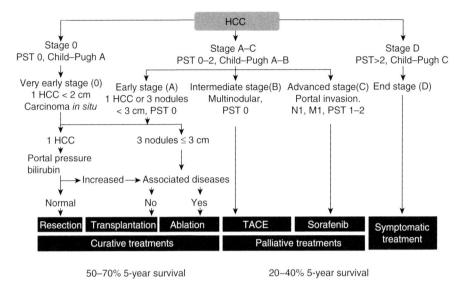

Fig. 7.3 Staging and treatment allocation of hepatocellular carcinoma according to the BCLC (Barcelona Cancer of the Liver Clinic) system. HCC, hepatocellular carcinoma; PST, performance status according to the Eastern Cooperative Oncology Group; TACE, transarterial chemoembolization.

patients not previously known to have liver disease. Ascites is usually the first clinical manifestation, followed or accompanied by weight loss and jaundice. Occasionally, an HCC may present with abdominal pain due to rupture into the peritoneum or intrahepatic bleeding. The diagnosis is confirmed radiologically in these patients.

Treatment
Treatment of HCC can be divided into three broad categories.[9] Curative therapy includes local ablation (either ethanol injection or radiofrequency ablation), resection, or transplantation. Palliative therapy includes chemoembolization or sorafenib, and, finally, late-stage disease requires only supportive care. A schematic representation of the types of patients who are suitable for the different types of treatment is shown in Fig. 7.3.

Liver transplantation
Liver transplantation is reserved for relatively early-stage disease. The standard criteria for transplant that are associated with good survival post transplant are the so-called "Milan criteria", that is a single tumor smaller than 5 cm in diameter, or up to three tumors none larger than 3 cm in diameter. Attempts to expand these criteria to larger tumors have not been adequately validated and are not widely accepted.

For patients with HCC transplanted within the Milan criteria the 5-year survival is about 70%, with a tumor recurrence rate that is less than 20%. However, in an intention-to-treat analysis of all patients listed for transplant, overall survival is about 65% at 5 years, that is similar to survival following resection. However, the recurrence rate is much better than for resection, in which the recurrence rate may be as high as 50% at 5 years. Thus liver transplantation has become the treatment of choice for HCC in the West. However, a lack of donor organs has meant that many patients on the waiting list for liver transplant are removed from the list because their tumors exceed listing criteria over time.

Resection

Treatment of HCC by resection has a long and venerable history. Recent improvements in patient selection and postoperative management has resulted in better survival—up to 70% at 5 years, but with a recurrence rate of about 50%. Patients with cirrhosis and poor liver function cannot tolerate resection. Thus resection is limited to patients with Child's A cirrhosis. Portal hypertension (esophageal varices, splenomegaly, portal–venous pressure gradient of more than 10 mmHg) or elevated bilirubin are contraindications to resection. Extensive resections, such as trisegmentectomy, are also usually not possible in cirrhotic patients.

Local ablation

This term refers to the local application of a noxious stimulus directly to the tumor. The initial studies were performed by injections of absolute alcohol directly into the lesion. More recently, application of heat using radiofrequency waves or microwaves has replaced alcohol injection. Radiofrequency ablation (RFA) provides more complete ablation than alcohol injection. RFA is usually restricted to tumors smaller than 4.5 cm, in order to achieve necrosis of the visible tumor and a margin of 0.5–1 cm around the lesion. Lesions smaller than 2 cm can be ablated completely in more than 95% of cases.[10] Lesions larger than 3 cm can be completely ablated in about 58% of cases. Since survival is related to the ability to achieve complete ablation, the smaller the tumor at diagnosis the more likely it is to be completely ablated, and the more likely is survival to be enhanced.[6] Some tumor locations preclude RFA, but it is possible, usually, to separate a lesion at the edge of the liver from neighboring organs by introduction of saline between the liver and the adjacent organ. Exophytic lesions need to be approached through a rim of non-tumor tissue, because direct puncture and RFA runs the risk of causing tumor seeding.

Chemoembolization

In this technique a chemotherapeutic agent, usually doxorubicin or cisplatin, is injected directly into an artery feeding the tumor. The drug is mixed with lipiodol to create an emulsion. Lipiodol is a viscous, oily, radiographic contrast agent. Following injection into HCC the lesion takes up lipiodol, so that the lesion is intensely white on CT scan. The lipiodol probably has its effect by slowing down the flow of blood, or even stopping the flow of blood completely, creating some local ischemia. Following the injection of the lipiodol–drug mix the artery feeding the tumor is embolized with gelfoam, polyvinyl alcohol, or other embolic agent. The induction of ischemia in the tumor cells appears to enhance the killing effect of the chemotherapeutic agent.

Two randomized controlled trials and a meta-analysis confirm that chemoembolization does prolong survival. Chemoembolization can only be given to patients with reasonably good liver function, Child's A cirrhosis. It is associated with some destruction of viable liver tissue, and is often associated with some degree of worsening of liver function. On average the 2-year survival after chemoembolization is about 60%, compared to about 30% in untreated controls.

Patients who have failed chemoembolization or whose disease is too far advanced for chemoembolization (either vascular invasion or extrahepatic disease) can be treated with sorafenib, a multikinase oral agent that has recently been approved. The gains in life expectancy are modest, but this is the first agent that has been approved for the treatment of HCC.

Other therapy for HCC
There are a large number of other, different forms of therapy that have been applied to patients with HCC. Unfortunately, none have been tested in randomized controlled trials against standard of care and therefore cannot be recommended. Combination of chemoembolization and local ablation seems a logical approach, but this has not been shown to be superior to either alone. Although the liver is radiosensitive, external beam conformal radiotherapy has been used to limit the exposure of uninvolved liver to radiation. Enhanced survival has not been demonstrated. Internal radiotherapy using ^{99}yttrium-labelled glass beads injected into the feeding artery is a promising therapy, but this has also not yet been shown to enhance survival. Intra-arterial chemotherapy or systemic chemotherapy has been shown in controlled trials to enhance survival only by a matter of a few weeks, but at the cost of a significant decrease in quality of life.

Practice point. The management of HCC is complex and may involve several different specialties. No single specialty has the necessary expertise to provide the most appropriate treatment for all patients. Therefore patients with suspected or confirmed HCC should be referred to multidisciplinary centers with expertise in the management of this disease.

Intrahepatic cholangiocarcinoma

This is a disease of the fifth and sixth decades, and occurs equally in males and females. Intrahepatic cholangiocarcinoma (ICC) is a tumor arising in the bile duct radicals within the liver. This is a relatively common tumor in some parts of the world, and often has recognized predisposing causes. These include infestations with liver flukes, such as *Clonorchis sinensus* or *Opisthorchis viverini*, hepatolithiasis, Caroli disease, a diet high in nitrosamines, or exposure to Thorotrast. *Opisthorchis viverini* infection is a major cause of ICC in parts of Thailand, where this tumor is very common. Hilar cholangiocarcinoma has a slightly different demographic distribution, and is more common in males, and more often associated with inflammatory bowel disease and sclerosing cholangitis.

The incidence of intrahepatic cholangiocarcinoma is rising alarmingly, whereas the incidence of extrahepatic cholangiocarcinoma is falling. This may be related to the modern high rate of cholecystectomy, and a significant decrease of gall bladder carcinoma. The causes of the increased incidence of intrahepatic cholangiocarcinoma are not known. It has been suggested that it may be related to cirrhosis due to hepatitis C and hepatitis B. The demographics of the populations that have HCC and cholangiocarcinoma are different, suggesting that they do not really have a common etiology. However, it is clear that cirrhosis is a risk factor for the development of ICC.

Diagnosis

Intrahepatic cholangiocarcinoma is usually clinically silent until late, and it often presents with cancer symptoms of weight loss, malaise, and abdominal pain, and decreased performance status, rather than symptoms that bring attention to the liver. Lesions that obstruct the bifurcation of the common hepatic duct present with obstructive jaundice and marked weight loss.

The diagnosis is primarily radiological.[11] Ultrasound may show a peripheral mass lesion in the liver or will show dilated intrahepatic bile ducts with a hilar carcinoma. Thickening of the bile duct wall may also be identified. For hilar cholangiocarcinoma MRI has become the investigation of choice because of its superior ability to identify the level of bile duct obstruction, and ability to delineate tumor anatomy and to determine resectability. It does not require injection of contrast, and thus there is no need to leave a drain *in situ* to prevent cholangitis in the obstructed duct. MRI, however, does under-stage disease in about 20% of cases. Endoscopic ultrasound allows fine-needle biopsy of the lesion. This is much more accurate than obtaining brushings at endoscopic retrograde cholangiopancreatography (ERCP). It also allows identification of local involved lymph nodes. Positron emission tomography (PET) scanning has also been used to assist with the staging and planning of therapy of cholangiocarcinoma. It is less specific than CT scanning for the primary lesion, but is better at detecting regional and distant lymphadenopathy. Although both CEA and CA 19-9, either alone or in combination, have been described as tumor markers of cholangiocarcinoma, neither is sufficiently sensitive or specific for routine use as diagnostic tumor markers.

Pathology

The lesion is an adenocarcinoma and may demonstrate a tubular appearance set in fibrous stroma; occasionally, the cells may be very pleiomorphic. In tumors arising in the larger ducts the tumor is usually surrounded by a wide zone of biliary epithelial cell dysplasia.

Treatment

Despite advances in treatment, the prognosis of intrahepatic cholangiocarcinoma remains poor, with most patients dying within 5 years, and 90% dying with the first 2 years.[12] Although reports from single centers suggest that resection improves survival, mortality data do not support this conclusion. Nonetheless, surgical resection remains the only chance of curative therapy. Intrahepatic cholangiocarcinoma spreads to local lymph nodes early in the course of the disease. This results in a high recurrence rate after surgery. The location of the tumor may also limit the ability to resect the lesion. Lesions involving the hilum may not be resectable, particularly if the tumor extends into the second order branches of the right and left hepatic ducts. Adjuvant radiotherapy and chemotherapy have not been shown to extend life. For tumors that obstruct the hepatic duct and cause biliary obstruction insertion of a stent to drain the duct may be required if the patient has uncontrollable pruritus. This can be placed by endoscopy at ERCP, or percutaneously under ultrasound guidance. Liver transplantation is usually associated with a 90% recurrence rate. Recently, an aggressive management protocol for early tumors, developed at the Mayo Clinic, has allowed post-transplant survival of 85% at 5 years. However, few patients are suitable for this protocol.

Other liver tumors

There are about 20 other mass-like lesions that may develop in the liver. Benign lesions include bile duct adenomas, and cystadenomas, hemangioendothelioma, lymphangioma, angiomyolipoma, and other rare benign soft tissue tumors. Of the malignant lesions that occur in the liver not discussed above, metastatic cancer is the most common and the colon is the most common primary site. The radiological appearances of metastases are similar wherever the source, but in the setting of a previous known carcinoma elsewhere the diagnosis is not difficult. Metastases from neuroendocrine tumors merit special mention. These are often slow growing, and may present with symptoms of the carcinoid syndrome, or phaeochromocytoma. However, the majority of the tumors are non-secreting, and present commonly during surveillance for metastatic disease after treatment of a primary neuroendocrine tumor, or in patients in whom a primary has not been diagnosed as an incidental finding on an ultrasound. These are usually very vascular tumors that may be mistaken for hepatocellular carcinoma. However, they do not usually display the typical "washout" that characterizes HCC. Tissue from a needle biopsy may be difficult to interpret, and often special stains for either hepatocyte markers or neuroendocrine markers, such as synaptophysin or chromogranin, may be necessary.

In addition, malignancies can arise from any component of liver tissue. Endothelium can give rise to angiosarcoma or malignant hemangioendothelioma; muscle can give rise to rhabdomyosarcoma. Other primary tumors include sarcomas and primary lymphoma of the liver. These are all exceptionally rare and all require tissue diagnosis.

Liver masses in children

Although many of the masses that are seen in adults are also rarely seen in children, such as hemangioma, the presence of a liver mass in a child is very worrying. However, the epidemiology of liver masses in children is different from that in adults, and differs at different ages. The evaluation of these masses is difficult, and frequently requires a biopsy. Therefore the diagnosis and management of the lesions is best reserved for expert pediatric gastroenterologists.

Case study 7.1

A 28-year-old body builder underwent an abdominal ultrasound for abdominal pain. The ultrasound showed several mass lesions in the liver. He admitted to anabolic steroid use. A CEUS confirmed the presence of at least five liver lesions. These were hypervascular in the arterial phase and venous phase of the examination and more or less isointense compared to the normal liver in the delayed phase. These features are not diagnostic for any specific lesion, but are compatible with hepatic adenoma. A biopsy was ordered to confirm the diagnosis and to test for markers of the potential for malignant transformation. Unfortunately, the liver bled after the biopsy. The bleeding required embolization for control. However, the embolization led to infarction of a significant proportion of the right lobe of the liver. The patient had severe pain, but did not develop liver failure. The necrotic area became infected with the development of a hepatic abscess. The biopsy showed alterations in the staining pattern of β-catenin, suggesting that there was a potential for malignant transformation. Eventually, after a lengthy recuperation the patient did well. However, even after more than a year since stopping the anabolic steroids liver masses remain and surveillance for HCC is ongoing.

Practice point. Liver biopsy carries risks and should only be used if radiology does not provide a confident diagnosis.

Case study 7.2

A 45-year-old Chinese man known to be chronically infected with hepatitis B had been under medical follow-up for years. His serum transaminases were never more than 1.2 times the upper limit of normal and were most often below the upper limit of normal. The viral load was always in the range of 100 000 to 250 000 IU/mL. Ultrasound did not suggest the presence of cirrhosis. He had never received treatment for his hepatitis B. He was being screened for HCC by measuring α-fetoprotein levels every 6 months. Seven years later he developed abdominal pain. An ultrasound showed a 10-cm hepatocellular carcinoma. The lesion was hypervascular in the arterial phase and washed out in the venous phase. There was portal vein invasion with tumor. No treatment could be offered. The patient died 6 months later.

Practice point. α-fetoprotein is not a reliable screening test for HCC. It is negative in about 40% of all HCCs, and in more than 90% of all HCCs below about 2 cm. Ultrasound at 6-monthly intervals is the recommended HCC screening test.

Multiple choice questions

1. A 55-year-old man presents with fever and right upper quadrant pain. There is no history of prior travel. An ultrasound demonstrates a cystic lesion in the liver and stones in the gall bladder. A diagnosis of hepatic abscess is made. The abscess is drained percutaneously, yielding pus, and the fever deffervesces on antibiotics. Further management should include:
   A. Colonoscopy
   B. Cholecystectomy
   C. Magnetic resonance cholangiopancreatography (MRCP)

2. A patient presents with a 3-cm mass lesion in the liver, found incidentally on ultrasound during an investigation for abdominal pain. The radiologist comments that this is likely a hemangioma. The pain is diagnosed as irritable bowel syndrome. Your approach should be:
   A. Order a nuclear red blood cell scan
   B. No further follow-up needed
   C. Order a CT scan
   D. Order an MRI
   E. Repeat the ultrasound in 6 months to determine stability

3. A 30-year-old woman who has chronic hepatitis B has a 2-cm mass lesion identified incidentally during an ultrasound examination of a pregnancy. She is at the end of the first trimester. The patient is taking tenofovir to suppress hepatitis B viral replication. There is a family history of hepatitis B and liver cancer. Your approach should be:

A. Order a CT scan
B. Order an MRI
C. Observe and repeat the ultrasound in 6 months
D. Order a CT scan when she is no longer pregnant

4. The most likely diagnosis in the case described in Question 3 is:
A. Hepatic adenoma
B. Hemangioma
C. Hepatocellular carcinoma

5. A 56-year-old man with cirrhosis due to hepatitis C is undergoing routine surveillance for HCC. An ultrasound shows a new lesion 1 cm in diameter. A CT scan shows arterial hypervascularity but no venous washout. The next step is:
A. Order a biopsy
B. Order an MRI
C. Repeat the CT scan in 3 months

6. For the patient described in Question 5, an MRI has the same features as the CT scan, i.e. the appearances are atypical. An ultrasound-guided biopsy is done, which shows only normal-looking hepatocytes and fibrosis. The follow-up should include:
A. CT scan in 3 months
B. CT scan in 6 months
C. An ultrasound in 3 months
D. Another biopsy

Answers

1. A and C. Diverticular disease or colon cancer may be sources for portal bacteremia leading to hepatic abscess. Stones in the gall bladder are unlikely to be the source of hepatic abscess unless there is biliary obstruction and/or cholangitis. MRCP is necessary to exclude the possibility of sclerosing cholangitis as a cause of hepatic abscess.
2. B. Red blood cell scans are obsolete. The typical ultrasound appearances of hemangioma are highly specific.
3. B. With a personal history of chronic hepatitis B and a family history of hepatocellular carcinoma, she has an above average risk of HCC. Delaying investigations may result in the cancer growing to an incurable stage.
4. B. Hemangioma remains the most common mass lesion found in the liver, even in the presence of risk factors for HCC. However, the presence of risk factors should prompt a more intensive investigation to exclude HCC.
5. B. Two different imaging techniques are required before a lesion is characterized as atypical and before a biopsy is ordered. Delaying investigation may result in the lesion progressing to a stage where the likelihood of cure is reduced.

6. Either C or D. If the clinical suspicion of HCC is high, another biopsy should be done because the first might have missed the lesion. Alternatively, a growing lesion warrants additional investigation. Because the ultrasound initially identified the lesion, further ultrasound follow-up will show if and when growth occurs. This would trigger re-investigation. Further CT scan or MRI would also show growth, but is expensive and unnecessary.

References

1. Birnbaum BA, Weinreb JC, Megibow AJ, et al. Definitive diagnosis of hepatic hemangiomas: MR imaging versus Tc-99m-labeled red blood cell SPECT. Radiology 1990; 176: 95–101.
2. Di Stasi M, Caturelli E, De Sio I, et al. Natural history of focal nodular hyperplasia of the liver: an ultrasound study. J Clin Ultrasound 1996; 24: 345–50.
3. Rooks JB, Ory HW, Ishak KG, et al. Epidemiology of hepatocellular adenoma. The role of oral contraceptive use. JAMA 1979; 242: 644–8.
4. Bosch FX, Ribes J, Diaz M, et al. Primary liver cancer: worldwide incidence and trends. Gastroenterology 2004; 127 (5 Suppl. 1): S5–S16.
5. Zhang BH, Yang BH, Tang ZY. Randomized controlled trial of screening for hepatocellular carcinoma. J Cancer Res Clin Oncol 2004; 130: 417–22.
6. Sala M, Llovet JM, Vilana R, et al.; Barcelona Clinic Liver Cancer Group. Initial response to percutaneous ablation predicts survival in patients with hepatocellular carcinoma. Hepatology 2004; 40: 1352–60.
7. Trevisani F, D'Intino PE, Morselli-Labate AM, et al. Serum alpha-fetoprotein for diagnosis of hepatocellular carcinoma in patients with chronic liver disease: influence of HBsAg and anti-HCV status. J Hepatol 2001; 34: 570–5.
8. Bruix J, Sherman M; Practice Guidelines Committee, American Association for the Study of Liver Diseases. Management of hepatocellular carcinoma. Available on the AASLD website. http://www.aasld.org/practiceguidelines/Documents/Bookmarked%20Practice%20Guidelines/HCCUpdate2010.pdf. Accessed Jan 2012.
9. Bruix J, Llovet JM. Prognostic prediction and treatment strategy in HCC. Hepatology 2002; 35: 519–24.
10. Livraghi T, Meloni F, Di Stasi M, et al. Sustained complete response and complications rates after radiofrequency ablation of very early hepatocellular carcinoma in cirrhosis: Is resection still the treatment of choice? Hepatology 2008; 47: 82–9.
11. Anderson CD, Pinson CW, Berlin J, et al. Diagnosis and treatment of cholangiocarcinoma. Oncologist 2004; 9: 43–57.
12. Khan SA, Davidson BR, Goldin R, et al.; British Society of Gastroenterology. Guidelines for the diagnosis and treatment of cholangiocarcinoma: consensus document. Gut 2002; 51 (Suppl. 6): VI1–9.

Chronic portosystemic encephalopathy and its management

CHAPTER 8

Leslie B. Lilly[1] and Binita M. Kamath[2]

[1] Multi Organ Transplant Program, Toronto General Hospital, University Health Network, Toronto, Ontario, Canada

[2] University of Toronto, and Division of Gastroenterology, Hepatology and Nutrition, The Hospital for Sick Children, Toronto, Ontario, Canada

---

Key points

- Acute episodes of hepatic encephalopathy are usually triggered by a potentially reversible cause, and identification of this precipitant is key in successful management.
- Measures used in the management of hepatic encephalopathy are primarily directed at reducing circulating levels of ammonia, whether via laxatives, alterations in stool pH, or modification of enteric flora.

Introduction

Alterations in mental status, ranging from subtle neurocognitive deficits (minimal hepatic encephalopathy) to hepatic coma, commonly complicate end-stage liver disease. The pathogenesis is thought to be linked to elevated serum ammonia levels, attributable to the shunting of blood directly from the portal circulation into the venous system without exposure to hepatocytes that line the sinusoids. Thus the term portosystemic encephalopathy (PSE) is often used to reinforce the notion that shunting plays a key role. Low-grade cerebral edema is likely the underlying brain injury; however, unlike the hepatic encephalopathy of fulminant hepatic failure, PSE is not associated with significant elevations in intracranial pressure and is therefore not directly associated with mortality.

This section outlines a practical approach to PSE, both acute in onset and in patients who are chronically affected by this challenging problem.

Hepatology: Diagnosis and Clinical Management, First Edition. Edited by E. Jenny Heathcote.
© 2012 John Wiley & Sons, Ltd. Published 2012 by John Wiley & Sons, Ltd.

Clinical presentations of portosystemic encephalopathy

Following a 1998 consensus conference, hepatic encephalopathy has been clas-sified into three types: acute, recurrent, or persistent. This classification is based on the underlying etiology. As most episodes of encephalopathy occur in patients with known cirrhosis, the focus will be on the recognition of this par-ticular subtype.

Precipitating factors and their management

Clinicians are commonly presented with the situation where a stable cirrhotic patient, often well-compensated, presents with the relatively rapid onset of neurological disturbance (as described above), which come under the umbrella of "hepatic encephalopathy". In the majority of these instances a specific pre-cipitant can be identified and treated; in only rare situations is PSE attributable to sudden worsening of the underlying chronic liver disease. As ammonia remains the leading candidate for a role in PSE, it is useful to start with condi-tions that may affect its serum levels.

Increased ammonia load

Ammonia remains the leading candidate as the agent implicated in hepatic encephalopathy, and serum levels are often measured as a result. While the information gained may be of some use in patients not already known to have liver disease, knowledge of the exact ammonia level rarely alters clinical deci-sion making. Further, venous ammonia levels are of little use due to degrada-tion of red blood cells; an arterial sample shipped on ice to the lab for prompt measurement should be obtained if the information is to be useful.

A sudden increase in arterial ammonia levels can be caused by gastrointes-tinal bleeding, dehydration, renal insufficiency, or, in relatively rare cases, dietary indiscretions (high protein intake). These conditions frequently coexist, and can be determined by history, physical examination, and blood tests, and appropriate treatments instituted (which are beyond the scope of this chapter).

Constipation

Constipation alone can precipitate PSE, and in patients with a history of well-controlled encephalopathy this may be due to non-compliance with lac-tulose therapy. In addition, medications that cause constipation (narcotics, for example) can aggravate PSE in addition to worsening it through direct central nervous system effects (see below).

Infections

Bacterial infections are the most common cause of death in patients with cir-rhosis and they are implicated in PSE. In sepsis, hemodynamic disturbances with associated renal dysfunction may further worsen PSE. In patients present-ing with the abrupt onset of encephalopathy, even if a fever is absent, investiga-tions should include an ascitic tap with fluid analysis for cell count and cultures, as well as urine and blood cultures, sputum cultures if appropriate, and chest X-ray. A low threshold for the introduction of broad-spectrum antibiotics should be observed until a specific etiology has been determined.

Electrolyte disturbances

Cirrhotic patients commonly receive diuretics, which can precipitate hyponatremia, hyperkalemia, and acid–base disturbances. The former is particularly associated with new onset or worsening of already present PSE, thus regular monitoring of renal function and electrolyte levels in patients receiving diuretics is very important.

Medications

Any medication that can cause sedation is more likely to do so in patients with cirrhosis. These include benzodiazepines, opioids, antihistamines, some antin-auseants, cough suppressants (which contain codeine), and drugs such as chlordiazepoxide. Patients with cirrhosis and their care-givers should be cautioned to avoid or minimize the use of such medications.

Acute brain injury

Although focal neurological symptoms or signs are certainly seen in patients with PSE, such as a transverse myelitis or a parkinsonian-like illness, they are relatively uncommon. CT of the brain should be performed if focal deficits are present. Intracranial bleeding may occur spontaneously or in response to minor trauma in coagulopathic cirrhotic patients. Many patients with alcoholic cirrhosis have a history of falls, and a chronic subdural hematoma may present with symptoms difficult to distinguish from PSE. In such patients, brain computed tomography should be performed if a clear precipitant of PSE has not been readily identified.

Worsening liver disease

Although an uncommon cause of PSE, patients with established cirrhosis may have sudden deterioration in liver function. This can be due to a toxic injury (alcohol, drugs), to portal vein (or, less commonly, hepatic vein) thrombosis (and one must think of a complicating hepatocellular carcinoma in this scenario), or following a general anesthetic for what would ordinarily be considered "minor" surgery (a hernia repair is a common example). A thorough history and the appropriate imaging should help to exclude these possibilities.

Specific measures to treat portosystemic encephalopathy

Diet

Dietary protein restriction was at one time commonly instituted in patients with PSE. It is now clear that it can worsen nutritional status in cirrhotic patients, and is no longer recommended. Protein intake of 0.8 to 1.0 g/kg/day is generally sufficient to maintain normal nitrogen balance. It may be appropriate to recommend reduction in protein from more dense sources (red meats, for example) and their substitution with vegetable proteins, that is protein "modification" rather than restriction.

Drug treatment

Lactulose has been the mainstay of PSE treatment for many years (Box 8.1). It works to reduce ammonia both via a direct osmotic laxative effect and via the lowering of stool pH. It is typically given at a dose of 20 g once or twice daily and titrated to achieve two to three loose bowel motions per day. In patients whose level of consciousness or state of agitation does not permit oral dosing, lactulose can be given in enema form, typically as a 30% solution (300 mL of lactulose brought up to a liter with tap water). Lactulose should not be given by a nasogastric tube in comatose patients as lactulose can cause severe lung damage if it is aspirated.

Antibiotics are often added in patients whose PSE is not responsive to lactulose. Recent evidence supports the use of rifaximin, a non-absorbed derivative of rifamycin, with a large study demonstrating its efficacy when added to lactulose. It is not yet available, however, in all countries. Other antibiotics have also been used. Metronidazole, usually at a dose of 250 mg every 12 h, may be

---

Box 8.1 Treatment of hepatic encephalopathy

Identification and management of the precipitating cause
1 Increased ammonia load, including constipation, renal dysfunction
2 Sepsis
3 Electrolyte disturbances
4 Medications, e.g. those that induce constipation
5 Acute brain injury
6 Worsening of underlying liver disease

Specific measures
1 Diet (protein "modification" rather than restriction)
2 Drug
   (i) Lactulose
   (ii) Antibiotics, including rifaximin
3 Other medical options
   (i) Flumazenil
   (ii) L-Ornithine L-aspartate
   (iii) Branched-chain amino acids
   (iv) Sodium benzoate, sodium phenylacetate
4 Artificial liver support
5 Liver transplantation

similar in effectiveness to neomycin (which is no longer used), but is limited in long-term use by gastrointestinal intolerance and potential neurotoxicity.

Flumazenil, a γ-aminobutyric acid (GABA) antagonist, produces at best a transient improvement in patients with PSE; its routine use cannot be recommended.

Other agents and measures

L-Ornithine L-aspartate (LOLA) serves to provide substrates involved in deammination, and has been shown to reduce serum ammonia levels in animals and humans. The typical dose is one or two sachets administered three times daily. It is not clear if it adds any benefit to patients already receiving lactulose and antibiotics for their PSE.

Branched-chain amino acid (BCAA) levels are often depressed in patients with advanced liver disease, and oral supplementation has been studied. Results have been inconsistent, but there have been reports of a reduction in complications in patients with cirrhosis, and of improved nutritional status.

Sodium benzoate and **sodium phenylacetate** have been used in urea cycle disorders to reduce serum ammonia levels. However, they both contribute sodium to the patient's diet, which may be undesirable in advanced liver disease, and there is little evidence supporting their use in patients with chronic PSE.

Artificial liver support (extracorporeal albumin dialysis), while studied in the setting of hepatic encephalopathy due to fulminant hepatic failure, has not been systematically examined in chronic PSE. Reviews of randomized control trials in the intermediate condition of acute-on-chronic liver failure have yielded inconsistent results.

Liver transplantation represents definitive management of chronic PSE, as it both corrects the shunts attributable to cirrhosis and restores a functional mass of healthy hepatocytes. However, the MELD (Model of End-stage Liver Disease) system that is currently in wide use for the allocation of deceased donor organs does not include PSE, and those patients with significant shunting who have well-preserved liver synthetic and renal function are unlikely to be transplanted using this algorithm.

Case study 8.1

Mr. JD is a 55-year-old man with established cirrhosis on the basis of alcohol, with ascites, which is well controlled on spironolactone 100 mg daily and furosemide 40 mg daily. He has no prior history of encephalopathy and has small esophageal varices noted on upper endoscopy 1 year earlier, for which he was placed on nadolol 40 mg daily.

He was in his usual state of health until last night, when he had complained about being unusually fatigued, and had gone to bed early. This morning he was difficult to rouse, and then was disoriented to place and time. His wife brought him to the emergency department.

On examination he had a temperature of 37.7°C. Blood pressure was 105/70 mmHg, heart rate 62 beats/min and regular. He could not identify the day or the month, and did not know what hospital he was in. Asterixis was present. He was mildly jaundiced. The remainder of the examination was remarkable for a slightly distended, non-tender abdomen, mild peripheral edema, and numerous stigmata of chronic liver disease. A diagnostic workup was commenced.

Diagnostic workup
Routine blood work was done, including complete blood count, creatinine, electrolytes, liver biochemistry, and INR. Cultures of blood and urine were drawn. Chest X-ray was obtained. A bedside diagnostic paracentesis was performed, and fluid was sent for cell count as well as inoculated into blood culture bottles.

Outcome
Pending the results of the investigations above, the patient was started on lactulose, which he was able to take by mouth. His diuretics were withheld. He was started empirically on antibiotics (third-generation cephalosporin). He was admitted to hospital for further management.

WBC 7.8×10^9/L	Platelets 62×10^9/L	
Hb 135 g/L	Albumin 22 g/L	INR 1.7
Na 129 mmol/L	K 5.5 mmol/L	Cl 110 mmol/L
AST 62 IU/L	ALP 110 IU/L	ALT 32 IU/L
Creatinine 145 μmol/L	Total bilirubin 75 μmol/L	
Chest X-ray within normal limits		
Ascitic fluid:	WBC 550×10^6/L	80% PMN

A diagnosis of spontaneous bacterial peritonitis was made, along with moderate renal insufficiency attributable to diuretic usage, infection, and third spacing of fluid into the peritoneal cavity. Hyponatremia was present, which could also be aggravating the hepatic encephalopathy.

The patient was started on 25% albumin, 200 mL i.v. every 12 h × 48 h. Urine sodium was ordered.

Ascitic fluid cultures grew *E. coli* that was pan sensitive. Antibiotics were continued.

In 24 h, the patient's mental status had normalized and his creatinine had improved, along with serum Na. His low-grade fever had disappeared. Urine Na was 42 μmol/L, not consistent with hepatorenal syndrome. Blood and urine cultures were negative.

Five days of intravenous antibiotics were administered; the patient improved and was discharged home in stable condition on no diuretics. He was started on prophylactic ciprofloxacin 750 mg once weekly.

Liver transplant referral was initiated (MELD 23 on presentation).

Multiple choice question

1. Which of the following factors is the LEAST likely to account for the abrupt
   onset of encephalopathy in a patient with previously well-compensated cir-
   rhosis due to chronic hepatitis C infection?
   A. Renal insufficiency secondary to dehydration
   B. Upper gastrointestinal bleeding from portal hypertensive gastropathy
   C. Progression of the underlying liver disease
   D. Urosepsis
   E. Institution of antiviral therapy 4 weeks earlier with pegylated interferon
   and ribavirin

Answer

1. C

Further reading

Bass NM, Mullen KD, Sanyal A, et al. Rifaximin treatment in hepatic encephalopathy. N
Eng J Med 2010; 362: 1071–81.

Cash WJ, McConville P, McDermott E, et al. Current concepts in the assessment and
treatment of hepatic encephalopathy. Q J Med 2010; 103: 9–16.

Charlton M. Branched chain amino acid enriched supplements as therapy for liver
disease. J Nutr 2006; 136: 295S–8S.

De Brujin KM, Blendis LM, Zilm DH, et al. Effect of dietary protein manipulation in
subclinical portal-systemic encephalopathy. Gut 1983; 24: 53–60.

Ferenci P, Lockwood A, Mullen K, et al. Hepatic encephalopathy—definition, nomencla-
ture, diagnosis and quantification: final report of the working party at the 11th World
Congresses of Gastroenterology. Hepatology 2002; 35: 716–21.

Haussinger D, Schliess F. Pathogenetic mechanisms of hepatic encephalopathy. Gut 2008;
57: 1156–65.

Zafirova Z, O'Connor M. Hepatic encephalopathy: current management strategies and
treatment, including management and monitoring of cerebral edema and intracranial
hypertension in fulminant hepatic failure. Curr Opin Anaesthesiol 2010; 23: 121–7.

Indications for liver transplantation in adults and children

CHAPTER 9

Nazia Selzner[1] and Vicky L. Ng[2]

[1] Division of Gastroenterology, Toronto General Hospital, University Health Network, Toronto, Ontario, Canada
[2] University of Toronto, and Division of Gastroenterology, Hepatology, and Nutrition, The Hospital for Sick Children, Toronto, Ontario, Canada

---

Key points

- Patients should be considered for liver transplantation if they have evidence of fulminant hepatic failure, a life-threatening systemic complication of liver disease, or a liver-based metabolic defect.
- Organ allocation is currently based on a risk-projection system using the Model for End-stage Liver Disease (MELD) score, which accurately predicts short-term mortality of patients while waiting for a transplant.
- Transplantation of patients with low MELD score (<15) has been associated with higher mortality than would be expected without transplantation and is not the ideal use of donor organs.
- Evaluation includes a detailed assessment to make sure that transplantation is technically feasible, medically appropriate, and in the best interest of both the patient and society.

End-stage liver disease (ESLD) is a major health problem worldwide. It has become clear over the last two decades that liver transplantation (LT) is an effective and life-saving intervention for patients with ESLD. Thomas E. Starzl performed the first liver transplantation in 1963, in a 3 year old with biliary atresia.[1,2] Since that landmark case, continuous advances in surgical techniques, intensive care, and immunosuppression, have permitted LT to evolve into an effective and widely accepted therapy for adults and children with ESLD. The advent of cyclosporine A in 1978 transformed the field and allowed LT to become standard-of-care therapy for patients with end-stage liver failure. The

Hepatology: Diagnosis and Clinical Management, First Edition. Edited by E. Jenny Heathcote.
© 2012 John Wiley & Sons, Ltd. Published 2012 by John Wiley & Sons, Ltd.

survival outcome of LT recipients has significantly improved over the last decade. According to the US Organ Procurement and Transplantation Network (OPTN)/Scientific Registry of Transplant Recipients (SRTR) data, the 1-year patient survival rate is 83–91%, and 5-year patient survival is also excellent, ranging from 82 to 84%. The Studies in Pediatric Liver Transplantation (SPLIT) Research Group is another important source of data regarding pediatric LT in North America, now representing 46 pediatric LT centers across the USA and Canada and reflects the results of programs with a strong pediatric emphasis. According to the SPLIT data, patient and graft survival mirrors OPTN/SRTR results, with the most recent review of the SPLIT database revealing patient survival rates of 91.4% and 86.5% at 1 and 5 years post pediatric LT, respectively.

As a result of the excellent survival outcome, the number of patients awaiting LT had grown proportionally. The transplant community is currently faced with a major organ shortage, which has led to the establishment of guidelines for selection of the candidates keeping in view that LT is potentially a life-saving operation yet with limited resources. This chapter will provide an over-view of the indications and contraindication for LT for both adults and children.

Indications for liver transplantation in adults

Patients should be considered for LT only if the procedure is considered to extend their life expectancy beyond the natural history of the liver disease. Today organ allocation is essentially based on a risk-projection system using the Model for End-stage Liver Disease (MELD) score or Pediatric End-stage Liver Disease (PELD) score for candidates younger than 12 years.[3] This math-ematical regression model, which incorporates serum creatinine, bilirubin, and prothrombin time (INR), allows accurate prediction of short-term mortality of the patients waiting for a transplant. The formula for the MELD score and 3-month mortality is available on the Internet at www.mayoclinic.org/meld/mayomodel6.html. Calculated MELD scores range from 6 to 40. Transplanta-tion of patients with low MELD score (<15) has been associated with higher mortality after transplantation than would be expected without transplantation on the waiting list, indicating that transplantation of patients with low MELD score is not the ideal use of the donor organs.[4]

Since the MELD score is based on short-term mortality risk, it might not be appropriate for some patients who are not at imminent risk of death but none-theless derive benefit from LT. The best example is the patient with compen-sated cirrhosis and hepatocellular carcinoma (HCC). Although the risk of death within 6 months might be quite low, the chance that the tumor might progress and therefore preclude LT is reasonably high. Thus, patients with stage T2 HCC are provided an exception score that offers them a reasonably high chance of receiving an organ offer before their tumor progresses to a point that would require them to be removed from the transplant waiting list.

Patients should be considered for LT if they are thought to be capable of surviving the perioperative period, that is have no competing comorbidities and complying with the follow-up post LT, including refrain from addictive behavior such as recidivism of alcohol or drug abuse. To qualify for listing, the patients expected survival rate should be 90% or more within the first year post LT. Referral for LT evaluation should be considered for irreversible hepatic failure regardless of cause, complications of decompensated cirrhosis, liver cancers, or liver-based metabolic conditions causing systemic disease. As a general rule, the following complications of cirrhosis warrant LT:

- recurrent variceal bleeding
- intractable ascites
- following first episode of spontaneous bacterial peritonitis
- refractory encephalopathy
- hepatorenal syndrome.

The common etiologies and indications for LT in adults are presented in Table 9.1. Cirrhosis accounts for more than 80% of transplants performed in adults. The most important indications for LT in the North America are hepatitis C (30%), alcoholic liver disease (10–20%), cholestatic liver disease including primary biliary cirrhosis and sclerosing cholangitis (17%). Other indications are chronic hepatitis B, generally only when complicated by HCC, autoimmune hepatitis, metabolic disease (Wilson disease, hereditary hemochromatosis, and α_1-antitrypsin deficiency), vascular disease (Budd–Chiari syndrome), fulminant hepatic failure (5–6%), and non-metastatic HCC.

Table 9.1 Indication for liver transplantation in adults	
Primary diagnosis	**Frequency (%)**

Viral hepatitis (not complicated by HCC)
    hepatitis C virus
    hepatitis B virus
	30–40

Alcohol	10–15
Non-alcoholic steatohepatitis (NASH)	10
Cholestatic liver diseases Primary sclerosing cholangitis, primary biliary cirrhosis	15

Metabolic disease
    Wilson disease, α_1-antitrypsin deficiency, tyrosinemia,
    cystic fibrosis, etc.
	5

Acute liver failure	10
Liver tumors	10
Other	10

For alcoholic liver disease, the prerequisites for transplantation in most centers are alcohol abstinence for at least 6 months, assessment by an addiction specialist, and active treatment for alcohol dependency prior to transplantation.[5] The rational for requiring a period of 6 months abstinence before liver transplantation is based on: (1) ensuring that the patient's liver will not recover sufficient function as a result of abstaining from alcohol; and (2) identifying the patients who are at high risk for recidivism.

In patients who experience a relapse, the pattern of drinking post transplantation is variable, but patients who return to occasional drinking rarely experience graft loss. A minority of patients return to abusive drinking, which may result in graft loss and decreased survival.[6]

Hepatitis C virus (HCV) remains a leading cause of end-stage liver disease but recurrence following LT is universal and often follows an accelerated post-transplant course and the issue of retransplanting patients with graft failure remains controversial. As a result, long-term survival of patients who undergo transplantation for chronic hepatitis C is inferior to that of patients who undergo transplantation for other indications. Patients can be treated for HCV after LT; however, the rate of response to antiviral therapy is usually lower than when instituted pretransplantation.

In contrast, availability of prophylactic therapies for hepatitis B virus has revitalized liver transplantation for this indication. Viremic individuals with cirrhosis due to hepatitis B were not eligible for transplantation in the past because of the high risk of recurrence after transplantation, with consequent rapid graft loss. Since the availability of antiviral medication, all degrees of viremia are treatable and transplantation has become a more realistic option with excellent graft and patient survival, which is even superior to that of many other indications. In those with chronic hepatitis B, liver transplant is almost always needed for complicating HCC now that their "hepatitis" can be controlled.

Fulminant hepatic failure or rapid onset of coagulopathy, jaundice, hepatic encephalopathy leading to coma, in patients without history of liver diseases is an indication for LT after the onset of stage 2 encephalopathy. Transplantation indications are usually based on King's College criteria,[7] and/or Clichy[8] criteria. Timely referral of these patients to the transplant center is critical since death from sepsis and/or cerebral edema may occur within days of onset of stage 3 or 4 hepatic encephalopathy (Fig. 9.1).

Contraindications for liver transplantation in adults

Table 9.2 provides some absolute and relative contraindications to LT accepted by most programs. Absolute contraindications are conditions where the outcomes of liver transplantation are so poor that it should not be offered. Relative contraindications are conditions that have a negative impact on survival, but not to the extent that the patient should be categorically withheld.

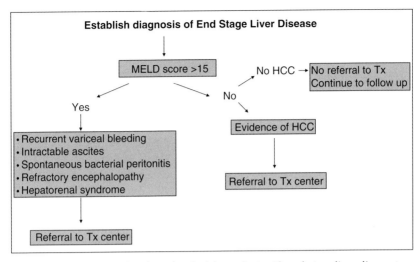

Fig. 9.1 Proposed algorithm for referral of the patient with end-stage liver disease to a transplant center.

Table 9.2 Contraindication for liver transplantation in adults
Absolute contraindications
Uncontrolled systemic sepsis
Severely advanced cardiopulmonary disease
Extrahepatic malignancy
Active alcohol or substance abuse
Inability to comply with immunosuppression protocols due to psychosocial situation
Multisystem organ failure
Relative contraindications (needing individual evaluations)
Advanced age > 70 years
Infection with human immunodeficiency virus (HIV)
Significant anatomic anomalies such as portal vein thrombosis extending throughout the mesenteric venous system

Advanced age (>70 years old) and individuals infected with HIV in the absence of acquired immune deficiency syndrome are currently considered as relative contraindication for liver transplantation.

Indications for liver transplantation in children

The most common clinical presentations prompting transplant evaluation in children are:[9,10]

1 progressive primary liver disease, with the anticipation of incipient of hepatic failure;
2 stable or non-progressive liver disease with remarkable morbidity and/or a predicable early mortality;
3 hepatic-based metabolic disease;
4 acute liver failure (or fulminant hepatic failure).

Table 9.3 illustrates the most common primary diagnoses leading to pediatric LT.[11,12] Further details on the specificities of diagnoses of biliary atresia, Alagille syndrome, genetic causes of intrahepatic cholestasis, and metabolic liver diseases are discussed elsewhere in this handbook.

Contraindications for liver transplantation in children

It is rare and devastating to exclude a pediatric candidate. Table 9.4 provides some absolute and relative contraindications to LT in children. The timing of LT is determined by weighing the relative risk/benefit of other forms of

Table 9.3 Primary diagnoses of children undergoing liver transplantation	
Primary diagnosis	**Frequency (%)**
Cholestatic liver diseases	
Biliary atresia	48
Other: Alagille syndrome, familial cholestasis, primary sclerosing cholangitis, idiopathic neonatal hepatitis, etc.	15
Metabolic disease	13
Primary hepatic disease: Wilson disease, α_1-antitrypsin deficiency, tyrosinemia, cystic fibrosis, etc. Primary non-hepatic disease: ornithine transcarbamylase deficiency, primary hyperoxaluria type 1, organic acidemia	
Acute liver failure	11
Liver tumors	4
Other	9

Table 9.4 Potential contraindications to liver transplantation in children

Absolute contraindications

  Primary extrahepatic unresectable malignancy

  Malignancy metastatic to the liver

  Simultaneous progressive terminal non-hepatic disease

  Uncontrolled systemic sepsis

  Irreversible neurological injury

Relative contraindications (needing individual evaluations)

  Advanced or partially treated systemic infection

  Advanced encephalopathy

  Severe psychosocial status

  Significant anatomic anomalies such as portal venous thrombosis extending throughout the mesenteric venous system

  Infection with human immunodeficiency virus (HIV)

treatment, the anticipated availability of a donor, and the likely outcomes. Hence, early referral to a pediatric liver transplant program is encouraged to allow for the earliest assessment of liver transplant candidacy.

Listing and evaluation

The appropriate selection and evaluation of a potential candidate for LT is fundamental in order to achieve the level of liver transplant success described above. The evaluation begins with a thorough patient history and physical examination, including a psychiatric and psychosocial evaluation. Patients should be evaluated by not only a transplant hepatologist and a transplant surgeon, but also by the transplant nurse, dietician, social worker, occupational and physical therapists, among others. The goals of the evaluation are presented in Table 9.5. The PELD score was introduced in the United States in 2002, and ranked children on a waiting list according to their probability of death and/or move to the intensive care unit within 3 months of listing. Hence, the PELD score was calculated from a formula based on the following predictive factors: international normalized ratio (INR), total bilirubin, serum albumin, age less than 1 year, and height less than 2 standard deviations from the mean for age and gender.

In addition, various specialists are often consulted to give their impressions and recommendations regarding patient suitability. Table 9.6 illustrates the

Table 9.5 Goals and objectives of pretransplantation evaluation of a potential candidate by a skilled multidisciplinary team

Confirm etiology of liver disease

Establish severity of liver disease and determine the necessity for liver transplantation

Consider feasibility of strategic management options
  Non-transplantation options
  1. Maximizing medical therapy for treatable metabolic liver disease
  2. Prognosticating natural history of the liver disease (i.e. non-progressive vs. progressive nature)
  Transplantation options
  1. Availability and suitability of available live donor candidates
  2. Deceased donor options

Recognize potential contraindications to liver transplantation

Establish plan for interim management
  Review childhood vaccination status
  Nutritional rehabilitation
  Maximize developmental progression

Education of patients and parents on preoperative and postoperative issues

detailed transplant work-up of potential candidates. The work-up process is complex and time consuming, and, from the patient and family perspectives, it is often physically and psychologically stressful.

The decision whether or not to register a patient on the transplant waiting list will be made following assessment and after discussion within a multidisciplinary team. Patients placed on the transplant waiting list following assessment usually need to be registered on a national transplant list.

Retransplantation

Currently, retransplantation accounts for approximately 10–15% of all LT. The number of patients requiring retransplantation is likely to grow as transplant recipients survive long enough to develop graft failure due to disease recurrence. Early graft loss due to primary non-function of the graft or hepatic artery thrombosis accounts for the majority of graft loss during the first year and is routinely managed by early retransplantation. However, late graft loss due to disease recurrence or chronic rejection occurs in a subset of patients in whom the only option for survival is retransplantation. Survival following retransplantation is usually inferior to that for primary graft.

Table 9.6 Transplant evaluation and work-up (adults and children)

Evaluation
  Transplant hepatologist
  Transplant surgeons
  Social workers
  Psychiatry/addiction specialists

Laboratory tests
  Blood group and antibody screen
  Sodium, potassium, chloride, creatinine, magnesium, phosphate, albumin, total protein, AST, ALT, ALP, total bilirubin, amylase, fasting glucose, LDL cholesterol, triglycerides, HDL, LDL, hemoglobin A1c
  CBC, PT/INR, aPTT
  Hepatitis B surface antigen (HBsAg), hepatitis B surface antibody (HBsAb), hepatitis B core antibody total (HBcAb), HCV RNA (quantitative and genotype), HAV IgG, CMV IgG, toxoplasmosis IgG, EBV, HIV, varicella IgG, syphilis screening (serum)
  Urinalysis

Diagnostic tests
  ECG
  Chest X-ray, PA and lateral
  TB skin test, performed by physician on ward/family doctor (record results on chart)
  Abdominal ultrasound with Doppler
  2D echocardiogram
  Pulmonary function test with arterial blood gases
  Triphasic abdominal CT
  Chest CT
  Gastroscopy: check for varices, band if large
  Colonoscopy (>50 years of age)
  Stress MIBI, abnormal echo (>50 years of age)

Consults
  Social worker, alcohol risk evaluation
  Anesthesia
  Dental
  Dietician
  Psychiatry
  Oncology (incidental findings)
  Cardiology
  Nephrology (hepatorenal syndrome)

ALP, alkaline phosphatase; ALT, alanine aminotransferase; aPTT, active partial thromboplastin time; AST, aspartate aminotransferase; CBC, complete blood count; CMV, cytomegalovirus; CT, computed tomography; EBV, Epstein–Barr virus; ECG, electrocardiogram; HAV, hepatitis A virus; HDL, high-density lipoprotein; HIV, human immunodeficiency virus; LDL, low-density lipoprotein; PT/INR, prothrombin time/international normalized ratio; TB, tuberculosis.

Case study 9.1

A 50-year-old Caucasian female with a diagnosis of cirrhosis attributed to non-alcoholic steatohepatitis was referred to our liver transplant assessment clinic for a liver transplant consultation. The patient reported intermittent nausea, weakness, and confusion, which had increased in frequency during the previous year, and abdominal swelling and lower extremity edema beginning 6 months earlier. While undergoing a cholestectomy for gallstones 3 years previously, the patient was noted to have a cirrhotic-appearing liver. Results of routine laboratory tests and an abdominal ultrasound performed at that time were consistent with cirrhosis. Gastroscopy did not show any varices.

The patient denied any history of drug or alcohol use and reported never having received a blood transfusion. She was accompanied by her husband and her 22- and 25-year-old sons. She was working as a librarian up to 6 months ago. She had no history of childhood liver disease and was unaware of any family history of liver disease. Her mother died from the complications of diabetes. The patient's medical history was remarkable for lifelong obesity, gastroesophageal reflux disease, recurrent urinary tract infections, and systemic hypertension. She had been an insulin-dependent diabetic for the last 5 years.

Physical examination was unremarkable, with the exception of mildly icteric sclera, spider nevi on the anterior chest wall, and bilateral lower extremity edema (on diuretics and Na restriction). Moderately decreased breath sounds in her lower left lung were also noted yet her chest X-ray and spirometry were within normal limits.

Laboratory data revealed a hemoglobin of 111 g/dL, platelet count 128×10^9/L, 35×10^9 WBC, creatinine 152 mol/L, AST 80 IU/L, ALT 45 IU/L, alkaline phosphatase 129 IU/L, total bilirubin 60 mmol/L, plasma albumin 27 g/L, INR 1.9.

Comments. This 50-year-old lady has end-stage liver disease due to non-alcoholic fatty liver disease, which has progressed to cirrhosis. She has clinical evidence of hepatic decompensation in that she has hepatic encephalopathy, ascites, and leg edema. Her calculated MELD score is 23. She has no obvious medical or psychosocial contraindications and her 1- and 5-year survival with a liver transplantation are higher than without. She was considered as a potential candidate and began her work-up for liver transplantation. Because of her comorbidities (i.e. diabetes, obesity, and hypertension) she will require a meticulous cardiologic work-up including cardiology consult, a 2D echo, a stress test, and an angiography.

Case study 9.2

A 3-year-old Caucasian female with no previously known medical concerns presents to the Emergency Room with a chief complaint of jaundice and abdominal pain for 3 days. History is notable for a viral-like illness (fever and coryza) in the preceding 3 weeks. Father was similarly unwell the week prior. Parents report a total of three (appropriate for age) doses of acetaminophen during the intercurrent illness, with the last dose given about 3 weeks ago. Otherwise, parents deny any recent use of over-the-counter medications or prescribed antibiotics. There are no concerns with neurocognitive or developmental milestones, she is growing well, and review of systems is unremarkable. Physical examination reveals a well-nourished, jaundiced but co-operative girl with stable vital signs. Liver edge is palpable 2 cm below the right costal margin, and a spleen tip is palpable. There are no rashes and no stigmata of chronic liver disease. The remainder of the physical exam is normal. Results of first laboratory investigations in the ER include AST 623 IU/L, ALT 815 IU/L, GGT 210 IU/L, total bilirubin 168 μmol/L, conjugated bilirubin 90 μmol/L, serum albumin 40 g/L, INR 2.3, Hb 89 g/dL, and platelet count 149×10^9/L. Ultrasound shows coarse hepatomegaly and mild splenomegaly.

Comment. In children, acute liver failure may be present without clinical evidence of hepatic encephalopathy. However, coagulopathy is an important, consistent, and reliable finding in children with acute liver failure. An international consensus definition for pediatric acute liver failure (PALF) involves the summation of clinical and biochemical parameters as follows: (1) the acute onset of liver injury/disease with no known evidence of chronic liver disease; *and* (2) severe liver dysfunction defined as either (a) hepatic-based uncorrectable coagulopathy with INR >1.5 (despite the use of vitamin K) *plus* clinical concern of encephalopathy; *or* (b) INR >2.0 (despite the use of vitamin K) *even without* hepatic encephalopathy.

There are recognizable clinical patterns for acute liver failure in childhood, including the school-aged child that presents with acute severe hepatitis that evolves to liver failure and aplastic anemia; the preschool-aged child that presents with abrupt onset of liver dysfunction often following a febrile illness; and infants that present within the first few months of life with hypoglycemia and steatosis.

In the ER, this child immediately received vitamin K 5 mg intravenously, and an INR repeated 2 hours after the vitamin K, which came back at 2.1. The Pediatric Gastroenterology/Hepatology service was consulted, and she was admitted to the GI ward with a diagnosis of pediatric acute liver failure for further diagnostic evaluation, supportive medical management, surveillance, and early consultation with the Pediatric Liver Transplant service—despite the fact that she clinically appeared well in the ER. After a complete investigative work-up for etiologies of pediatric acute liver failure, no specific diagnosis could be reached. The diagnosis of indeterminate PALF is given, which is the case in almost 50% of all infants and children meeting the consensus definition of acute liver failure. This observation is indeed sobering given that there are specific directed medical therapy applications as well as variations in short-term outcome of PALF amongst final diagnostic groups. Four days later, this child's clinical condition deteriorated with evidence of hepatic encephalopathy, concurrent with deterioration of liver function tests, with total bilirubin level increased to 257 μmol/L (conjugated proportion increased to 126 μmol/L), and INR increased to 2.8 despite daily intravenous vitamin K. She underwent liver transplantation the next day, with liver explants confirming massive necrosis and parenchymal collapse.

Multiple choice questions

1. Which of the following is not an indication for liver transplantation?
   A. Haemochromatosis
   B. Acute alcoholic hepatitis
   C. Hepatocellular carcinoma (single 4-cm lesion)
   D. Cirrhosis secondary to hepatitis B
   E. Budd–Chiari disease

2. Regarding retransplantation, which of the following is correct?
   A. The number of patients requiring retransplantation will remain unchanged over the next decade
   B. Primary non-function is a main indication for retransplantation
   C. Hepatic vein thrombosis is a solid indication for retransplantation
   D. All patients with severe HCV recurrence should be assessed for retransplantation
   E. Survival following retransplantation is identical to a first transplantation

Answers

1. B
2. B

References

1. Moore FD, Wheele HB, Demissianos HV, et al. Experimental whole-organ transplantation of the liver and of the spleen. Ann Surg 1960; 152: 374–87.
2. Starzl TE, Marchioro TL, Vonkaulla KN, et al. Homotransplantation of the liver in humans. Surg Gynecol Obstet 1963; 117: 659–76.
3. Wiesner R, Edwards E, Freeman R, et al. Model for end-stage liver disease (MELD) and allocation of donor livers. Gastroenterology 2003; 124: 91–6.
4. Brown RS, Jr., Lake JR. The survival impact of liver transplantation in the MELD era, and the future for organ allocation and distribution. Am J Transpl 2005; 5: 203–4.
5. DiMartini A, Day N, Dew MA, et al. Alcohol consumption patterns and predictors of use following liver transplantation for alcoholic liver disease. Liver Transpl 2006; 12: 813–20.
6. Pfitzmann R, Schwenzer J, Rayes N, et al. Long-term survival and predictors of relapse after orthotopic liver transplantation for alcoholic liver disease. Liver Transpl 2007; 13: 197–205.
7. O'Grady JG, Alexander GJ, Hayllar KM, et al. Early indicators of prognosis in fulminant hepatic failure. Gastroenterology 1989; 97: 439–45.
8. Bernuau J, Goudeau A, Poynard T, et al. Multivariate analysis of prognostic factors in fulminant hepatitis B. Hepatology 1986; 6: 648–51.
9. Balistreri WF. Transplantation for childhood liver disease: an overview. Liver Transpl Surg 1998; 4 (5 Suppl. 1): S18–S23.

10. Kamath BM, Olthoff KM. Liver transplantation in children: Update 2010. Pediatr Clin North Am 2010; 57: 401–14.
11. Ng VL, Fecteau A, Shepherd R, et al. Outcomes of 5-year survivors after pediatric liver transplantation: Report on 461 children from a North American multi-center registry. Pediatrics 2008; 122: e1128–35.
12. McDiarmid SV, Anand R, Lindblad AS. Development of a pediatric end-stage liver disease score to predict poor outcome in children awaiting liver transplantation. Transplantation 2002; 74: 173–81.

Management of fulminant hepatic failure

CHAPTER 10

Leslie B. Lilly

Multi Organ Transplant Program, Toronto General Hospital, University Health Network, Toronto, Ontario, Canada

---

Key points

- The precise cause of fulminant hepatic failure is often unclear; drugs, especially acetaminophen, are the most common identified cause in many centers.
- Fulminant hepatic failure is a multisystem disease, best managed in a center of expertise with access to liver transplantation.
- It is critical that patients unlikely to recover in spite of the introduction of specific and/or general measures of care be identified early, to permit liver transplantation in a timely manner with an excellent chance of full recovery.

Introduction

Fulminant hepatic failure (FHF) can be precipitated by a number of causes; the exact etiology varies in different parts of the world and, in many cases, is never precisely established. Thus, while every effort should be made to identify a specific cause, the focus has tended to be on the early identification and treatment of the associated complications. While many patients may recover with specialized care, frequent re-evaluation is essential to identify those factors that predict a poor prognosis without transplantation so that life saving surgery can be offered in a timely manner.

Diagnostic workup

Viral hepatitis remains an important cause of FHF, although the wide application of hepatitis B vaccination has reduced the numbers of patients seen with acute liver failure due to hepatitis B. Some patients with longstanding hepatitis

Hepatology: Diagnosis and Clinical Management, First Edition. Edited by E. Jenny Heathcote.
© 2012 John Wiley & Sons, Ltd. Published 2012 by John Wiley & Sons, Ltd.

B infection can present with acute liver failure, generally at the time of HBeAg seroconversion or as result of superinfection with hepatitis D or other hepatotrophic viruses. Hepatitis A is an infrequent cause of FHF in adults, although cases where an otherwise mild infection is aggravated by concomitant acetaminophen use are not uncommon. Acute hepatitis C infection virtually never precipitates FHF; however, hepatitis E is an important cause of FHF in the developing world, particularly in pregnant women, and should be considered in patients with a history of travel to those areas although serologic studies indicate that exposure to hepatitis E occurs in North America. Other viruses, such as herpes simplex, herpes zoster, and HHV-6, in addition to Epstein–Barr virus, cytomegalovirus, and parvovirus, are uncommon causes of FHF, but should be considered particularly in the immunocompromised or pregnant patient. The appropriate serologic investigations are outlined in Box 10.1.

Box 10.1 Diagnostic workup in fulminant hepatic failure

General investigations:
- CBC, electrolytes, INR, creatinine, glucose
- Liver biochemistry (total/direct bilirubin, AST, ALT, ALP, albumin)
- Serum lactate, serum amylase
- Arterial blood gases with pH
- Liver ultrasound with Doppler evaluation of portal and hepatic veins
- Chest X-ray, electrocardiogram
- Pregnancy test if applicable
- Toxicology screen with acetaminophen

Specific investigations:
- Viral serology
  - HAV-IgM, HBsAg, IgM anti-HBc, HCV-Ab
  - HIV, HBVDNA if HBV suspected, HDAg (PCR) and/or HDV-IgM if HBV present
  - HSV-IgM, EBV-IgM, HEV-IgM, CMV-IgM or PCR
- Autoimmune
  - ANA, SMA, quantitative immunoglobulins
- Metabolic
  - Ceruloplasmin, urine copper, and slit lamp examination for Kayser–Fleischer rings

Other investigations to be considered:
- CT brain
- EEG
- Transjugular liver biopsy

ALP, alkaline phosphatase; ALT, alanine aminotransferase; ANA, antinuclear antibody; AST, aspartate aminotransferase; CBC, complete blood count; EEG, electroencephalography; PCR, polymerase chain reaction; SMA, smooth muscle antibodies.

Box 10.2 Hepatotoxic herbal remedies

Artemisia	Hare's ear
Atractylis	Heliotropium
Black cohosh	Jin bu huang
Callilepsis	Kava kava
Chaparral leaf	LIV.52
Chaso	Ma huang
Chrysanthemum	Mistletoe
Comfrey	Onshido
Crotalaria	Plantango
Dai-saiko-to	Red peony root
Gardenia	Senecio
Germander	Skullcap
Greater celandine	Valerian root

Drugs, including prescription medications, over-the-counter preparations, and natural or herbal products (Box 10.2), are the principal identified cause of FHF in many Western centers. Acetaminophen, or paracetamol, is the leading cause in most published series, either as an overdose or in medicinal quantities in association with other precipitants, for example alcohol. Other classes of drugs, particularly anti-infectives, anticonvulsants, and anti-inflammatories, the latter because of their widespread use, are also relatively frequent causes of FHF, although it is difficult to find any drug that has not been associated with some degree of liver injury. A careful history, toxic screens, and, in some cases, a search of the patient's home, are essential in identifying the specific agent or agents involved.

A variety of other conditions may be associated with FHF, including hyperthermia, mushroom poisoning with *Amanita phalloides*, Wilson disease, ischemic hepatopathy (including cocaine-induced ischemic hepatitis), Budd–Chiari syndrome, autoimmune hepatitis, malignancy (usually lymphoma), and pregnancy. Reye syndrome, an acute microvesicular steatosis attributed to acetylsalicylic acid use in children and rarely seen today, is another precipitant of acute liver failure. Specific investigations designed to pursue these possibilities are also outlined in Box 10.2. It has also been reported that hematologic malignancies, including lymphoma (non-Hodgkin) and leukemia, may present as acute liver failure.

In some series, over a quarter of FHF cases have no identified cause. This has been referred to as seronegative or indeterminate disease, and tends to have a poorer prognosis than viral hepatitis-related disease.

Patient management

General principles: a multisystem disease (Box 10.3)

Hepatic encephalopathy

The development of hepatic encephalopathy is the hallmark of FHF. In contrast to the situation in chronic liver disease, where hepatic encephalopathy is frequently present with fluctuating severity, this complication is associated with a poor outcome in the fulminant setting. A rise in intracranial pressure can occur in a matter of hours following the onset of clinical encephalopathy, and the resultant herniation of brainstem structures may lead to irreversible brain injury that would not be corrected with transplantation. Thus, once hepatic encephalopathy has developed, liver transplantation should become an active consideration and the various models developed for prognosis can be applied.

While lactulose can be administered at the onset of encephalopathy, after colonic cleansing has been achieved its ongoing use achieves little benefit. Elevation in serum ammonia and other substances due to portosystemic

---

Box 10.3 Fulminant hepatic failure: a multisystem disease

- Central nervous system
  - Hepatic encephalopathy
  - Elevated intracranial pressure
- Renal
  - Acute tubular necrosis
  - Hepatorenal syndrome
- Respiratory
  - Aspiration pneumonia
  - Pulmonary edema
- Cardiovascular
  - Systemic hypotension
  - Tachycardia, hyperdynamic circulation
- Hematological
  - Coagulopathy
  - Disseminated intravascular coagulation
  - Aplastic anemia
- Gastrointestinal
  - Upper gastrointestinal bleeding
  - Pancreatitis
- Endocrine
  - Hypoglycemia
  - Adrenal insufficiency
- Other
  - Sepsis and its complications

shunting, the major mechanisms of encephalopathy in chronic liver disease, is not implicated in FHF. Additional measures include nursing the patient with the head up (15–30° from the horizontal), keeping the patient "dry" by administering only the amount of i.v. fluids necessary to maintain minimum (30 mL/h) urine output when renal function is still preserved and, in more severe cases, the use of intravenous mannitol, phenobarbital-induced coma, and hypothermia. Controversy remains as to whether the insertion of an intracranial pressure monitor is of value, particularly as neurosurgical intervention in this setting may carry a higher risk; some authorities recommend doing so in an effort to identify patients with intractably elevated intracranial pressure who may no longer be transplant candidates.

Renal dysfunction

With progressive hepatic insufficiency, renal dysfunction is common, with a profile reminiscent of hepatorenal syndrome as seen in chronic liver disease. The avoidance of potential nephrotoxins, including antibiotics, non-steroidal anti-inflammatory drugs (NSAIDs), and contrast agents, is important, along with treatment of causes of renal hypoperfusion, such as sepsis. However, systemic hypotension is common in FHF, and in an effort to minimize fluid infusions a lower threshold for the use of vasopressors is advocated. Renal replacement therapy is frequently required for the management of the profound acid–base disturbances seen in acute liver failure.

Pulmonary dysfunction

In addition to the airway and breathing challenges that can arise as patients slip into deepening levels of hepatic coma, primary pulmonary complications can develop, which can further compromise oxygenation. An acute respiratory distress syndrome (ARDS) picture is not infrequent, especially if sepsis is present, and renal failure may result in pulmonary edema. Pneumonia, often due to aspiration, is common in patients with FHF and can further affect pulmonary function.

Hemodynamic disturbances

As mentioned earlier, systemic hypotension is frequent, and is associated with tachycardia and increased cardiac output, the so-called "hyperdynamic circulation". Invasive monitoring, often including a pulmonary artery catheter, is usually required to navigate through this complication; diminishing cardiac performance can further exacerbate pulmonary function, and patients end up on maximal pressors and fractional inspired oxygen (FIo_2) as FHF progresses.

Coagulopathy/thrombocytopenia

A rapidly rising and highly elevated INR is the norm in patients with FHF. This is due both to the impaired production of clotting factors by the failing liver and, in many cases, to increased factor consumption attributable to disseminated intravascular coagulation, a common complication. While the administration of FFP to correct an elevated INR may be appropriate in the setting of active bleeding or prior to carrying out an invasive procedure, serial measurement of INR carries enormous prognostic information in its role as an index of liver function, and should not be manipulated without careful consideration.

Gastrointestinal complications

Upper gastrointestinal bleeding, usually due to gastritis, is often seen, and is of course exacerbated by the coexisting coagulopathy of FHF. Prophylaxis with proton pump inhibitors is recommended. Further, albeit rarely, bleeding esophageal varices can develop in the setting of acute liver injury, and aggressive intervention, with correction of coagulopathy, resuscitation and emergency endoscopy with variceal ligation, may be required. Acute pancreatitis has also been described in FHF, with unclear etiology, and should be managed as it would be in any other patient.

Hypoglycemia

While not included in any prognostic model, hypoglycemia is common in FHF, and should be sought out and corrected when present as it may complicate the interpretation of altered mental status and contribute to brain injury. Frequent glucometer readings are recommended, with the institution of intravenous dextrose supplementation when blood glucose readings begin to fall, especially in patients in deeper levels of hepatic encephalopathy.

Sepsis

The impaired level of consciousness of FHF, with its associated risks of aspiration, the insertion of intravenous and urinary catheters, the development of pulmonary edema, and the loss of hepatic Kupffer cell function, as well as other factors, contribute to high rates of bacterial and fungal sepsis in FHF. Broad-spectrum intravenous antibacterials are usually started as soon as hepatic coma begins to develop, with the subsequent addition of antifungals. Regular surveillance cultures of blood and urine are recommended, along with frequent chest radiographs, so that infections can be identified and managed early. They represent the next most important cause of death (second to elevated intracranial pressure) in FHF.

Etiology-specific measures
Viral hepatitis

There is no specific treatment for liver failure due to hepatitis A virus. In the case of hepatitis B, the use of lamivudine or other more potent nucleoside/nucleotide analogues has not been convincingly shown to improve prognosis. In the situation where a flare of chronic hepatitis B has precipitated liver failure, oral antiviral drugs may be used, perhaps not for immediate effect but to reduce viral load and lower the risk of recurrent hepatitis B following liver transplantation. Superinfection with delta virus suppresses HBV DNA.

When other viruses, such as herpesviruses (cytomegalovirus, herpes simplex, etc.) are involved, specific antiviral therapy can be administered. Acyclovir has been shown to be of benefit in herpes simplex virus-related FHF.

Acetaminophen intoxication

N-acetylcysteine (NAC), given either orally or intravenously, is the specific antidote for acetaminophen-related hepatic failure. It should be administered according to widely available algorithms as soon as the diagnosis is suspected, and many authorities recommend its continuation well beyond 16 hours, often until the INR has approached normal. Although the best evidence supports its use in the first 24 hours following acetaminophen ingestion, there is little harm in starting it beyond that window.

Fulminant hepatic failure related to pregnancy

Early delivery is recommended in almost all cases of pregnancy-related fulminant liver failure (acute fatty liver of pregnancy, HELLP syndrome, acute hepatitis E), not only for the safety of the fetus, but as treatment for the disease process itself. Hence, liver transplantation is rarely required for this indication.

Other etiologies

NAC is also often administered in FHF of non-acetaminophen etiology, as it is relatively non-toxic and may improve outcome in those situations as well. A recent randomized controlled trial did demonstrate improvement in transplant-free survival in patients with Stages I and II encephalopathy, although there was no survival benefit in the overall group.

There is no specific treatment for Wilson disease with a fulminant presentation, although there are case reports suggesting possible benefit of plasmapheresis and chelation therapy. These modalities may serve as a bridge to early transplantation, rather than directly affecting the natural history of the disease.

Corticosteroids or other immunosuppressive medications have not been established as effective treatment in fulminant autoimmune hepatitis; indeed, corticosteroids may be associated with a higher risk of sepsis, particularly fungal, and introduce potential complications if liver transplantation is being considered.

Prognosis and liver transplantation

Several models have been developed to assist in determining prognosis in patients with FHF (Box 10.4). The mostly widely used prognostic criteria are the King's College Hospital criteria, which incorporate the etiology of FHF along with a variety of biochemical markers. Those who fulfill criteria are highly unlikely to survive without urgent liver transplantation. Other widely used models include the Clichy criteria, which are based on the measurement of factor V levels. In addition, serum lactate has been proven to be an independent predictor of poor outcome in acetaminophen-induced liver failure, and MELD (Model for End-stage Liver Disease) may be of some value, although it is not currently in use for organ allocation in patients with FHF.

Box 10.4 Prognostic models in fulminant hepatic failure

King's College criteria

Acetaminophen:

List for transplant if arterial pH < 7.3

or if all 3 of the following occur within 24 h:

Grade III–IV hepatic encephalopathy

INR > 6.5

Serum creatinine > 300 µmol/L

Non-acetaminophen:

INR > 6.5 irrespective of grade of encephalopathy

or if any 3 of the following 5 are present:

Unfavorable (non-viral) etiology

Age < 10 years or > 40 years

Interval jaundice to encephalopathy > 7 days

INR > 3.5

Bilirubin >300 µmol/L

Clichy criteria

All etiologies:

Hepatic encephalopathy + factor V levels < 20% (age < 30) or <30% (age > 30)

Hepatic encephalopathy Grade III–IV + factor V < 20%

Serum lactate

Acetaminophen:

Arterial lactate > 3.5 mmol/L on admission

Model for End-stage Liver Disease (MELD)

Acetaminophen:

MELD > 33 at onset of hepatic encephalopathy

Non-acetaminophen:

MELD > 32

Case study 10.1

Ms. PA is a 17-year-old girl with no significant past medical history. She was out with her boyfriend two evenings prior to admission to hospital. They had a huge fight, and she came home crying. She missed school the next day, complaining of feeling unwell. On the morning of the visit to hospital, her mother became concerned when her daughter began vomiting and complaining of abdominal pain. She brought her to the hospital.

On examination she was afebrile, with normal vital signs except for a sinus tachycardia of 120. She was slightly icteric. There was no asterixis. Chest and cardiovascular examinations were non-contributory. She was tender in the RUQ. There was no ascites or edema, and no signs of chronic liver disease.

(Continued)

Initial laboratory data revealed: Hb 145g/L, WBC 12.0 × 10^9/L, platelets 140 × 10^9/L. Total bilirubin was 72μmol/L, AST 8055 IU/L, ALT 6350 IU/L, ALP 110 IU/L, creatinine 132μmol/L, electrolytes normal, INR 2.7.

A hepatology consult was requested.

Diagnostic workup/initial management

An acetaminophen overdose was suspected. A serum level of 800 μmol/L was determined, and therapy with intravenous *N*-acetylcysteine was initiated. Further blood testing revealed a pH of 7.33, and a serum lactate level of 2 mmol/L. Blood was sent off for viral and autoimmune serology, and a toxicology screen obtained, with no other substances detected. Vitamin K was administered parenterally, and the patient was transferred to a step down unit for close monitoring. A catheter was placed, and maintenance fluids with 2/3 + 1/3 at 75 mL/h initiated. Vital signs, including neurovitals, were determined every 4 h, along with glucometer values and urine output. Routine labs, including INR and serum pH and lactate levels, were repeated every 6 h. Strict instructions to avoid administration of narcotics and sedatives were placed in the chart.

The following morning, the INR had risen to 3.7, and asterixis was noted. The serum pH was 7.30, and serum lactate 4.0 mmol/L. Serum creatinine had risen to 175μmol/L. The patient remained hemodynamically stable. Abdominal ultrasound revealed a large liver with no ascites, patent vessels, and a normal spleen. *N*-acetylcysteine was continued, and urgent transfer to a specialized liver unit with access to transplantation was arranged.

Outcome

Upon arrival at the liver unit, the patient was noted to be drowsy, although she was still protecting her airway and oxygenating well, with normal hemodynamics. Empiric therapy with broad-spectrum antibiotics and a proton pump inhibitor was started, and additional investigations necessary to determine the patient's candidacy for transplantation arranged.

The patient, however, remained stable for the next 24 h, and the INR began to improve. Serum pH and serum lactate levels began to normalize, and the patient's drowsiness began to lift. Listing for transplantation was never required, and the patient was returned to her referring hospital with an INR <2.0, normal serum pH, and no neurological changes, for ongoing management including referral to psychiatric services.

Multiple choice questions

1. Fulminant hepatic failure may occur as a result of viral hepatitis. Which of the following viral infections is LEAST likely to present in this way?
   A. Hepatitis A
   B. Hepatitis B

   C. Hepatitis C
   D. Hepatitis D (superinfection)
   E. Hepatitis E

2. *N*-acetylcysteine is recommended for the treatment of acute liver failure due to acetaminophen intoxication. In which of the following situations would its use also be considered appropriate?
   A. *Amanita phalloides* poisoning
   B. Ischemic hepatopathy
   C. NSAID-induced acute liver failure
   D. HSV-related liver failure
   E. All of the above
   F. None of the above

Answers

1. C
2. E

Further reading

Bernal W, Auzinger G, Dhawan A, et al. Acute liver failure. Lancet 2010; 376: 190–201.

Craig DGN, Lee A, Hayes PC, et al. Review article: the current management of acute liver failure. Aliment Pharmacol Ther 2010; 31: 345–58.

Esfahani K, Gold P, Wakil S, et al. Acute liver failure because of chronic lymphocytic leukemia: case report and review of the literature. Curr Oncol 2011; 18: 39–42.

Ichai P, Duclos-Vallee JC, Guettier C, et al. Usefulness of corticosteroids for the treatment of severe and fulminant forms of autoimmune hepatitis. Liver Transpl 2007; 13: 996–1003.

Larson AM. Diagnosis and management of acute liver failure. Curr Opin Gastroenterol 2010; 26: 214–21.

Lee WM, Hynan LS, Rossara L, et al. Intravenous N-acetylcysteine improves transplant-free survival in early stage non-acetaminophen acute liver failure. Gastroenterology 2009; 137: 856–64.

Marudanayagam R, Shanmugam V, Gunson B, et al. Aetiology and outcome of acute liver failure. HPB (Oxford) 2009; 11: 429–34.

Stravitz RT. Critical management decisions in patients with acute liver failure. Chest 2008; 134: 1092–102.

Trotter JF. Practical management of acute liver failure in the intensive care unit. Curr Opin Crit Care 2009; 15: 163–7.

Management of the complications of liver transplantation

CHAPTER 11

Eberhard L. Renner[1] and Eve A. Roberts[2]

[1]GI Transplantation, Toronto General Hospital, University Health Network and University of Toronto, Toronto, Ontario, Canada
[2]Departments of Paediatrics, Medicine, and Pharmacology, University of Toronto, and Division of Gastroenterology, Hepatology and Nutrition, The Hospital for Sick Children, Toronto, Ontario, Canada

Key points

- Early complications after liver transplantation include bleeding, bile leaks, anastomotic and non-anastomotic biliary strictures, and hepatic artery or portal vein thrombosis (seen most often in children).
- Acute cellular rejection occurs in about 20% of liver transplant recipients, usually within the first 3 postoperative months; its diagnosis requires a liver biopsy and it usually resolves with increased immunosuppression.
- Liver transplant recipients are at increased risk of any type of infection, CMV infection/disease being among the most important ones.
- Many malignancies are more frequent in liver transplant recipients than in the normal population; liver transplant recipients, especially children who acquire EBV post transplant, are at high risk of developing EBV-associated lymphoma (post-transplant lymphoproliferative disorder).
- Calcineurin inhibitors (cyclosporine A, tacrolimus) form the backbone of maintenance immunosuppression and are, among other side effects, associated with nephrotoxicity.
- Obesity, hypertension, dyslipidemia, and insulin resistance/diabetes are common in liver transplant recipients; the risk for fatal and non-fatal cardiovascular events is therefore threefold increased compared to a normal population.
- The underlying disease may recur with varying frequency after liver transplantation and may impact on survival outcome, such as recurrent hepatitis C.
- Internist/family physician and transplant hepatologist share the long-term care for the liver transplant recipient; the internist/family physician is best qualified to

Hepatology: Diagnosis and Clinical Management, First Edition. Edited by E. Jenny Heathcote.
© 2012 John Wiley & Sons, Ltd. Published 2012 by John Wiley & Sons, Ltd.

manage cardiovascular risk factors and many conditions common in the non-transplant population, which may occur also in the liver transplant recipient (including respective screening and preventative measures); the transplant hepatologist's expertise is best utilized to manage immunosuppression, recurrent disease, and other directly graft-related issues.

• In the pediatric population, the age at transplantation can lead to many long-term issues with regard to social and intellectual functioning.

Table 11.1 Early postoperative complications of potential long-term importance

Event/complication	Long-term sequelae
Anastomotic biliary stricture	Need for repeated endoscopic or percutaneous intervention or re-operation
Hepatic artery malperfusion (due to stenosis, subacute thrombosis, or transplant with a liver donated after cardiac death)	Ischemic type diffuse intrahepatic biliary structuring, cholangitis, biliary liver abscess, secondary biliary cirrhosis, and graft failure

Introduction

Complications of liver transplantation are manifold. They not only include surgical issues that typically manifest in the early postoperative period, such as bleeding, bile leaks, or hepatic artery thrombosis, but also allograft rejection, and complications intrinsic to long-term immunosuppression (such as infections and malignancies). They also include renal dysfunction and metabolic long-term sequelae such as obesity, hypertension, dyslipidemia, insulin resistance, and diabetes, which translate into an increased risk for cardiovascular diseases. Recurrence of the underlying liver disease may, in a strict sense, not be regarded as a complication of liver transplantation, but adds to the long-term morbidity and mortality post transplant and is briefly discussed at the end of this chapter. In the pediatric population, depending on the age at transplantation, issues related to education and socialization need to be addressed.

Early postoperative period

Early postoperative complications mostly occur during the initial hospital stay and are dealt with by the multidisciplinary transplant team. A detailed review of these complications is beyond the scope of this chapter. However, a few are worth mentioning because they may pertain to the longer-term course and therefore be of importance for the internists or family physicians involved in the long-term care of liver transplant recipients (Table 11.1).

Usually, graft function resumes immediately with normalization of coagulation parameters and improvement of bilirubin within the first couple of days, that is, return of liver function to normal. Delayed graft function, primary non-function (i.e. when the graft never regains function), and hepatic artery thrombosis are rare but serious conditions, which may require early re-transplantation. As with any large hepatobiliary surgery, bleeding and bile leaks can occur and may require surgical re-intervention. Bile duct problems occur in 10–20% of cases. Early bile leaks are secondary to ischemia, sepsis, or rarely to severe rejection. Anastomotic biliary strictures may develop and require endoscopic intervention (dilatation and/or stenting) or re-operation. Any compromised arterial blood supply to the graft may lead to ischemic type diffuse intrahepatic biliary stricturing, which is difficult to manage, often results in secondary biliary cirrhosis (with associated cholangitis and/or abscess formation), and may require late re-transplantation.

Most patients are extubated within 24 hours post transplant (and some immediately after surgery). Some recipients, particularly when severely deconditioned prior to transplant, or those with delayed graft function, large pleural effusions, pulmonary infiltrates, and/or diaphragmatic dysfunction/paralysis, may require extended ventilator support (with the risk of acquiring a ventilator-associated pneumonia). Resolution of pre-existing severe encephalopathy, particularly as seen in fulminant hepatic failure, often requires prolonged ICU care. Confusion and seizures related to metabolic disturbances and the calcineurin inhibitors used for immunosuppression may occur. Renal dysfunction, fluid overload requiring diuretics, and temporary renal replacement therapy are not uncommon complications. Typically, these issues have all resolved or are medically controlled by the time the patient is discharged.

Rejection

Having an enormous functional reserve and a unique regeneration potential, the liver is a privileged organ for transplantation. Thus, destruction of hepatocytes by rejection will not affect long-term outcome, provided the rejection process can be stopped, which is almost always possible with today's medications. It is therefore safer to err on the side of under-immunosuppression and risk rejection, than over-immunosuppress and run the risk of life-threatening infections and, in the long-term, malignancies (Table 11.2).

Acute cellular rejection (ACR) develops in about 20% of liver transplant recipients, most frequently in the first 3 months after transplantation. Late ACR, that is rejection episodes occurring more than 3 months post transplant, is usually attributable to under-immunosuppression caused by compliance issues, therapeutic misadventures (drug interactions, see below), or drug malabsorption (nausea/vomiting, diarrhea). ACR is often clinically asymptomatic but can be accompanied by a low-grade temperature, and some malaise and right upper quadrant discomfort. ACR is accompanied by (and needs to be considered when routine blood work shows) rising liver enzymes in an entirely non-specific pattern that can either be hepatitic (high serum concentrations of

Table 11.2 Balance of immunosuppression	
Immunosuppression level	Sequelae
Too little immunosuppression	Acute cellular rejection
Too much immunosuppression	Infections (bacterial, viral, fungal)
	Malignancies in general, especially: EBV-associated post-transplant lymphoproliferative disorder Non-melanoma skin cancers

aspartate aminotransferase (AST) and alanine aminotransferase (ALT)), or cholestatic (high bilirubin and alkaline phosphatase (ALP)), or mixed. The clinical suspicion of ACR, therefore, requires confirmation by liver biopsy. This typically shows a mixed cellular periportal inflammation with mononuclear cells, neutrophils and eosinophils, bile duct injury, and endothelialitis, that is (sub)endothelial inflammatory changes in small portal and/or central veins. Using the Banff rejection activity index (RAI, maximum 9 points),[1] ACR is graded into mild (RAI ≤ 3), moderate (RAI 4–6), and severe (RAI ≥ 7). Mild ACR usually responds to increased maintenance immunosuppression alone. Moderate and severe ACR, typically resolve with i.v. bolus steroids (500 mg methylprednisolone i.v. daily for 3 consecutive days), followed by a gradual oral prednisone taper. Steroid-resistant rejection requiring therapy with an antilymphocyte globulin preparation has become extremely rare.

Failure of ACR to respond to immunosuppressive therapy, in conjunction with other ill-defined mechanisms, may result in **chronic ductopenic rejection** (CDR). CDR leads to obliteration of medium-sized arteries (that are typically not sampled by liver biopsy) by lipid laden, hyperplastic endothelial cells (foamy cell obliterative arteriopathy). This results in disappearance of small interlobular bile ducts and eventually evolves into biliary cirrhosis. CDR causes late graft loss, that is, the need for re-transplantation or death, in 2–5% of all liver transplanted recipients.

Side effects of immunosuppression

Lifelong immunosuppression to prevent rejection is required in all liver transplant recipients. There are general complications associated with the extent and duration of immunosuppression per se, such as infections and malignancies, and the specific side effects associated with each individual immunosuppressive drug.

General

Infectious complications are the single most important cause of mortality early after liver transplantation. The risk of infection is associated with surgical problems, for example bile leaks, as well as the degree of immunosuppression, and endogenous/exogenous exposure to pathogens. Immunosuppressed patients are at risk for all types of infections; bacterial, viral, fungal, and parasitic. In the early postoperative period, the typical postsurgical bacterial infections prevail (e.g. wound infection, line infection, pneumonia). More rarely, bacterial infections present more than 1–2 months post transplant; this includes reactivation of latent tuberculosis. Viral infections are common and typically occur at or later than 6 weeks post transplant. Cytomegalovirus (CMV) infection, often presenting as a high spiking fever and neutropenia, is the most important one. The diagnosis of CMV disease is accomplished by demonstrating viremia (CMV PCR) or tissue invasion (biopsy). In the absence of CMV prophylaxis, seronegative recipients of organs from seropositive donors have a greater than 50% risk of developing symptomatic disease. Patients with a CMV mismatch (and those who receive T-cell depleting antilymphocyte products as induction immunosuppression post transplant) must receive prophylaxis with i.v. ganciclovir followed by oral valganciclovir for at least 3 months post transplant. Other viral infections include herpes simplex virus (HSV), Epstein–Barr virus (EBV), varicella zoster virus (VZV), and adenovirus. Fungal infections are diagnosed in up to 20% of liver transplant recipients and carry significant mortality. At particular risk are patients transplanted for fulminant hepatic failure. As in other immunocompromised hosts, *Pneumocystis jirovecii* (formerly called *Pneumocystis carinii*) can cause pneumonia in liver transplant recipients and it is associated with a high mortality. Thus, prophylaxis with co-trimoxazole during the first 6–12 months post transplant is routine in most programs.

Most **malignant tumors** are more frequent in liver transplant recipients than in the general population. Tumor risk seems to be associated with the degree and the duration of immunosuppression. The risk for most solid tumors is moderately increased (approximately twofold). Liver transplant recipients with PSC (with or without ulcerative colitis) have an increased risk for colon cancer; many programs recommend annual screening colonoscopies in these patients and sometimes prophylactic colectomy. Patients transplanted for alcoholic cirrhosis have an increased risk of oropharyngeal, esophageal, and lung cancer. This is presumably due to a long-term smoking history that typically accompanies alcohol misuse. Solid organ transplant recipients are at high risk for EBV-associated, typically CD21 positive, B-cell lymphoma, also termed post-transplant lymphoproliferative disorder (PTLD). Malignant transformation of an EBV-induced polyclonal B-cell proliferation is more likely with a primary EBV infection than with reactivation of a latent infection. Thus, children who are EBV negative at time of transplant and acquire EBV infection after transplantation while on immunosuppression are at particularly high risk for PTLD.

Non-melanoma skin cancers (squamous cell carcinoma and basal cell carcinoma) are also particularly common in solid organ transplant recipients. It is, therefore, recommended that solid organ transplant recipients avoid sun

Table 11.3 Side effects of commonly used immunosuppressive drugs

Drug	Common side effects
Steroids: prednisone, methylprednisolone	Impaired wound healing, psychosis, weight gain, hypertension, insulin resistance and diabetes, dyslipidemia, acne, osteoporosis and aseptic bone necrosis, cataract
Calcineurin inhibitors: cyclosporine A, tacrolimus	Tremor, headaches, weight gain, hypertension, insulin resistance and diabetes, dyslipidemia, impaired renal function, hyperuricemia, hypomagnesemia, hyperkalemia, gingival hyperplasia, hirsutism, hair loss, potential for drug interactions due to extensive metabolism via CYP3A4
Antimetabolites: azathioprine, mycophenolate preparations	Bone marrow suppression (in particular leukopenia), diarrhea
mTOR inhibitors: sirolimus, everolimus	Hypertriglyceridemia, impaired wound healing, anemia, nephrotic syndrome, lymphedema, interstitial pneumonitis

bathing and use sunscreen when outside. Many programs also recommend annual screening for premalignant actinic keratoses by a dermatologist. Diagnosis and therapy of all these malignancies is not different from that in the non-transplant population and should be carried out by a respective specialist. However, malignancies are generally more aggressive and carry a guarded prognosis in the immunosuppressed host.

Individual immunosuppressive agents (Table 11.3)

Corticosteroid. The vast majority of programs use high-dose methylprednisolone perioperatively for the first week, followed by oral prednisone (20 mg/day) that is subsequently tapered and discontinued within 3 to 6 months. Major side effects include impaired wound healing, psychosis with the high perioperative doses, an increased incidence of infections (bacterial and fungal), insulin resistance/diabetes mellitus, weight gain, dyslipidemia, and osteoporosis.

Cyclosporine A (CsA, available in the microemulsified form as Neoral). The introduction of the calcineurin inhibitor cyclosporine A was a milestone in liver transplantation, leading to dramatically improved results. The drug has a narrow therapeutic index (efficacy vs. toxicity) and therapeutic drug monitoring is routinely performed lifelong to guide its dosage. CsA undergoes extensive hepatic metabolism though the cytochrome P450 system (CYP3A4). Drugs that induce the cytochrome P450 system, such as rifampicin, carbamazepine, and phenytoin, accelerate its metabolism and lead to decreased CsA exposure and immunosuppression. Drugs that inhibit the cytochrome P450 system, such as macrolide antibiotics (e.g. clarithromycin) and antifungals (e.g. fluconazole), inhibit its metabolism, leading to increased CsA exposure and toxicity. Possible drug interactions have to be kept in mind when starting CsA-treated transplant recipients on any new drug. Common side effects of CsA include renal dysfunction, tremor, headaches, arterial hypertension, dyslipidemia, weight gain, and insulin resistance/diabetes mellitus. Hirsutism and gingival hyperplasia are less frequent.

Tacrolimus (FK506; Prograf). Tacrolimus is the newer of the two calcineurin inhibitors, but has a similarly narrow therapeutic index and also requires therapeutic drug monitoring. At clinically used doses, tacrolimus seems to be at least equally, and possibly slightly more, immunosuppressive compared to CsA. As for CsA, tacrolimus is extensively metabolized by the hepatic cytochrome P450 system and the same considerations regarding drug interactions apply. Both calcineurin inhibitors also share a qualitatively similar side effect profile. However, insulin resistance/diabetes mellitus seems more frequent with tacrolimus, and hirsutism as well as gingival hyperplasia more frequent with CsA.

Azathioprine (Imuran). Azathioprine is a purine synthesis inhibitor, and inhibits the proliferation of all rapidly dividing cells such as leukocytes (including T and B cells). Its side effects include bone marrow suppression.

Mycophenolate. The mycophenolate preparations mycophenolate mofetil (MMF/Cellcept) and mycophenolate sodium (MPA/Myfortic) block the production of guanosine nucleotides and inhibit T- and B-cell proliferation. Their main side effect is bone marrow suppression and gastrointestinal symptoms such as diarrhea.

Other immunosuppressive agents are less frequently used and include antilymphocyte preparations (ALG, ATG, thymoglobulin), which convey an increased risk for CMV re-activation, and possibly EBV associated lymphoproliferative disorder; the mTOR inhibitors sirolimus (Rapamune) and everolimus (Certican), which inhibit growth factor-dependent proliferation of hematopoetic and non-hematopoetic cells (both impair wound healing and may cause anemia, as well as lymphedema, nephrotic syndrome, and interstitial pneumonitis); and, finally, the interleukin-2 (IL-2) receptor antagonist basiliximab (Simulect), which inhibits T-cell proliferation.

Long-term complications

The long-term complications of liver transplantation include renal dysfunction and an increased risk for fatal and non-fatal cardiovascular events. Table 11.4 and Fig. 11.1 summarize the role of the internist/family physician and of the

Table 11.4 Role of the internist/family physician and of the transplant hepatologist in the shared care of the liver transplant recipient

Internist/ family physician	Annual check-up, screening for common diseases/malignancies (including colon cancer screening) and other prophylactic measures (e.g. influenza vaccination)
	Management of cardiovascular risk factors including overweight/ obesity, high blood pressure, dyslipidemia, insulin resistance/ diabetes
	Management of other conditions including, but not limited to, gout and osteoporosis
	Management of social and intellectual development in pediatric liver transplant subjects
Transplant hepatologist	Management of immunosuppression (including diagnosis/ treatment of rejection)
	Management of graft dysfunction (diagnosis/therapy of underlying cause, including biliary complications and recurrent disease)
	Prophylaxis/therapy of immunosuppression related conditions such as infections (CMV, EBV, *Pneumocystis jirovecii*), certain malignancies (e.g. post-transplant lymphoproliferative disorder) and renal dysfunction that require adaptation of immunosuppression as part of their management

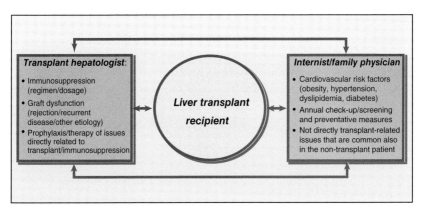

Fig. 11.1 Practice points/management algorithm: shared management of complications in the liver transplant recipient—communication between internist/ family physician and transplant hepatologist is essential.

transplant hepatologist in the shared long-term care for the liver transplant recipient in which communication between all parties involved is essential.

Renal dysfunction

Renal dysfunction is common in all organ transplant recipients. Calcineurin inhibitors lead to a dose-dependent glomerular vasoconstriction associated with an initially reversible decrease in renal plasma flow and glomerular filtration rate (GFR). If this persists, anatomically fixed and irreversible glomerular damage, the so called calcineurin inhibitor-induced nephropathy, ensues. Once an ill-defined "point of no return" has been passed, renal function progressively deteriorates, irrespective of interventions, and results in end-stage renal disease, eventually requiring renal replacement therapy. It has been estimated that up to 25% of liver transplant recipients develop severe renal dysfunction (defined as GFR < 29 mL/min) within 10 years post transplant.[2] The first step in managing renal dysfunction post liver transplant is awareness. Delaying the postoperative start of calcineurin inhibitor dosing by using other immunosuppressive strategies is common practice in the patient with transiently impaired renal function immediately after surgery. Later on, early calcineurin minimization (or even discontinuation) by adding another immunosuppressant, such as a mycophenolate preparation, can be effective in preserving renal function. In the liver transplant recipients with impaired renal function, it is of utmost importance to avoid any additional nephrotoxic insult. Renal function is very sensitive to intravascular volume depletion by diuretics, which should thus be dosed with caution. Similarly, vomiting and/or diarrhea can precipitate renal failure. Tight control of blood pressure and blood glucose is mandatory (see below). Nephrotoxic drugs such as aminoglycosides should be avoided. In patients taking calcineurin inhibitor therapy, renal perfusion is heavily dependent on renal prostaglandin synthesis. Thus, the use of non-steroidal anti-inflammatory drugs can precipitate acute renal failure and should be avoided (Table 11.5).

Cardiovascular risk factors

Cardiovascular risk factors are frequently present in liver transplant recipients. Steroids and calcineurin inhibitors predispose to obesity, aggravate pre-existing and trigger *de novo* post-transplant insulin resistance and overt diabetes

---

Table 11.5 Preservation of renal function in the liver transplant recipient

Do *not* use non-steroidal anti-inflammatory drugs
Use diuretics with caution
Avoid nephrotoxic drugs such as aminoglycosides
Minimize calcineurin inhibitor (CNI) exposure (if possible)
Optimize blood pressure control
Optimize blood sugar control

Table 11.6 Treatment targets for cardiovascular risk factors in the liver transplant recipient

Risk factor	Treatment target
Blood pressure	≤140/80 mmHg
LDL cholesterol	<2–2.5 mmol/L
Fasting blood glucose	Within normal limits
HbA1c	<7%

mellitus, arterial hypertension, and dyslipidemia. One or a combination of these cardiovascular risk factors is present in 60% or more of liver transplant recipients who survive for more than 1 year post transplant. It is therefore not surprising that the incidence of non-fatal and fatal cardiovascular events is around threefold higher in liver transplant recipients than in a comparable normal population.[3] In fact, cardiovascular conditions and malignancy are the most frequent causes of death late after liver transplantation. Liver transplant recipients are therefore regarded as at a high cardiovascular risk and the respective intervention thresholds and the therapeutic targets for control of blood pressure,[4] low-density lipoprotein (LDL) cholesterol,[5,6] and blood sugar[7] apply (Table 11.6).

Weight gain is common and leads to an average BMI increase of 3–4 units during the first 1–2 years after liver transplantation when more than 20% of pre-transplant non-obese patients have become overtly obese.[8] In the years to come, these prevalence rates will likely increase due to increasing numbers of obese patients transplanted for non-alcoholic fatty liver disease and the increasing prevalence of overweight and obesity in the general population. Overweight/obesity is a risk factor for insulin resistance/diabetes, arterial hypertension, dyslipidemia, and, thus, cardiovascular risk. In addition, overweight/obesity predisposes to non-alcoholic fatty liver disease that can *de novo* occur in the graft. Life style counseling (diet, exercise), prophylactically in all patients and therapeutically in those developing overweight/obesity, seems intuitively to make sense. Many patients find it difficult, however, to adhere to these measures. The efficacy and safety of other therapies for morbid obesity, such as orlistat and bariatric surgery, have not been systematically evaluated in liver transplant recipients but may affect absorption of immunosuppressive drugs.

Forty to eighty percent of liver transplant recipients develop **arterial hypertension** within months to years after transplantation. The target blood pressure in liver transplant recipients is at or below 140 mmHg systolic and at or below 80 mmHg diastolic. Lifestyle modification (weight loss, adopting a healthy diet, and increasing physical activity) is effective in decreasing blood pressure, but difficult to adhere to for many patients. Pharmacotherapy of high blood pressure in the liver transplant recipient is not different from that in the non-transplant patient. Some specifics should, however, be mentioned. Thus, tapering and withdrawing steroids can improve blood pressure. Calcineurin inhibitors frequently increase uric acid plasma levels and concomitant use of thiazide diuretics may further increase hyperuricemia and precipitate gout. Calcineurin inhibitors increase plasma potassium levels; concomitant use of angiotensin-converting enzyme (ACE) inhibitors and angiotensin-II (AT-II) blockers may lead to clinically relevant hyperkalemia. Calcium channel blockers, except for nifedipine and amlodipine, interfere with calcineurin inhibitor metabolism and lead to increased cyclosporine and tacrolimus exposure; nifedipine and amlodipine protect against calcineurin inhibitor nephrotoxicity in animal models and are therefore considered by some transplant physicians as first-line blood pressure therapy in liver transplant recipients.

Insulin resistance and diabetes are common in liver transplant recipients and are most frequent in patients with hepatitis C virus related liver disease. Conceptually, one distinguishes between pretransplant pre-existing diabetes and post-transplant new-onset or *de novo* diabetes. Ten to fifteen percent of liver transplant recipients have pre-existing diabetes; new onset post-transplant diabetes develops in 10–40%. As in the non-transplant population, diabetes in liver transplant recipients is the cause of significant morbidity and mortality, in particular due to cardiovascular, infectious, and renal diseases. In addition, insulin resistance/diabetes accelerates fibrosis progression in the graft, particularly in those with hepatitis C and likely also decreases response rates (SVR) to interferon-based antiviral therapy post transplant. Diagnostic criteria, intervention thresholds, and therapeutic targets have been summarized by the American Diabetes Association[9] and include an HbA1c of more than 6.5% as diagnostic of diabetes mellitus. New-onset post-transplant diabetes has been recently reviewed by an international expert panel[7] and is felt to resemble type 2 diabetes and managed accordingly.

Dyslipidemia is common after liver transplantation, with hypercholesterolemia occurring in one-third to two-thirds of liver transplant recipients. In 2006, the Canadian Cardiovascular Society put forward updated, more stringent, evidence-based guidelines recommending a primary target LDL of less than 2.0 mmol/L for high-risk individuals, such as is the case in the typical adult liver transplant recipient (i.e. in his/her mid-fifties, hypertensive, overweight/obese, and/or insulin resistant/diabetic). Statins seem safe in liver transplant recipients, pravastatin and cerivastatin having been formally tested in controlled clinical trials. Pravastatin is devoid of drug interactions with calcineurin inhibitors, having little affinity to CYP3A4.

Other long-term complications

Osteoporosis of the lumbar spine and hip (T-score in dual X-ray absorptiometry (DEXA) < –2.5, i.e. bone mineral density > 2.5 standard deviations below the mean for young healthy adults) is present in around one-third of liver transplant recipients. An additional proportion of patients has severely reduced bone mineral density (osteopenia with Z-scores between −1 and −2.5). Typically, bone mineral density decreases in the first 3–6 months post transplant (when fractures may occur) but subsequently stabilizes and later increases again, reaching pretransplant levels 1 year after transplant.[10] Predisposing factors include pre-existing bone loss attributable to end-stage liver disease (in particular of cholestatic etiology), perioperative immobilization, and immunosuppressive therapy with steroids and calcineurin inhibitors. In most programs, a bone density measurement (DEXA) is performed during transplant evaluation and patients are counseled regarding lifestyle measures (exercise and smoking cessation), and vitamin D (800–1000 IU daily) and calcium (1–2 g daily) supplements. Bisphosphonates are often prescribed in patients with bone density measurements within the osteoporotic range and/or with a history of osteoporotic fractures. In osteoporotic liver transplant recipients, corticosteroids should be tapered and withdrawn as soon as possible; vitamin D and calcium supplements, as well as bisphosphonates, are continued post transplant in appropriate patients. Repeating a bone mineral density measurement 1 year after transplant seems reasonable in order to decide on further therapy.

Hyperuricemia develops in 50–80% of liver transplant recipients, but manifests as gout in less than 10%; it is attributable to calcineurin-inhibitor-induced impairment of renal uric acid handling. Treatment is indicated only for symptomatic gout (not for asymptomatic hyperuricemia) and does not differ from that in the non-transplant patient, colchicine being the treatment of choice for an acute attack and allopurinol for prevention of future attacks. Of note, non-steroidal anti-inflammatory drugs should never be used in the liver transplant recipient (see above, renal dysfunction) and allopurinol is contraindicated in patients on azathioprine because of the risk for severe bone marrow suppression due to accumulation of the myelotoxic azathioprine metabolite 5-mercaptopurine.

Recurrent disease

After cardiovascular events and malignancies, the third most important long-term issue in managing liver transplant recipients is recurrent disease. Certain underlying liver diseases cannot recur after liver transplantation such as **Wilson disease** where the causative defect has been removed with the explant; others may recur, the frequency depending on the etiology of the disease. **Autoimmune hepatitis** recurs infrequently (10%) but may develop *de novo* post transplant—it is treated with steroids as in the non-transplant setting. **Primary biliary cirrhosis** recurs in about 20%, is usually treated with ursodeoxycholic acid, as in the non-transplant setting, and hardly ever leads to significant liver disease in the graft during the life time of the recipient. About 20% of patients transplanted for **primary sclerosing cholangitis** develop recurrent PSC in the graft; there is no therapy of proven efficacy and some patients develop graft failure and need a re-transplantation. Patients with **alcoholic liver disease** selected for transplantation according to current criteria often consume alcohol again post transplant, but rarely resume harmful drinking and have overall one of the best long-term survival rates. **Non-alcoholic fatty liver disease** recurs not infrequently but seems only rarely to cause graft cirrhosis/failure again in the lifetime of the patient. **Hepatitis B** recurrence is successfully prevented by administration of anti-HBs immunoglobulin and an anti-HBV nucleoside/nucleotide analogue. Some programs continue both medications lifelong, others stop the expensive anti-HBs immunoglobulin after a year and continue only the anti-HBV nucleoside/nucleotide analogue for life. Even if HBV recurs, despite these measures, it is easily controlled with the potent anti-HBV nucleoside/nucleotide analogues available today. **Hepatitis C** recurs universally post transplant, runs an aggressive course in 10–30% of patients, leading to progressive fibrosis and graft cirrhosis in less than 5 years. The life expectancy of HCV-positive liver transplant recipients is therefore overall impaired; life expectancies will normalize if antiviral therapy with pegylated interferon-α and ribavirin is successful, that is, if SVR is achieved.[11] This occurs infrequently but new, directly targeting antivirals for hepatitis C are likely to improve the SVR following a liver transplant.

Special considerations in children with a liver transplant

Management in the immediate postoperative period for children who undergo liver transplantation is broadly similar to that for adults.[12] Most young children receive a reduced graft, which usually consists of the left lateral segments (II and III). Modifications of surgical technique are required if the child has had biliary atresia and a Kasai portoenterostomy previously; because a duct-to-duct anastomosis cannot be performed, the enterostomy loop is reused. In small children the rate of hepatic artery thrombosis is higher than in adults, and it occurs in approximately 5–10% of children.[13,14] Perioperative management to prevent this complication includes treatment with platelet inhibitors. Portal vein thrombosis occurs less commonly than hepatic artery thrombosis. Biliary complications are relatively common and are usually due to biliary leaks, which can be managed conservatively. Overall outcomes with a reduced liver graft are as good as with a size-matched, whole liver graft.[15] Acute cellular rejection usually occurs in the first few months after the transplant, but it can occur at any time after the transplant.[16]

Among the later complications of liver transplantation in children, CMV infection and post-transplantation lymphoproliferative disorder (PTLD) deserve special comment. Both occur more often in children because children are frequently CMV-negative and/or EBV-negative at the time of transplantation. The risk of clinically significant CMV infection is directly associated with the CMV-negative recipient receiving a CMV-positive liver graft, although CMV-positive recipients can also develop clinically significant CMV reactivation. Prophylaxis with antivirals may prevent serious disease, and treatment with high-dose intravenous ganciclovir is standard; CMV hyperimmune globulin may be added. PTLD is a major issue for children undergoing liver transplantation, occurring in up to 15%.[17] The typical setting for PTLD is that the child who was EBV-negative before transplant develops a primary EBV infection after transplant. Clinical severity and presentation can be highly variable, including tonsillar enlargement, chronic diarrhea, or unexplained fever/weight loss. Early detection of PTLD is important for best outcome. Proactive surveillance of EBV levels is routine. Treatment includes reducing immunosuppression and/or high-dose ganciclovir; chemotherapy is reserved for those patients who develop very severe disease. Other late complications include biliary strictures, which may develop as a consequence of hepatic artery thrombosis and are treated by balloon dilation of the bile duct or surgical correction. Finally, an entity currently known as plasma cell hepatitis (previously called *"de novo* autoimmune hepatitis"*) is a late hepatic problem which seems to occur more often in children than in adults. This disorder clinically resembles autoimmune hepatitis (elevated serum aminotransferases, positive autoantibodies such as antinuclear antibody and smooth muscle antibody) and occurs in children who did not have an autoimmune disease before the transplant. Whether it is a peculiar pattern of chronic rejection remains disputed. Treatment is the same as for autoimmune hepatitis.

Dealing with childhood infections is a problem encountered much more frequently in the pediatric age bracket than with older liver transplant recipients. Administration of standard childhood immunizations may be incomplete at the time of transplant. Some infants will have had the transplant before getting, or completing, their "baby shots" for diphtheria, tetanus, pertussis, and polio (DPTP). Many will have been transplanted before receiving the measles, mumps, rubella (MMR), which as a live attenuated vaccine becomes contraindicated after transplant. In general, the immunization schedules for infants obviously headed for transplant are compressed in the pretransplant period. Immunizations for *H. influenzae* and *Pneumococcus* are also provided pretransplant, if possible. Immunization against hepatitis A and B is also provided when time permits pretransplant. With the recent availability of varicella zoster (chickenpox) vaccination, children get this protection; however, it is another live attenuated virus vaccine which must be administered well before the transplant. It is vital to assess and record the immunization history of each patient. After transplant, live-virus vaccines are contraindicated and non-live vaccines may not be effective.[18] Children not protected against chickenpox (by virtue of previous natural infection or immunization) require prophylaxis against acute chickenpox whenever they may have been exposed to it. Parents need to identify any potential exposure to chickenpox and know the importance of reporting it to their child's health-care provider.

General health issues relate to renal and cardiovascular function, as with adults.[19] Renal dysfunction occurs commonly as a result of immunosuppression with calcineurin inhibitors. In children serum creatinine and urea nitrogen levels may not reflect the degree of renal dysfunction accurately, and direct measurement of glomerular filtration rate by nuclear medicine scanning is required. Late renal failure requiring dialysis or renal transplant may occur.

Hypertension persists in approximately one-quarter of children a decade after transplant, and it can be managed with standard therapies. Cardiomyopathy has been found in children treated with tacrolimus, but it is rare. Hyperlipidemia may be transient in children after liver transplantation, but there is increasing evidence of significant coronary artery disease in these patients over the long term. This may be associated with late development of overweight/obesity in these children. Chronic anemia occurs in some children, and its etiology is uncertain, not obviously due to iron deficiency nor chronic disease.

A major issue for children after liver transplantation is nutritional status. Wherever possible, good nutritional status should be maintained in the pre-transplant period; however, problems of nutrient absorption and utilization associated with cholestasis or inherited metabolic disease are often difficult to solve. Recent studies indicate that many, but not all, children will regain normal growth patterns and body habitus after a successful liver transplant.[20,21] However, children whose liver disease is due to a genetic disorder character-ized by growth failure, such as Alagille syndrome, may not achieve complete catch-up growth. Immunosuppressive regimens that wean corticosteroids fairly rapidly and utilize calcineurin inhibitor monotherapy enhance nutri-tional recovery. Especially with good nutrition status re-established, prepuber-tal children may be expected to progress through puberty normally. Nutritional issues of note include general under-nutrition and disruption of vitamin D physiology resulting in osteopenia. Vitamin D deficiency requires immediate and effective treatment because of the increased risk for fractures. Other fat-soluble vitamin stores and essential fatty acid stores may also be depleted despite absence of symptoms of deficiency. The post-transplant diet should be nutritionally complete, well-balanced, and palatable, though not heavy on junk food (table sugar and trans fats). Dietary supplements geared to children may be used. Infants who were dependent on tube-feeding for dietary adequacy may actually need to learn the motor skills of how to eat, best accomplished through teamwork between occupational therapists and clinical nutritionists.

Long-term social and intellectual functioning in children seems to be favo-rable. Infants who fall off their normal neurodevelopmental curve pretrans-plant, possibly because of nutritional deficiencies, may not attain their projected neurodevelopmental curve after transplant. Indeed, after fully recovering from the liver transplant, many children end up in the lower range of a broadly normal IQ. Evaluating and enhancing quality of life after liver transplant remain priorities of long-term management.[22] Some children regard their general well-being as being like that of other children with a severe health problem (such as childhood cancer) or an ongoing chronic disease (such as type 1 diabetes mellitus), but others describe themselves as being really normal, just like their friends and classmates. Children report some distress over unpleas-ant medical procedures, which are a routine part of long-term follow-up (blood work, liver biopsy, diagnostic imaging) and they worry about missing school, both for academic and social reasons, whereas parents tend to worry about broader problems relating to drug side effects, complications involving infection or rejection, and their child's future as an adult functioning independently in society. From the family's point of view, liver transplantation for a child is extremely stressful and can result in marital disharmony or divorce, or in more generalized dysfunction within the family unit. Many of these issues play out in adolescence, when accumulated simmering anxieties and emotional injury can become prominent.[23] Resentment for the intrusion of medical routines and minor life-style restrictions can become an important problem, which may result in non-adherence to the medical regimen. This is a serious problem, resulting in graft loss or rejection in a substantial proportion of liver transplant recipients, particularly in teenagers.[24] Management of the adolescent liver transplant patient should anticipate these challenges by being broadly supportive and educational, and it should recognize that the transition years from adolescence to young adulthood are particularly challenging for these patients.

Case study 11.1

You see a 48-year-old farmer in your office for the first time after his liver transplant. You know that he received a deceased donor organ 4 months ago for cryptogenic cirrhosis. Based on the fact that he was known for type 2 diabetes and obesity (BMI around 35) for 10 or more years prior to hepatic decompensation, his cirrhosis is likely to have been caused by non-alcoholic fatty liver disease. You learned from the transplant center's discharge summary, that the postoperative course was complicated by a bile leak on the fourth postoperative day that required surgical revision and conversion from a duct-to-duct to a Roux-en-Y biliary anastomosis. After the re-operation his renal function temporarily declined and his tacrolimus dose was therefore decreased; his liver enzymes had almost normalized by that time. Over the subsequent days he developed a secondary increase in his liver enzymes in a mixed pattern (ALT 154 IU/L, ALP 203 IU/L). On the 10th postoperative day, a liver biopsy was performed and revealed a moderate acute cellular rejection (RAI 4/9). His tacrolimus dose was increased back up again (the renal function had fortunately recovered) and he was started on 500 mg methylprednisolone daily on three consecutive days. The patient's liver enzymes promptly normalized and remained within the normal range since that time while taking just tacrolimus and tapering doses of prednisone. However, the patient's blood sugar was no longer controllable without insulin. He was discharged home on the 17th postoperative day with prescriptions for tacrolimus, prednisone 15 mg daily, and insulin. Since then he was closely followed by the transplant team. Their report tells you that there were no further complications, the incision healed nicely, prednisone was weaned and completely stopped 2 weeks ago, and the patient is now on monoimmunosuppression with tacrolimus and he still requires insulin.

 The patient tells you that he feels great and has already started doing some work on the farm. According to the patient's self-monitoring, his blood sugar varies between 6 and 10 mmol/L. His body weight has increased by 3 kg compared to your

(Continued)

last weight prior to transplant when he still had ascites (which has now completely resolved). His blood pressure is 150/90. A brief physical exam is unremarkable. You order some laboratory tests including an HbA1c and a lipid profile and arrange for a follow-up, 1 month later. The laboratory results show normal liver enzymes and normal graft function (bilirubin, albumin, INR), the creatinine is with 95 μmol/L at the upper limit of normal, the HbA1c is 7.5% and the lipid profile shows an LDL cholesterol of 4.0 mmol/L.

When the patient returns for his follow-up you start discussing with him his cardiovascular risk (obesity, elevated blood pressure, dyslipidemia, diabetes) and counsel him regarding lifestyle measures. You discuss with him intensifying his insulin regimen to achieve better blood sugar control. You explain to him why he should be on an antihypertensive (because he is diabetic an ACE inhibitor is recommended with a need to follow the potassium closely) and on a statin (you suggest atorvastatin 10 mg daily). You also feel that as a diabetic he should be on a baby aspirin (does not impair renal function). The patient seems understandably somewhat overwhelmed and asks you "I feel great, give me one good reason why I should do all this?"

Case study 11.2

Your practice as a family physician includes a family where one of the children, a girl now 14 years old, has had a liver transplant. This liver disease has been hard on the family. The little girl presented with unexplained jaundice as a toddler, and it took a few years to figure out that she was suffering from a rare genetic liver disease affecting bile formation. It was confirmed as an autosomal recessive disorder. Then there were several years of trying various treatments, all of which were unsuccessful. Finally she was listed for transplant, deteriorated over the 2 years of waiting on the list, and had a prolonged stormy recuperation. The family has suffered financially and emotionally, and the parents are on the brink of divorce, currently in therapy with a marriage counselor. The girl's younger brother has been checked genetically and is only a carrier for this disorder, but he has become a shy, introverted child through this ordeal.

However, for the past 3–4 years your transplant patient has been doing pretty well. She is brought to your clinic today for a non-routine visit by her mother. Before you can ask anything, her mother blurts out angrily: "She has gone and gotten a tattoo! And she is skipping school and acting out at home!" Without stopping to ask about where and how she got the tattoo, you look at your young teenaged patient. In addition to her discreet nose stud, she does indeed have a large multicolored (actually quite attractive) tattoo of a bouquet of flowers on her upper chest, in the "bodice" area. It looks as if it is healing well. She says: "I wanted something pretty. I'm already covered with scars." You ask her mother to step out and your nurse to step in: in chatting together you hear that schoolwork is hard just now, and tiring, and that the other kids tease her a lot saying that she has a spare-parts liver, and that she is fed up with hearing her parents argue over who caused this "genetic mess". You order some blood tests for various viral infections and tacrolimus level. You arrange consultation with a psychologist specializing in adolescent adjustment disorders.

The tacrolimus level comes back undetectable and the serum aminotransferases are elevated 50% over normal. You call the patient back to the clinic and discuss her immunosuppressive medication. In consultation with her transplant hepatologist, you start her back on a higher dose of tacrolimus and monitor her closely. The liver test abnormalities resolve, and weekly tacrolimus levels show that she is taking her medication regularly. She seems pretty happy and rather interested in taking responsibility for her medication.

A few months later you see her for a routine visit. She has no specific complaints, but you notice that she looks thinner and her weight has dropped 6 kg. She denies fevers, fatigue, or gastrointestinal problems, but she admits that her periods, which have never been very regular, are more irregular than ever. In fact she has not had one for a couple of months. Physical exam is essentially negative, apart from a prominent tattoo: in particular there is no lymphadenopathy, liver enlargement, or abdominal tenderness. You send tests for a broad spectrum of viral infections, thyroid function, as well as a pregnancy test and liver function tests. She is not pregnant and also not hypothyroid. You arrange an urgent consultation for her with her transplant hepatologist, and an extensive assessment for PTLD is negative. Likewise, she has no evidence of a new viral infection. A serum carotene level is elevated, and consequently you talk to her about her diet. It turns out that she has been eating less and less and exercising a lot. You discuss the problem of an eating disorder in the anorexia nervosa/bulimia spectrum with her psychologist. Obviously this young lady's post-transplant psychological problems are going to be more complicated than was first apparent. On the positive side, her school performance has become quite good and she is graduating to the next grade.

Multiple choice questions

1. Which of the following is correct?
   A. Late acute cellular rejection (>3 months post transplant) is often caused by under immunosuppression secondary to non-compliance or a therapeutic misadventure.
   B. Renal dysfunction is frequent after liver transplantation and related to mycophenolate preparations used for immunosuppression.
   C. Cardiovascular risk factors such as obesity, hypertension, dyslipidemia, and insulin resistance/diabetes occur in 30–60% of liver transplant patients and lead to a threefold increased risk for non-fatal and fatal cardiovascular events in the long term.
   D. Answers A and C are correct.
   E. All of the above are correct.
   F. None of the above are correct.

2. A 4-year-old child who had a liver transplant as a toddler for biliary atresia starts having loud snoring and otherwise rather persistent mouth-breathing. Diagnostic considerations include:
   A. Strep throat
   B. Sleep apnea associated with obesity
   C. PTLD in the tonsils
   D. Seasonal allergies
   E. Thyroid nodule

Answers

1. D
2. C

Further reading

1. Banff schema for grading liver allograft rejection: an international consensus document. Hepatology 1997; 25: 658–63.
2. Ojo AO, Held PJ, Port FK, et al. Chronic renal failure after transplantation of a non-renal organ. N Engl J Med 2003; 349: 931–40.
3. Johnston SD, Morris JK, Cramb R, et al. Cardiovascular morbidity and mortality after orthotopic liver transplantation. Transplantation 2002; 73: 901–6.
4. Chobanian AV, Bakris GL, Black HR, et al. Seventh report of the Joint National Committee on Prevention, Detection, Evaluation, and Treatment of High Blood Pressure. Hypertension 2003; 42: 1206–52.
5. Grundy SM, Cleeman JI, Merz NB, et al., for the Coordinating Committee of the National Cholesterol Education Program. Implications of recent trials for the National Cholesterol Education Program Adult Treatment Panel III Guidelines. Circulation 2004; 110: 227–39.
6. McPherson R, Frohlich J, Fodor G, et al. Canadian Cardiovascular Society position statement—recommendations for the diagnosis and treatment of dyslipidemia and prevention of cardiovascular disease. Can J Cardiol 2006; 22: 913–27.
7. Davidson JA, Wilson A, on behalf of the International Expert Panel on New-Onset Diabetes after Transplantation. New-onset diabetes after transplantation 2003 international consensus guidelines. Diabetes Care 2004; 27: 805–12.
8. Everhart JE, Lombardero M, Lake JR, et al. Weight change and obesity after liver transplantation: incidence and risk factors. Liver Transpl Surg 1998; 4: 285–96.
9. American Diabetes Association. Diagnosis and classification of diabetes mellitus. Diabetes Care 2010; 33 (Suppl. 1): S62–9.
10. Leslie WD, Bernstein CN, Leboff MS. AGA technical review on osteoporosis in hepatic disorders. Gastroenterology 2003; 125: 941–66.
11. Selzner N, Renner EL, Selzner M, et al. Antiviral treatment of recurrent hepatitis C after liver transplantation: predictors of response and long-term outcome. Transplantation 2009; 88: 1214–21.
12. Kamath BM, Olthoff KM. Liver transplantation in children: update 2010. Pediatr Clin North Am 2010; 57: 401–14.

13. Martin SR, Atkison P, Anand R, et al. Studies of pediatric liver transplantation 2002: patient and graft survival and rejection in pediatric recipients of a first liver transplant in the United States and Canada. Pediatr Transpl 2004; 8: 273–83.
14. Warnaar N, Polak WG, de Jong KP, et al. Long-term results of urgent revascularization for hepatic artery thrombosis after pediatric liver transplantation. Liver Transpl 2010; 16: 847–55.
15. Otte JB, de Ville de Goyet J, Reding R, et al. Pediatric liver transplantation: from the full-size liver graft to reduced, split, and living related liver transplantation. Pediatr Surg Int 1998; 13: 308–18.
16. Ng VL, Fecteau A, Shepherd R, et al. Outcomes of 5-year survivors of pediatric liver transplantation: report on 461 children from a North American multicenter registry. Pediatrics 2008; 122: e1128–35.
17. Kamdar KY, Rooney CM, Heslop HE. Posttransplant lymphoproliferative disease following liver transplantation. Curr Opin Organ Transpl 2011; 16: 274–80.
18. Allen U, Green M. Prevention and treatment of infectious complications after solid organ transplantation in children. Pediatr Clin North Am 2010; 57: 459–79.
19. Avitzur Y, De Luca E, Cantos M, et al. Health status ten years after pediatric liver transplantation—looking beyond the graft. Transplantation 2004; 78: 566–73.
20. Superina RA, Zangari A, Acal L, et al. Growth in children following liver transplantation. Pediatr Transpl 1998; 2: 70–5.
21. Alonso EM, Shepherd R, Martz KL, et al. Linear growth patterns in prepubertal children following liver transplantation. Am J Transpl 2009; 9: 1389–97.
22. Nicholas DB, Otley AR, Taylor R, et al. Experiences and barriers to health-related quality of life following liver transplantation: a qualitative analysis of the perspectives of pediatric patients and their parents. Health Qual Life Outcomes 2010; 8: 150.
23. Kaufman M, Shemesh E, Benton T. The adolescent transplant recipient. Pediatr Clin North Am 2010; 57: 575–92.
24. Falkenstein K, Flynn L, Kirkpatrick B, et al. Non-compliance in children post-liver transplant. Who are the culprits? Pediatr Transplant 2004; 8: 233–6.

Acute viral hepatitis in adults and children: hepatitis A, B, C, D, E, and others

CHAPTER 12

Hemant A. Shah[1] and Eve A. Roberts[2]

[1] Division of Gastroenterology, Toronto Western Hospital, University Health Network, Toronto, Ontario, Canada

[2] Departments of Paediatrics, Medicine, and Pharmacology, University of Toronto, and Division of Gastroenterology, Hepatology and Nutrition, The Hospital for Sick Children, Toronto, Ontario, Canada

Key points

- Any acute viral hepatitis may present in three main ways: asymptomatic, symptomatic, or as a fulminant hepatitis.
- There are five well-characterized hepatitis viruses (HAV, HBV, HCV, HDV, HEV), and each of these viruses is distinct. HBV is a DNA virus; the others are RNA viruses, and HDV is an incomplete virus.
- Serological markers are used to differentiate individuals with acute viral hepatitis from those with chronic viral hepatitis.
- Treatment consists mainly of general supportive measures although some virus-specific therapies are available.
- Vaccinations are available for protection against HAV and HBV infection, and a vaccine against HEV is being developed. Immunity to HBV also provides protection against HDV infection. In North America, universal vaccination of infants/young children against HAV and HBV is the standard policy. There is no vaccine against HCV currently available.
- Standard public health measures such as clean water, single use of all medical/dental equipment that pierces the skin, and the practice of safer sex can impact global outcomes.

Introduction

Several viruses, such as adenovirus, cytomegalovirus, echoviruses, Epstein–Barr, herpes simplex, varicella, and rubella, may cause "hepatitis" as a component of a systemic disease, but certain viruses, namely hepatitis viruses A, B,

Hepatology: Diagnosis and Clinical Management, First Edition. Edited by E. Jenny Heathcote.
© 2012 John Wiley & Sons, Ltd. Published 2012 by John Wiley & Sons, Ltd.

Box 12.1 Serologic testing for acute hepatitis suspected to be viral in origin

Complete blood count, electrolytes, creatinine, INR, albumin
ALT, AST, ALP, conjugated/unconjugated bilirubin
Hepatitis A: anti-HAV Ab IgM
Hepatitis B: HBsAg, anti-HBc IgM, anti-HBs Ab, (HBV DNA if HBsAg positive)
Hepatitis C: HCV RNA RT-PCR, anti-HCV Ab
Hepatitis D: anti-HDV IgM, HDV RNA RT-PCR if positive
Hepatitis E: anti-HEV IgM, HEV RNA RT-PCR if positive
EBV: Monospot, EBV-specific IgM
CMV: anti-CMV IgM, CMV antigen, CMV PCR

Table 12.1 Definition of syndromes associated with acute viral hepatitis

Syndrome	Clinical manifestations	Biochemical manifestations
Asymptomatic infection	Absence of symptoms	Mild elevation in aminotransferases. Normal liver function (INR, bilirubin, albumin)
Acute hepatitis	Preicteric symptoms including fatigue, nausea, anorexia, flu-like symptoms. Hepatomegaly and liver tenderness. Can progress to icteric illness (more severe symptoms)	Mild–moderate elevation in aminotransferases. Mild–moderate elevation in bilirubin
Fulminant hepatitis	Initial symptoms resemble acute hepatitis but then rapid development of jaundice, edema, ascites, confusion (encephalopathy), bleeding	Presence of active infection. Moderate–severe elevation in aminotransferases. Markers of liver failure (high INR, high bilirubin)

C, D, and E, cause a hepatitis of variable severity as their primary effect (Box 12.1). Inoculation of a non-immune host with any of these five unrelated viruses results in one of three clinical syndromes: (1) asymptomatic disease; (2) acute hepatitis; or (3) fulminant hepatitis (Table 12.1). The risk for development of these different manifestations of acute viral hepatitis depends upon both virus and host factors.

Hepatitis A

Virology

Hepatitis A virus (HAV) was first characterized in 1973. HAV contains a single-stranded RNA molecule and lacks an envelope. Only one serotype of HAV is known, and there is no antigenic cross-reactivity with hepatitis B, C, D, or E. HAV can survive acidic environments (down to pH 3) and high temperatures (60°C for 60 min). HAV is capable of surviving in dried feces for up to 4 weeks.

Epidemiology

HAV transmission is by the fecal–oral route. It is primarily transmitted either person-to-person or by ingestion of contaminated food and water. Only very rarely does transmission take place by blood-to-blood contact such as via transfusion or injection drug use. It is also present in all bodily fluids of an infected person and can be transmitted via contact.

HAV infection follows one of three epidemiologic patterns.
1 In countries with poor sanitary conditions, most children are infected at an early age and thus epidemic outbreaks are unlikely.
2 In developed countries the prevalence of HAV infection is low (the sero-prevalence of anti-HAV antibodies in USA is approximately 10% in children and 37% in adults (Fig. 12.1)). Over 50% of cases in developed countries are the result of infection acquired while traveling to endemic areas.

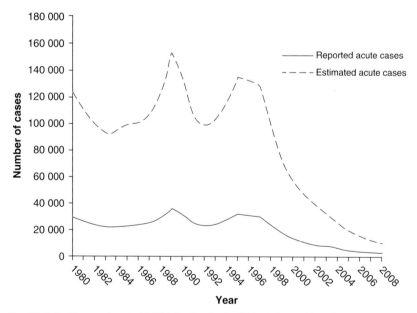

Fig. 12.1 Incidence of acute HAV infection in the United States (data from Centers for Disease Control and Prevention).

3 HAV infection within an isolated community can cause an epidemic since individuals will not have immunity from prior exposure. In these communities, future newborns remain susceptible until the virus is reintroduced.

Clinical features

HAV infection results in an acute self-limited episode of hepatitis and never results in chronic infection. There are usually five different clinical patterns:
1 asymptomatic without icterus;
2 symptomatic with jaundice and self-limited;
3 symptomatic and evolving to a cholestatic pattern lasting 10 weeks or more;
4 relapsing, with two or more bouts of acute hepatitis occurring from the one infection over a 2- to 3-month period;
5 fulminant hepatic failure.

The clinically silent incubation (preclinical) phase is usually 2 to 4 weeks during which time viral transmission is likely as HAV is readily detectable in stool and blood. A prodromal illness can include fatigue, anorexia, nausea, weakness, and right upper quadrant abdominal pain. Eventually, jaundice and dark urine may develop. Symptoms, if present, last from a few days to 2 weeks. Complete clinical recovery is observed in 60% of affected individuals in 2 months and nearly all individuals by 6 months. The overall prognosis is excellent. After full recovery the anti-HAV antibody is protective against reinfection.

In general, the severity of clinical illness increases with increasing age. Children under 2 years are typically asymptomatic and jaundice occurs in only 20%. After age 5 years, most (80%) infected individuals will experience symptoms. A relapsing course is observed in about 10% of patients with HAV infection. Profound cholestasis may complicate acute HAV infection especially in those taking estrogens (including the very-low-dose oral contraceptive formulations). Approximately one-third of individuals infected after age 60 years will require hospitalization. Women past middle age seem to be at greater risk for a more severe course of acute hepatitis A, including some predisposition to acute liver failure. Overall the risk for acute liver failure with acute hepatitis A is approximately 1%. In endemic areas, young children are at excess risk for acute liver failure from acute hepatitis A, despite the usual pattern of trivial or unapparent infection. Consequently, it has been a leading indication for liver transplantation in pre-school-aged children in these countries, for example, Argentina. Universal vaccination programs for young children have been established to eliminate this avoidable indication for liver transplant. A further, very rare, complication with acute hepatitis A is the development of aplastic anemia.

Making the diagnosis

Acute HAV infection cannot be clinically distinguished from other types of acute hepatitis (viral or otherwise). The diagnosis is based on detection of specific antibodies against HAV in serum. Diagnosis of acute infection is made

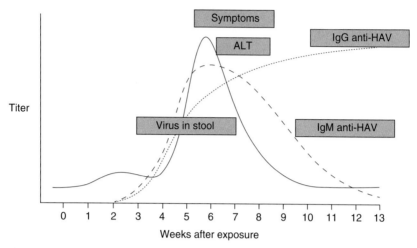

Fig. 12.2 Course of acute HAV infection (adapted from Hoofnagle JH, DiBisceglie AM. Serologic diagnosis of acute and chronic viral hepatitis. Semin Liver Dis 1991; 11: 73).

by the detection of IgM anti-HAV antibodies in serum. This test result is positive at the onset of symptoms (Fig. 12.2). IgM anti-HAV antibodies can be detectable at low level up to 1 year after infection. IgG anti-HAV antibodies are often also detectable at the onset of disease and usually remain present for life. Testing for HAV RNA is not widely available and is unnecessary. It is worth noting that in many parts of the world IgM and IgG anti-HAV antibodies are tested together so a specific request for IgM anti-HAV antibodies is necessary to test for acute disease. Relapse with or without cholestasis may recur.

Prevention and therapy

Because HAV is transmitted by the fecal–oral route, adherence to sanitary practices, including heating of foods, hand-washing, and avoidance of unsanitized water, in endemic areas is very effective for prevention of disease.

Vaccination

Several effective and safe vaccines are available for HAV. Live vaccines are available, but inactivated vaccines are highly effective and are used almost exclusively. These include HAVRIX (Smith–Kline Beecham), VAQTA (Merck Sharp Dohme), and TWINRIX (Glaxo Smith–Kline). While HAVRIX and VAQTA are single HAV vaccines, TWINRIX is a combination HAV and HBV vaccine. Inactivated vaccines have high immunogenicity and studies of efficacy report a nearly 100% seroconversion rate after a single course in healthy adults and children (Box 12.2).

The Advisory Committee on Immunization Practices of the Centers for Disease Control and Prevention has recommended HAV vaccination for adults

---

Box 12.2   Regimens for HAVRIX and VAQTA vaccination

Adult dosing
  HAVRIX : Initial 1 mL dose with 1 mL booster at 6–12 months
  VAQTA: Initial 1 mL dose with 1 mL booster at 6–18 months
Pediatric (>1 year old) dosing
  HAVRIX: Initial 0.5 mL dose with 0.5 mL booster at 6–12 months
  VAQTA: Initial 0.5 mL dose with 0.5 mL booster at 6–18 months

---

Table 12.2 Groups requiring HAV vaccination (adapted from Centers for Disease Control and Prevention)

Persons with chronic liver disease
Persons with close personal contact with an international adoptee from a country of high or intermediate HAV endemicity within first 60 days following arrival of adoptee
Persons working in day care, nursing home, or residential care for the mentally challenged
Persons traveling to countries with high or intermediate endemicity
Any person wishing to obtain immunity

with medical, occupational, and lifestyle risk factors (see Table 12.2 for a modified version of this table). Note that vaccine is contraindicated for children less than 12 months old because it is generally ineffective in young infants.

Pre-exposure prophylaxis
Passive immunization with polyclonal serum immunoglobulin can decrease the incidence of HAV infection by 90%. Passive immunity lasts up to 6 months. It should be considered for non-immune individuals who are at risk of HAV exposure or who are allergic to HAV vaccine.

Postexposure prophylaxis
Immediate postexposure prophylaxis should be considered in individuals (particularly those over age 60 years) who have been exposed to HAV infection and have not been previously immunized. These include individuals who are close personal contacts of an infected person, anyone present in child care centers where HAV is present, or who work with or persons have received food from a food handler with HAV infection. The immediate administration of HAV vaccine or immunoglobulin is equally effective for healthy individuals. For

children less than 12 months old, immunocompromised persons, or those with chronic liver disease, immunoglobulin (0.02 mL/kg) is preferred.

Hepatitis B

Virology

Hepatitis B virus (HBV) is a DNA virus that belongs to the Hepadnaviridae family. The HBV genome has a relaxed, circular, partially double-stranded configuration. Despite its being a DNA virus, replication occurs through an RNA intermediate. There are eight well-characterized genotypes with varying geographic distributions (classified by letters A to H). While HBV replicates primarily in hepatocytes, its presence is found in all body fluids of infected individuals.

Epidemiology

The prevalence of hepatitis B varies markedly around the world (Fig. 12.3). In highly endemic regions such as China, Africa, and Southeast Asia, over 8% of the population are chronically infected, with lifetime risk of infection between 60 and 80%. In these regions, perinatal transmission and horizontal spread amongst children are the major sources of spread leading to chronic infection. Areas of intermediate endemicity (2 to 8% of population chronically infected) include the Middle East, Japan, parts of Southern and Eastern Europe, the former Soviet Union, the Indian subcontinent, and Northern Africa. In these regions, the lifetime risk of infection is 20 to 60%. Spread is similar to that in high endemicity regions. Regions of low prevalence are North America,

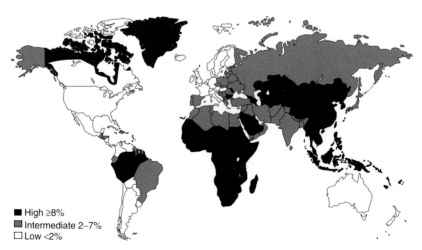

■ High ≥8%
■ Intermediate 2–7%
□ Low <2%

Fig. 12.3 Worldwide prevalence of hepatitis B (data from Centers for Disease Control and Prevention, http://wwwnc.cdc.gov/travel/yellowbook).

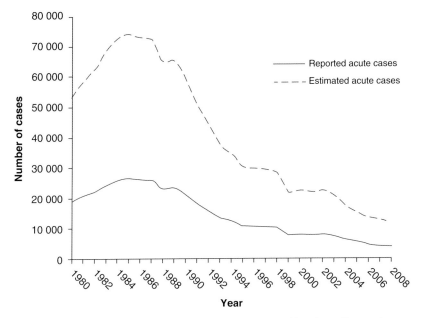

Fig. 12.4 Rates of acute HBV infection in the United States (data from Centers for Disease Control and Prevention).

Box 12.3 Recommended testing for chronic hepatitis

Hepatitis B (after diagnosis confirmed):
  Every 3 to 6 months: CBC, ALT, AST, ALP, bilirubin, INR, albumin, HBV DNA
  At 6 to 12 months: HBsAg, HBeAg, anti-HBe Ab to check for clearance
Hepatitis C (after diagnosis confirmed):
  Every 3 to 6 months: CBC, ALT, AST, ALP, bilirubin, INR, albumin

---

Western Europe, and parts of South America; sexual contact and injection drug use are the main modes of transmission in these areas.

Although hepatitis B virus (HBV DNA) can be detected in most body fluids, it is spread by blood and sexual exposure only. HBV is 100 times as infectious as human immunodeficiency virus (HIV) and 10 times as infectious as hepatitis C virus. Rates of acute HBV infection are decreasing since the 1990s in the United States, attributed to routine childhood vaccination (Fig. 12.4).

Clinical features

The age at which an individual is infected with HBV is the primary determinant of the clinical outcome (Box 12.3). Infection prior to age 1 year is highly likely to result in chronic infection (see Chapter 13). Infection in adults is likely to cause clinically apparent acute hepatitis B but only 1 to 5% of these individuals become chronically infected, though this is higher in those who are immunosuppressed.

The incubation period of HBV is 1 to 4 months. In adults, the incubation period may be followed by a prodromal serum-sickness-like syndrome, which consists of constitutional symptoms, anorexia, arthralgias, nausea, and right upper quadrant discomfort. However, 70% of individuals infected with HBV as an adult have a subclinical (non-icteric) course and only 30% develop icteric hepatitis. Laboratory testing during this acute phase reveals alanine aminotransferase (ALT) and aspartate aminotransferase (AST) elevations up to 1000 to 2000 IU/L. In patients who clear the virus, the serum aminotransferases normalize over 1 to 4 months. A serum sickness illness syndrome may accompany (albeit rarely) acute infection with hepatitis, which can include severe generalized arthralgias that last no more than a few weeks.

Fulminant hepatic failure is unusual, occurring in approximately 0.5 to 1% of individuals with acute hepatitis B. Fulminant hepatitis B results from massive immune-mediated destruction of infected hepatocytes and thus affected patients may have no evidence of HBV replication at the time of presentation as they seroconvert to anti-HBs (IgM) very rapidly. The reasons for developing fulminant HBV are not well understood. Fulminant disease should always prompt testing for a superinfection with hepatitis D virus ("delta virus"). "Fulminant" hepatitis may also occur at time of HBeAg seroconversion in someone with a chronic hepatitis B infection.

During recovery from non-fulminant acute hepatitis B, normalization of biochemical tests (ALT and AST) occurs prior to loss of hepatitis B surface antigen (HBsAg) and the development of anti-HBs antibodies. However, complete eradication of HBV within hepatocytes does not occur and profound immunosuppression (e.g. with rituximab) can lead to reactivation of virus.

Making the diagnosis

After infection, hepatitis B surface antigen (HBsAg) and HBV DNA become detectable within days. Several weeks later, hepatitis B core antibodies (anti-HBc IgM) and hepatitis B e antigen (HBeAg) become detectable (Fig. 12.5). In cases where hepatitis B resolves after acute infection, HBsAg disappears after a few weeks. The disappearance of HBsAg is followed by the appearance of antibodies to surface antigen (anti-HBs). However, there may be a "window period" lasting several weeks to months before anti-HBs antibody is detected. During this time, the serologic diagnosis must be made by the detection of anti-HBc IgM antibody. As symptoms resolve, serum ALT improves over several weeks.

Treatment

Treatment of acute HBV is mainly supportive for the infected individual. While there is no clear consensus on whether antiviral therapy with nucleotide/nucleoside analogues have any benefit, some practitioners recommend their

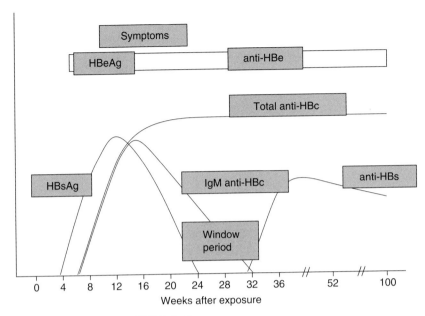

Fig. 12.5 Course of acute HBV infection.

use in individuals with early evidence of liver failure, such as marked hyper-bilirubinemia (>171 μmol/L) or coagulopathy (INR > 1.5). Additionally, patients who are immunocompromised, are coinfected with hepatitis C virus, have pre-existing liver disease, or are elderly should be strongly considered for therapy as their baseline risk for developing liver failure is high. Coinfection with hepatitis D virus inhibits HBV DNA replication and there is no treatment for this superinfection.

Moreover, appropriate measures should be taken to prevent infection in exposed contacts by immediate administration of HBV vaccine and hepatitis B immune globulin (HBIG).

Vaccination

Universal infant vaccination with recombinant vaccines has revolutionized the nature of chronic hepatitis B in childhood (Box 12.4). In Taiwan, childhood universal vaccination against HBV has already lowered the incidence of HCC in childhood, making the vaccine effectively an anticancer vaccine. An effective multivalent vaccine against HBV is given concurrently with routine infant immunizations. Infants born to mothers who are chronically infected with HBV should receive an accelerated vaccination schedule, which includes administration of the first dose of vaccine plus a dose of HBV immune globulin at separate sites within 12 hours of birth. The next doses are given at 1 and 6 months of age. The efficacy of this regimen is greater than 90%. Infants who fail this regimen may have been infected *in utero*. Some children and adults are

> **Box 12.4 Serologic patterns of immunity to hepatitis A and B**
>
> Hepatitis A:
>   Anti-HAV IgG positive
> Hepatitis B:
>   HBsAg negative, anti-HBs positive, anti-HBc IgG negative = immunity after vaccination
>   HBsAg negative, anti-HBs positive, anti-HBc IgG positive = natural immunity after prior exposure

non-responders to HBV vaccination, and thus revaccination protocols are being developed. There is as yet no firm recommendation about the need for booster vaccinations, but in general immune response to this vaccine appears highly durable.

Hepatitis C

Virology

Hepatitis C virus (HCV) is a single-stranded RNA virus of the Flaviviridae family. The viral genome codes for a number of structural (nucleocapsid and envelope) and non-structural proteins. HCV has a high mutation rate, which results in marked genomic heterogeneity. There are six major genotypes (designated by numbers) with similarities of 50 to 70%. There are more than 50 subtypes with similarity between 77 and 80%. Within a single infected individual, genotype only needs to be measured once as it does not change over time unless reinfection occurs. However, each individual will harbor multiple quasispecies of the virus (with closely related yet heterogeneous sequences) due to mutations that occur during replication. One of the major impediments to research on HCV is the lack of adequate animal and tissue culture models.

Epidemiology

Worldwide seroprevalence of HCV is estimated to be 3%. Marked geographic variation exists, with North African rates estimated to be between 10 and 20% and North American rates between 0.4 and 1.1%. Worldwide, there are three epidemiologic patterns of HCV infection. In Egypt and developing countries, high rates of infection are observed in all age groups, suggesting an ongoing acute infection. In Japan and southern Europe, rates are highest in the older population, suggesting a past risk of HCV transmission. In North America, peak prevalence is between 30 and 49 years old, suggesting maximal transmission in the 1980s and 1990s.

HCV is transmitted predominantly via the percutaneous routes (needlestick inoculation and blood transfusion), contaminated medical equipment (e.g. EEG needles, infusion therapy) and much less frequently via non-percutaneous routes (sexual and mother-to-infant transmission). After a single needlestick

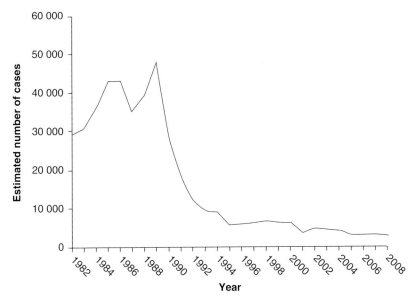

Fig. 12.6 Incidence of acute HCV infection in the United States (from Centers for Disease Control and Prevention).

exposure, health-care workers have a risk of acquisition of HCV between 0 and 7%. The frequency of HCV infection in injection drug users is 50 to 90%. Most injection drug users become positive for HCV seromarkers within 6 months of i.v. drug use. As a result of blood donor screening in most countries, the risk of transfusion-associated HCV has decreased substantially. Rates of HCV in sexual partners of low-risk infected individuals varies between 0 and 7%, and transmission typically occurs during traumatic sex. Rates of vertical transmission of HCV are on the order of 5 to 7%, higher in mothers coinfected with HIV. Infants born to infected mothers should not be tested prior to 18 months of age due to the possible transfer of maternal anti-HCV antibodies. When tested, infants should have an HCV RNA RT-PCR performed.

Acute hepatitis C is difficult to diagnose but fortunately the incidence is falling (Fig. 12.6). In the USA, the incidence rate peaked in the mid-1980s and has declined steadily since then. Factors contributing to falling incidence rates are widespread blood donor screening, needle exchange programs, use of universal precautions and human immunodeficiency virus prevention programs. As no protective immunity follows viral clearance, reinfection may occur in those at high risk.

Clinical features
Symptomatic acute hepatitis C occurs in approximately 15% of individuals after infection. Most of these individuals have a clinically mild course. Symptoms could include nausea, fatigue, malaise, and right upper quadrant pain.

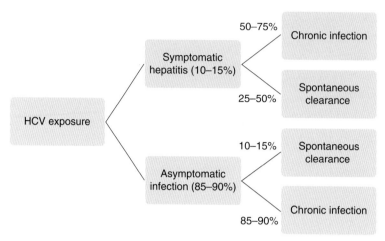

Fig. 12.7 Sequelae of HCV exposure in adults.

An icteric illness develops in fewer than 25% of symptomatic individuals, but it may be indistinguishable from that of acute HAV or HBV infection. Fulminant hepatic failure from acute HCV infection is very rare.

In adults who experience symptoms, the illness typically lasts for 2 to 12 weeks. The possible outcomes of acute HCV infection are shown in Fig. 12.7. Outcome is dependent on a number of viral and host factors. Viral factors associated with spontaneous resolution include genotype 3 infection, lower peak viral load, and viral load decline in the first 4 weeks. Host factors associated with viral clearance include a strong Th-1 type immune response, the presence of jaundice, female sex, age at infection, and possibly being Caucasian. It should be noted that this is observational data from small studies and needs to be confirmed with larger cohorts.

There are many extrahepatic manifestations of chronic HCV infection, such as cryoglobulinemia, vasculitis, membranous glomerulonephritis, and porphyria cutanea tarda (see Chapter 14), but they are not seen with acute HCV infection.

The risk of acute infection becoming chronic varies by age. In adults, spontaneous clearance rates are about 20%. In infants and young children, spontaneous clearance rates may be higher.

Making the diagnosis
After acute infection with HCV, the presence of HCV RNA is the first evidence of infection (Fig. 12.8) and is detectable by RT-PCR within days to 8 weeks of infection, depending upon the size of the inoculum. Serum aminotransferases subsequently become elevated, approximately 6 to 12 weeks after exposure. The development of anti-HCV antibodies can be delayed; most studies find that approximately 50% of individuals with acute infection have detectable antibodies at the time of presentation. Fluctuations of serum ALT and HCV RNA levels are common during acute infection.

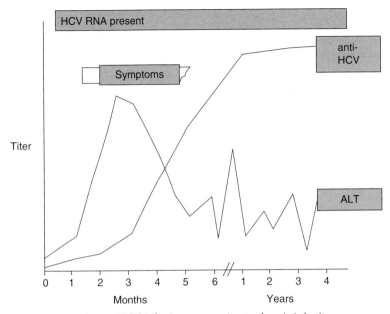

Fig. 12.8 Course of acute HCV infection progressing to chronic infection.

There is no definitive diagnostic test for acute HCV infection. The timing of acute infection is usually unknown or missed unless there is an identifiable single exposure to HCV. The finding of positive serology for HCV infection in an individual found to have marked increases in concentrations of liver enzymes (10 times normal commonly seen), in whom other acute liver diseases have been excluded does not indicate whether the hepatitis C is acute or chronic. Positive serology in an individual previously known to be negative is the only method to conclusively diagnose acute infection. In an individual suspected of being exposed to HCV within the last 8 weeks, both anti-HCV antibodies and HCV RNA RT-PCR should be tested. However, if potential exposure took place less than 2 weeks prior then anti-HCV antibodies could be undetectable.

Routine periodic testing for HCV is generally not recommended, but can be considered in high-risk groups (such as active injection drug users or patients on hemodialysis) to identify acute asymptomatic infection which responds better to treatment than chronic (see below). Unfortunately, no preventative vaccine is available.

Treatment
Rationale for the treatment of acute HCV infection comes from observational studies showing that sustained virological response (SVR) rates are very high in the acute setting. This observation is biologically plausible since it is early after infection when the immune response to HCV is most vigorous and immune-modulating therapies such as interferon may be most effective.

Published studies on treatment of acute HCV infection demonstrate significant heterogeneity in patient populations, treatment onset relative to time of infection, and treatment methods.

The optimum timing of treatment is unclear. Generally, it is recommended to wait at least 12 weeks after infection before initiating antiviral treatment, especially in symptomatic individuals. This strategy will minimize treatment of patients who may spontaneously clear the virus. Special considerations must be given to individuals identified with acute HCV based on postexposure testing (i.e. after a needlestick injury); because these individuals are often asymptomatic, earlier treatment may increase SVR rates.

The most favorable duration of therapy for acute HCV is also unclear. Studies have demonstrated that high SVR rates (71 to 100%) can be achieved with varying length of interferon-α or pegylated interferon-α monotherapy between 4 and 48 weeks. In all studies, early responders (negative HCV RNA RT-PCR by 4 weeks) have the highest sustained response rates. A reasonable strategy is to treat all patients with 12 weeks of therapy but extend therapy to 24 weeks in those who did not test negative for HCV RNA RT-PCR at week 4 of treatment. Note that, in general, monotherapy with pegylated-interferon-α is sufficient and addition of ribavirin should be considered only for patients with predictably lower response rates (HIV coinfection; genotype 1 infection).

Hepatitis D (Delta)

Virology

Hepatitis D virus (HDV), also known as delta virus, is classified in the Deltaviridae family. It is a defective particle that requires presence of coexistent HBV infection. HDV is an RNA virus and encodes for an inner ribonucleic protein but requires the outer lipoprotein protein to be the HBV surface antigen. There are three known genotypes of HDV (I, II, III). Genotype I is the most prevalent.

Epidemiology

HDV is distributed worldwide although prevalence is very variable. It is estimated that worldwide at least 5% of individuals with HBV infection are infected with HDV. The mode of HDV transmission mirrors that of HBV, with the parenteral route being the most common. Sexual transmission has also been reported.

The highest prevalence is seen in South America, the Mediterranean Basin, Mongolia, and Sudan. In North America and Northern Europe, the prevalence is low and confined mostly to injection drug users. Rates of HDV infection peaked in the 1970s and have been steadily declining since.

Because of the necessary relationship between HDV and HBV, two types of HDV infection are possible. One is co-primary infection, in which there is simultaneous infection of HDV and HBV. This type of infection is most commonly seen in injection drug users, and since HBV usually resolves in the

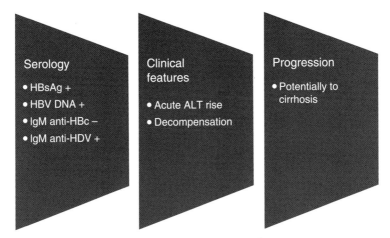

Fig. 12.9 Serologic and clinical features of HDV superinfection.

majority of these patients, HDV also usually disappears. The second type of HDV infection is superinfection of a person already chronically infected with HBV and the superinfection with HDV causes a flare of their hepatitis.

Clinical features
Superinfection of HDV in a person infected with HBV can lead to an acute decompensation of pre-existing liver disease (Fig. 12.9). Chronic HDV infection ensues in approximately 70%. HDV infection has a varying effect on the clinical course of HBV, and several factors (viral genotypes, host factors) may impact the severity of disease.

Making the diagnosis
The diagnosis of HDV superinfection can usually be made serologically. Markers detectable at the time of superinfection include anti-HDV IgM and HDV RNA. Serum hepatitis D antigen (HDAg) assays are not readily commercially available but if testing is available, HDAg is only positive in approximately 40% patients acutely infected with HDV. Differentiating HDV superinfection from HDV/HBV co-primary infection can be done historically (known chronic HBV with new HDV markers) or serologically. Co-primary infection patients will be positive for anti-HBc IgM while superinfected patients will only test positive for the IgM antibody to HDV.

Superinfection can cause a decline in serum HBV DNA levels, since HDV replication inhibits HBV replication. HDV should be suspected in someone with ongoing chronic hepatitis known to be infected with hepatitis B but whose HBV DNA is undetectable. Rarely, HDV superinfection can result in disappearance of HBsAg. Chronic HDV is characterized by the persistent presence of anti-HDV antibodies, HDV RNA, and HBsAg.

Treatment

There are no known effective and proven therapies for acute HDV. In patients chronically infected with HDV long term (>1 year), prolonged treatment with interferon-α (1 to 10 years) has been shown to improve aminotransferase levels and histologic findings. However, it is not effective in most patients and has many side effects. Nonetheless, in the patient with chronic progressive disease it should be attempted. Nucleoside/nucleotide analogues do not affect HDV replication and are not recommended for HDV infection. Additionally, as patients with decompensated HDV hepatitis lack HBV DNA replication, their outcomes following liver transplant are good.

Hepatitis E

Virology

The first documented epidemic of hepatitis E virus (HEV) was from India in 1955 and the virus was first identified in 1983. It is a small RNA virus classified in a genus named hepatitis E-like viruses. There are at least four genotypes and they are geographically distributed. Genotype 1 is found most commonly in Asia (east, central, and south), genotype 2 in Mexico, genotype 3 in the USA, and genotype 4 in parts of China and Taiwan. Outbreaks have occurred on the Indian subcontinent, southeast and central Asia, Africa, the Middle East, and Mexico.

Epidemiology

HEV is transmitted via the fecal–oral route. It is primarily transmitted through water and person-to-person transmission is rare. HEV can be transmitted via blood transfusion in endemic areas. Overall attack rates during an outbreak vary between 1 and 15% and are higher for adults than children. HEV is the second most common cause of sporadic hepatitis in North Africa and the Middle East.

Seroprevalence studies in the USA have placed HEV exposure at 21% of the non-Hispanic white population but clinically apparent disease in the USA is either missed or unusual.

HEV may be transmitted from mother to infant; there are case reports where infants born to mothers with HEV developed clinical, serological, or virological evidence of fulminant infection shortly after birth.

Clinical features

HEV generally causes a self-limited, acute hepatitis. Chronic hepatitis does not develop. After infection with HEV, the incubation period lasts 15 to 60 days. Following incubation, a typical acute hepatitis clinical picture can develop with elevation in aminotransferases to greater than 10 times normal. In addition to malaise, anorexia, nausea, and abdominal pain, HEV can be accompanied with diarrhea, arthralgias, pruritus, and rash. Up to 60% of individuals develop prolonged cholestasis, lasting months. Aminotransferases return to normal within 1 to 6 weeks after the illness. Overall case fatality rate is approximately 0.5 to 3% in hospital surveys, and between 0.07 and 0.6% in population surveys.

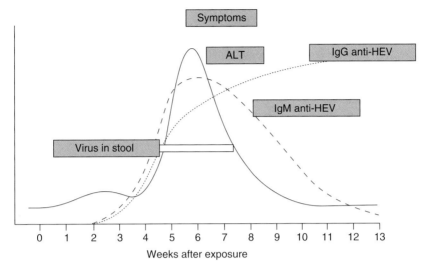

Fig. 12.10 Course of acute HEV infection.

Fulminant hepatitis can develop. For reasons that are not well understood, fulminant disease seems to occur more frequently in pregnant women, resulting in mortality rates of 15 to 25% in pregnant women. Pregnant women with acute HEV infection also have worse fetal outcomes.

Making the diagnosis

To make the diagnosis of an individual suspected to have acute hepatitis E, identification of virus is necessary in stool or serum (Fig. 12.10). HEV antibodies are not as useful since they are frequently associated with false positive and negative results. However, HEV antibodies as a result of prior infection do confer immunity to the host.

HEV can be detected in the stool approximately 1 week before the onset of illness and for up to 2 weeks after onset. HEV RNA can be detected in serum for 2 weeks after the onset of illness. HEV RNA has also been isolated from serum, bile, and feces a few days prior to the onset of illness. HEV Antigen (HEVAg) can be detected in liver tissue but is not a useful serum test. Anti-HEV antibodies appear at the onset of serum ALT elevations.

Anti-HEV IgM appears in the early phase of clinical illness and lasts 4 to 5 months. If tested early (within 40 days of symptom onset), positive rates approach 100%. However, if tested late (6 to 12 months after onset of jaundice), rates fall to 40% or less. Anti-HEV IgG appears in serum a few days after anti-HEV IgM. The sensitivity of assays for antibody detection varies widely.

Histopathology is similar to other forms of acute hepatitis except that up to 60% of individuals with HEV will have a cholestatic hepatitis, characterized by canalicular bile stasis and gland-like transformation of parenchymal cells.

Treatment

Since HEV is usually self-limited, treatment is supportive. Prevention is critical; measures that improve water quality quickly can resolve an epidemic. There are no vaccines available for HEV though they are in an advanced stage of development.

Other viruses

Systemic viral infections of Epstein–Barr virus (EBV), cytomegalovirus (CMV), herpes simplex virus (HSV), and varicella zoster virus (VZV) can all lead to an acute hepatitis.

Epstein–Barr virus

Up to 90% of patients with EBV infection develop elevation in their serum aminotransferases of two to three times the upper limit of normal. The enzyme levels peak over a 1 to 2-week period and then return to normal within 1 month. Acute myositis may also contribute to elevated serum AST. EBV hepatitis tends to be more severe in individuals older than age 30 years. A severe presentation can lead to jaundice. In jaundiced patients, a simultaneous autoimmune hemolytic anemia must be ruled out. All women on oral contraceptives at the time of any acute hepatitis should stop them as they may promote cholestasis.

The diagnosis is based on clinical features of systemic EBV infection. Monospot test is sensitive for the detection of heterophile antibodies but is not specific. EBV-specific IgM antibody titers peak early in serum and are present for months before the development of IgG antibodies. Imaging may demonstrate hepatosplenomegaly. A liver biopsy is not necessary to make the diagnosis but, if performed, it shows portal and sinusoidal mononuclear cell infiltration. Treatment is supportive. Acyclovir does inhibit viral replication but its administration does not change the clinical course.

X-linked lymphoproliferative disorder (Duncan syndrome) is associated with a focal immune defect directed toward EBV. Though rare, it can be associated with extremely severe hepatitis and/or aplastic anemia, mainly in the pediatric age bracket. Diagnosis requires special laboratory tests. Obviously, it occurs only in boys.

Cytomegalovirus

CMV persists lifelong in a latent state after primary infection. Thus, an acute presentation can be the result of primary infection or, more commonly, reactivation of latent infection. In immunocompetent children and adults, CMV infection is usually subclinical. Liver involvement is common and characterized by a mild elevation of serum aminotransferases and a rise in ALP. Rarely, CMV causes a fulminant hepatitis or granulomatous cholestatic hepatitis with or without jaundice. CMV is a common cause of neonatal hepatitis. In patients with impaired cell-mediated immunity, life-threatening and disseminated CMV infection can develop. Hepatobiliary involvement is common and can manifest as hepatitis, pancreatitis, or acalculous gangrenous cholecystitis. HIV-infected persons and organ transplant recipients are at risk for aggressive CMV hepatitis.

Diagnosis is usually based on serologic studies or liver biopsy. In acute primary infection, IgM antibodies to CMV are present. With reactivation of CMV infection, CMV antigens or CMV virus by PCR can be detected. Liver biopsy shows multinucleated inflammatory infiltrates, cholestasis, and large nuclear inclusions in hepatocytes ("owl's eye inclusions"). Treatment is not indicated for mild disease in immunocompetent adults as the disease never becomes chronic. In the immunodeficient patient, ganciclovir can be used as a first-line therapy.

Herpes simplex virus

HSV infection does not usually cause hepatitis. However, HSV hepatitis does occur in neonates, pregnant women, and immunocompromised individuals. In these subgroups it can be serious and life-threatening. In most neonates the clinical pattern is one of acute liver failure. Infection can be due to exposure to infected genital secretions during delivery (HSV-2) or to an active fever blister (HSV-1). In pregnant women, HSV hepatitis usually has a fulminant course and occurs most commonly in the third trimester. In pregnant women, the typical mucocutaneous lesions are present in only 50%. Maternal and perinatal mortality approach 40%.

The diagnosis usually requires biopsy. Hemorrhagic or coagulative necrosis with few inflammatory infiltrates can be seen. Intranuclear inclusions may be identified in hepatocytes at the margin of necrotic areas. In addition, a ground-glass appearance of some hepatocytes can suggest viral inclusion. Electron microscopy, immunohistochemistry, and PCR can be used to confirm the diagnosis. A confirmed diagnosis constitutes an emergency such that high-dose intravenous acyclovir should be initiated immediately. Acyclovir is effective and safe in pregnancy. In infants with acute-pattern neonatal liver failure, acyclovir may be started pre-emptively; dosing must take the potential for renal damage into consideration.

Varicella zoster virus

VZV infection occasionally causes hepatitis. Liver enzymes can be elevated in up to 3 to 4% of children with "chickenpox"; however, clinically significant hepatitis is exceptionally rare. In adults, VZV reactivation can rarely lead to hepatitis. If visceral involvement is suspected, then treatment with acyclovir is indicated.

Other special issues in children

Acute-pattern neonatal liver failure typically occurs in the first 1 to 8 weeks of life and is usually due to infection, which is almost always viral. However, severe bacterial infection can also produce a similar clinical picture. The acute liver failure pattern is evident with extremely elevated serum aminotransferases, severe coagulopathy, and jaundice. Liver involvement may dominate the clinical picture but is often part of severe systemic infection. Lethargy, metabolic instability, and meningitis may be other prominent features. Apart from HSV, enteric viruses are the most common causes of acute-pattern neonatal liver failure: adenovirus, echovirus, and Coxsackie viruses. With Coxsackie viruses, myocarditis may be apparent and if present helps to make the diagnosis. The prognosis for enteroviral neonatal liver failure is very poor although meticulous supportive care contributes importantly to survival. Antiviral medication may be effective; pleconaril has been used with some success, but close monitoring is required.

Parvovirus B19 (now renamed erythrovirus) and human herpesvirus-6 have been reported as causing severe hepatitis in infants. CMV is one of the agents in the TORCH mnemonic for congenital infectious causes of infantile liver disorders with conjugated hyperbilirubinemia, often called "neonatal hepatitis". CNS involvement may be evident with clinical neurological disorder or intracranial calcifications on sonography. Clinical resolution of the liver involvement is usually spontaneous and complete. These children are at increased risk for deafness and definitely require hearing tests before kindergarten. By contrast, rubella is rarely a cause of neonatal hepatitis nowadays, due to widespread and effective vaccination.

A certain proportion of children present with acute liver failure that has all the clinical features of a viral hepatitis but for which no virus (nor any other etiology) can be identified. Not infrequently, the acute hepatitis is severe and may progress to acute liver failure. Anecdotally, such non-A-E hepatitis is often complicated by aplastic anemia, which may not become evident until after liver transplantation for acute liver failure has been performed. Children with apparently severe acute viral hepatitis should be checked after the hepatitis has resolved to be certain that bone marrow function remains intact.

Case study 12.1

A 27-year-old man who was previously healthy returned to Canada after visiting India. After 1 week, he began complaining of fatigue, malaise, and anorexia. After 2 weeks, he presented to the emergency room as a family member noted he was jaundiced. His temperature was 37.8°C, BP was 105/70mmHg, and his heart rate was 104bpm. Physical examination demonstrated scleral icterus, but no other focal findings. Initial laboratory tests revealed Hb 148g/L, WBC 8.6×10^9/L, platelets 452×10^9/L, ALT 1254 IU/mL, AST 1465 IU/mL, ALP 224 IU/mL, bilirubin 88 μmol/L, and INR 1.04.

Further history revealed no previous hepatitis A or B immunization, and no sick contacts. Two of four members of his family that traveled with him developed a mild gastrointestinal illness upon return.

Because of his jaundice, he was admitted to hospital for observation and supportive care. Bloodwork for hepatitis A, B, C, and E were sent. Within 24 hours, it was known that his anti-HAV IgM was negative, anti-HBc IgM was negative, and anti-HCV was negative. Sonography with Doppler studies of his liver was normal. Complete toxicology screen was negative.

After 48 hours, he began to improve clinically and biochemically. ALT fell to 548 IU/mL, AST to 662 IU/mL, INR remained normal and bilirubin was 80 μmol/L. He was discharged home. During outpatient follow-up, it was found that his anti-HEV IgM sent at the time of the acute illness was positive. He recovered completely after 2 months.

Comment

In many cases of acute hepatitis, a cause is not immediately identifiable especially in Western countries where access to HEV testing is only via centralized laboratories. However, clinical improvement without worsening of liver function was reassuring. Note, his ill family members were likely also infected with HEV but presented with different clinical syndromes. Obviously this patient was not pregnant, but pregnant woman with this presentation must be monitored closely. The diagnosis of acute hepatitis E must be entertained early as a fulminant course of disease can develop and serial monitoring of bilirubin and INR are required. After his recovery, he can safely return to India without concern for hepatitis E reinfection, as previous exposure is believed to confer lifelong immunity.

Case study 12.2

Your patient is a 16-year-old boy with rather brittle type 1 diabetes mellitus. It is early May and he presents with the acute onset of anorexia, fatigue, and "just not feeling well" for the past week. On physical examination he has scleral icterus and a slightly enlarged, tender liver. You suspect that he has acute hepatitis. He denies being sexually active, using drugs, getting a tattoo, or body-piercing (his parents would not allow it anyway), and he had not been able to go to a Caribbean resort for a March break trip. In fact he was in hospital a few weeks before the March break because his diabetes was out of control. Now in May, laboratory data show that AST and ALT are both in the 2000 IU/L range. Total bilirubin is elevated at 74 μmol/L, but CBC and INR are normal. You send viral markers which are reported as follows: anti-HAV IgM negative, anti-HAV negative, HBsAg positive, anti-HBs negative, anti-HBc IgM positive. You are a little surprised until you remember that the boy's parents refused the HBV vaccination offered to grade 7 schoolchildren because they believed that it might make the diabetes mellitus worse and no one could convince them otherwise. You are highly perplexed as to the source of this acute hepatitis B, but on a hunch you have the boy's glucose tester checked. The dried blood on it tests positive for HBV DNA. It turns out that your patient had let some of his friends try it out just for fun. The acute hepatitis B runs an uncomplicated course, and your patient recovers and develops natural protective anti-HBs.

Multiple choice questions

1. Which of the following tests are not useful in differentiating acute from chronic hepatitis B?
   A. Anti-HBc IgM antibodies
   B. HBV DNA
   C. HBsAg
   D. Anti-HBs antibodies
   E. C and D

2. Which of the following viruses does not cause a fulminant hepatitis?
   A. Epstein–Barr virus
   B. Hepatitis B virus
   C. Hepatitis E virus
   D. Hepatitis A virus
   E. Hepatitis C virus

3. Your young female patient is thinking ahead to having a baby. What is the best thing she can do to minimize the risk of acute hepatitis in her infant?
   A. Get vaccinated against HAV and HBV
   B. Avoid traveling to India during her pregnancy
   C. Check that her MMR was effective
   D. Start taking folic acid supplements
   E. Both A and C

Answers

1. E
2. E
3. E

Further reading

Aggarwal R, Naik S. Epidemiology of hepatitis E: current status. J Gastroenerol Hepatol 2009; 24: 1484–93.

Ni YH, Chen DS. Hepatitis B vaccination in children: the Taiwan experience. Pathol Biol (Paris) 2010; 58: 296–300.

Rizzetto M. Hepatitis D: clinical features and therapy. Dig Dis Sci 2010; 28: 139–43.

Shiffman ML. Management of acute hepatitis B. Clin Liver Dis 2010; 14: 75–91.

Yeung LT, Roberts EA. Current issues in the management of pediatric viral hepatitis. Liver Int 2010; 30: 5–18.

Chronic viral hepatitis in adults and children: hepatitis B

CHAPTER 13

Jordan J. Feld

Division of Gastroenterology, Toronto Western Hospital, University Health Network, University of Toronto, Ontario, Canada

---

Key points

- Country of birth is the most important risk factor for HBV infection.
- Age at acquisition is strongly associated with the risk of chronic infection (95% of infants develop chronic infection, 5% of immunocompetent adults develop chronic infection).
- Patients progress through the clinical stages of chronic hepatitis B (CHB) over their lifetime (immunotolerant, immune clearance, immune control, HBeAg-negative chronic hepatitis B).
- Treatment is indicated in the immune clearance phase, chronic HBeAg-negative hepatitis B with active disease, prior to receiving immunosuppressive therapy, and possibly in other select circumstances.
- Treatment options include peginterferon or nucleoside/nucleotide analogues.
- Hepatocellular carcinoma may develop in the setting of CHB infection even in the absence of cirrhosis. Screening for hepatocellular carcinoma in patients with CHB is based on age, sex, ethnicity, family history, and the presence of cirrhosis.
- HDV may complicate HBV with coinfection or superinfection. HDV worsens the course of both acute and chronic HBV infection and there are limited treatment options.

Background

Hepatitis B virus (HBV) has a unique genomic structure and lifecycle. Despite being a DNA virus, HBV has a very compact genome of just 3.2 kb, much smaller than either HIV or hepatitis C virus (HCV) (both ~ 9.6 kb). The genomic DNA of HBV is partially double stranded, meaning that the inner (positive) strand of the DNA is shorter than the outer (negative) strand. HBV infects hepatocytes and upon entering the nucleus of the cell, the inner strand is

Hepatology: Diagnosis and Clinical Management, First Edition. Edited by E. Jenny Heathcote.

completed by cellular polymerases to form so-called covalently closed circular or cccDNA. cccDNA serves as the template for HBV replication but also remains in infected cells for the life of the cell, possibly even surviving cell replication. The fact that small amounts of cccDNA remain in hepatocytes indefinitely has important implications for the possibility of reactivation of HBV even after long-term quiescence.

Epidemiology

Approximately 2 billion people have been exposed to HBV infection (i.e. test anti-HBc positive) worldwide and nearly 400 million remain chronically infected (HBsAg positive). The prevalence varies widely with the highest rates occurring in east (China, Taiwan) and southeast Asia (Vietnam, Cambodia, Laos, Korea) as well as sub-Saharan Africa. In highly endemic countries, prevalence of HBsAg ranges from at least 8% to as high 20% of the adult population. However, exposure to HBV is much more common with up to 80% of adults testing positive for the presence of anti-HBc in endemic regions.

Intermediate endemic countries (prevalence 2–8%) include South Asia (India, Pakistan), eastern and southern Europe (Italy, Turkey, Greece), the Middle East and most of South America. Low endemic countries (prevalence <2%) include North America (excluding the Canadian North), western and northern Europe, Australia, and New Zealand. However, large urban centers in low endemic countries may have intermediate prevalence of HBV due to large foreign-born populations (e.g. New York, London, Toronto).

Risk factors

HBV is spread parenterally via blood and body fluids and is the most infectious of the blood-borne chronic viral infections. HBV is not spread by saliva, insect bites, or by casual contact. The age at acquisition largely determines the outcome of HBV infection. Approximately 95% of neonates infected with HBV will develop chronic infection. In contrast, 95% of immunocompetent adults will spontaneously clear infection (with or without symptomatic acute infection). Rates of chronicity are higher in people with HIV infection and other causes of immunosuppression (Table 13.1). Vertical and very early horizontal transmission account for the vast majority of chronic HBV infections globally and hence country of birth is by far the most important risk factor for chronic HBV infection.

Vertical transmission generally occurs at delivery, with very low rates of intrauterine infection. Cesarean section has not been shown to reduce the rates of transmission. The risk of vertical transmission depends on the viral load and HBeAg status of the mother. Transmission to infants occurs in up to 90% of cases in which the mother is HBeAg positive because of the associated high viral loads (generally >10E7 IU/mL). In contrast, chronic infection occurs in

Table 13.1 Risk factors for HBV

Vertical transmission	Most common route of transmission worldwide
Early horizontal transmission	Precise mechanisms unclear; important that infants are vaccinated within 12 hours of birth if mother *or* father/siblings HBsAg positive
Sexual	95% spontaneous clearance
Injection drug use	High rate of spontaneous clearance
Blood transfusion	1 in 60000 in USA
Hemodialysis	Immunosuppressed patients are more likely to become chronically infected

less than 30% of infants born to HBeAg-negative mothers. In addition to the viral titer, the presence of HBeAg itself increases the risk of chronicity.

Early horizontal transmission occurs in children under the age of 5, particularly in sub-Saharan Africa. The direct modes of transmission are unknown. To prevent early horizontal transmission, it is important that children with known HBV-positive close contacts (siblings, father, other relatives) should also be vaccinated at birth. Other sources of transmission include: sexual (hetero- and homosexual), injection drug use, blood transfusion (1 in 60000 in USA), hemodialysis, and other parenteral exposures.

Postexposure prophylaxis

Infants of known HBsAg-positive mothers should receive HBV vaccine (10 μg) and hepatitis B immune globulin (HBIG) (0.06 mL/kg) at birth (within 12 hours) to reduce rates of transmission. These infants should then complete a full three or four-course vaccine schedule (1 and 6 months) or (1, 2, and 12 months). Even with appropriate vaccination and HBIG administration, transmission may occur in 5 to 10% of cases, particularly if mothers are HBeAg-positive and have viral loads above 10E7 IU/mL. It is important to explain to HBsAg-positive mothers that vaccination and HBIG are not 100% effective. For women with very high viral loads (>10E7 IU/mL), antiviral therapy with lamividuine, telbivudine or tenofovir in the final trimester of pregnancy may reduce the risk of transmission.

All infants must be tested at 9–12 months of age. Testing should not be done prior to 9 months as antibodies may still come from the mother prior this age.

Infants of mothers of unknown HBsAg status should receive HBV vaccine, but not HBIG, within 12 hours of birth, and complete a full HBV vaccination schedule. Infants of HBsAg-positive fathers (or other household members) should be vaccinated at birth (no HBIG) to prevent early horizontal transmission.

Unvaccinated individuals exposed to HBV should receive HBV vaccine and HBIG within 48 hours of exposure. Vaccinated individuals exposed to HBV should have HBsAb titers assessed. Those with anti-HBs titers less than 10 IU/mL should be treated as unvaccinated individuals. If protective titers (>10 IU/mL) are present, no action is required.

Serology

A number of serological markers have been identified that indicate different stages of HBV infection. The definition of each marker is described below and is shown in Table 13.2.

- **HBsAg** indicates ongoing infection. Still present even with complete viral suppression with therapy (the HBsAg protein is produced before DNA replication).
- **Anti-HBs** indicates immunity to HBV unless HBsAg also present (up to 10% of cases). May be acquired by vaccination or immune control of natural infection (if accompanied by anti-HBc).
- **Anti-HBc (IgG)** indicates exposure to HBV. All chronically infected (HBsAg-positive) will also be anti-HBc positive. Lone anti-HBc positive status may be a false positive if there are no risk factors for exposure. Anti-HBc generally remains positive life-long.

Table 13.2 Interpretation of viral markers in hepatitis B

Test	Full name	Significance
HBsAg	Hepatitis B surface antigen	Ongoing HBV infection
Anti-HBs	Anti-hepatitis B surface antibody	Immunity (natural or vaccine induced)
Anti-HBc (IgG)	Anti-hepatitis B core antibody (IgG)	Indicates current or resolved HBV infection
Anti-HBc (IgM)	Anti-hepatitis B core antibody (IgG)	Acute HBV infection or flare of chronic HBV
HBeAg	Hepatitis B e antigen	Active viral replication
Anti-HBe	Anti-hepatitis B e antibody (may persist after clearing HBsAg)	May indicate immune control but active viral replication may still occur
HBV DNA	Hepatitis B DNA	Direct measurement of viral particles: range 1–10 log IU/mL

- **Anti-HBc (IgM)** indicates either acute infection or flare of chronic HBV infection.
- **HBeAg** is a soluble protein produced by the virus that is not necessary for viral replication. Its presence is almost always associated with active viral replication and high viral load; however, the corollary is not true, i.e. absence of HBeAg does not imply low-level replication. HBeAg is also thought to act as a tolerogen, helping HBV evade the host immune response. HBeAg crosses the placenta and likely tolerizes the fetus to HBV prior to birth, increasing the risk of chronic infection.
- **Anti-HBe** indicates clearance of HBeAg (although both HBeAg and anti-HBe may be present simultaneously). The presence of anti-HBe is generally associated with lower viral loads than the HBeAg-positive state; however, active liver disease may be present.
- **HBV DNA:** direct measurement of viral particles in the blood. The titer of HBV DNA ranges vary widely, from less than 1 to more than $10 \log IU/mL$. The degree of liver disease associated with a given viral titer depends on the stage of disease (see below).

Stages of infection

Most chronically infected individuals are infected at birth or in early childhood and progress through a series of stages of infection over their lifetime. Although the stages are shown in the order in which they typically occur, patients may flip-flop between stages. The serological markers help determine the stage of infection; however, for a given patient, at a given moment, it may be difficult to determine the current stage of infection. As a result, longitudinal follow-up is necessary to clarify the stage of disease and pattern of progression for individual patients.

Adult-acquired HBV that becomes chronic may have a different natural history. The immunotolerant phase of infection is typically shorter and often does not occur at all, with patients moving directly into the immune clearance phase with active HBeAg-positive hepatitis. A similar scenario may occur in babies or young children infected from an HBeAg-negative mother or any other HBeAg-negative contact. Because of the absence of the tolerizing effects of the HBeAg protein, the risk of severe acute or even fulminant HBV infection is greater in infections occurring from an HBeAg-negative mother/contact.

Immunotolerant phase
Profile. *HBeAg positive, normal alanine aminotransferase (ALT), very high viral load (>8 log IU/mL), and normal liver biopsy (if performed).*

The immunotolerant phase is the initial stage of infection, typically lasting from birth into the third or fourth decade of life. However, in certain regions of the world, particularly sub-Saharan Africa, the immunotolerant phase may be much shorter, lasting only into the early teenage years. Differences in the duration of this phase of infection relate to the HBV genotype and possibly to host factors as well.

The immunotolerant phase is characterized by very high levels of viremia with no associated liver damage. HBV is not a cytopathic virus, with liver damage occurring due to the immune response targeting the virus. During this stage of infection, the virus is not recognized by the immune system and hence no liver damage ensues.

Management

During the immunotolerant phase of infection, therapy of all types is ineffective and also is unnecessary as there is no progressive liver disease. Therapy of immunotolerant patients is not currently advised and carries a high risk of leading to antiviral resistance. Patients who remain in the immunotolerant phase of infection until above age 40 may have an increased risk of hepatocellular carcinoma. Whether therapy is warranted for such patients is unknown.

Immune-active/immune-clearance phase

Profile. *HBeAg positive, anti-HBe negative, elevated ALT (range from mild elevation to into the 1000s), and active inflammation with or without fibrosis on liver biopsy.*

All patients eventually transition from the immunotolerant phase of infection to the immune-active/clearance phase. The transition typically occurs in the third or fourth decade of life, but may occur in childhood or early adolescence. The precipitant(s) for entering this active phase of HBV infection is unknown. Some patients remain in the immunotolerant phase until later in life and this is likely associated with an increased risk of development of hepatocellular carcinoma (HCC).

With immune recognition, flares of hepatitis occur as the immune system attempts to clear infected hepatocytes. The immune-active phase is characterized by recurrent flares of disease, with rises in ALT, accompanied by falls in viral load. Ultimately, patients eventually clear HBeAg and develop anti-HBe antibodies; however, the process of HBeAg seroconversion may take months to years to develop. The repeated flares of hepatitis lead to progressive liver disease with associated fibrosis and may ultimately progress to cirrhosis. Rarely, flares may be very severe, leading to jaundice and occasionally to liver failure. However, most flares are entirely asymptomatic, even with marked ALT elevation, and thus all patients require regular follow-up for their recognition, particularly those with ongoing viral replication. Symptomatic flares are more likely to lead to spontaneous HBeAg seroconversion. Patients may intermittently be positive or negative for both HBeAg and anti-HBe, particularly as they are transitioning from the immune-active to immune-control phase of infection.

Management

Before instituting therapy, patients should be followed for at least 3 to 6 months to allow for spontaneous HBeAg seroconversion. If the ALT remains elevated with elevated HBV DNA for longer than 6 months, therapy should be considered. Prior to starting therapy, a liver biopsy or non-invasive assessment of fibrosis is generally advised to clarify the degree of liver damage. Exclusion of other causes of liver disease is also important in the appropriate clinical scenario (alcohol, fatty liver, HCV coinfection, HDV etc.).

Immune control
Profile. *HBeAg negative, anti-HBe positive, HBV DNA less than 2000 IU/mL, ALT normal, and liver biopsy (if performed) shows minimal activity with variable degrees of fibrosis depending on previous course of infection.*

The phase of immune control is sometimes referred to as the "inactive carrier state"; however, this term is not preferred because patients may or may not remain inactive and all require long-term follow-up. Notably, some patients may even have developed cirrhosis during the previous HBeAg-positive stage of infection. Although many patients truly remain inactive lifelong, 40% of patients will go on to develop HBeAg-negative chronic hepatitis B.

The level of HBV DNA is useful for predicting subsequent short-term course:
- HBV DNA less than 2000 IU/mL, risk of flare in 12 months less than 10%—follow annually;
- HBV DNA 2000–20 000 IU/mL, risk of flare in 12 months 30–40%—follow every 6 months;
- HBV DNA more than 20 000 IU/mL, risk of flare in 12 months 70%—follow closely and consider antiviral therapy.

For patients with low or undetectable HBV DNA levels, HBsAg should be checked annually, as 0.5–1% of patients will clear HBsAg per year. HBsAg clearance prior to age 50 is associated with an excellent prognosis and, in the absence of cirrhosis, follow-up is no longer required. HBsAg clearance after age 50 is still associated with a risk of HCC and therefore ongoing ultrasound surveillance is recommended. Disease activity may flare significantly with immunosuppression (see below) but can be largely prevented with the use of pre-emptive antiviral therapy.

Management
In the immune-control phase, the immune system is adequately controlling viral replication with no ongoing liver damage. Provided the liver disease remains quiescent, no treatment is indicated; however, age and ethnicity-appropriate screening for HCC is indicated. Treatment should be considered prior to significant immunosuppression (e.g. cancer chemotherapy, organ transplantation, therapy with biologics) to avoid reactivation (see below).

HBeAg-negative chronic hepatitis B
Profile. *HBeAg negative, anti-HBe positive or negative, HBV DNA more than 2000 IU/mL, elevated ALT, and liver biopsy with activity and variable fibrosis.*

Because HBeAg is not necessary for viral replication, even after HBeAg clearance, viral replication may occur at high levels and this can lead to an associated hepatitis and progressive liver disease. HBeAg-negative chronic HBV is sometimes referred to as "pre-core mutant HBV" because many patients harbor virus with a mutation leading to a stop codon in the pre-core gene that is responsible for production of HBeAg. "HBeAg-negative CHB" is a preferable term because mutations other than the pre-core mutation may occur, most commonly in the promoter for the HBeAg gene (basic core promoter). In either scenario, viral replication occurs despite the absence of HBeAg. Mutations leading to the loss of HBeAg (pre-core or basic core promoter) do not impair viral replication.

Importantly, HBV-related liver disease may occur at much lower thresholds of viral replication, that is lower HBV DNA titers, because unlike during the immunotolerant phase, the immune system recognizes and responds to HBV and tolerizing effects of HBeAg are absent. Therefore, even small rises in HBV DNA (between 2000 and 20 000 IU/mL) can lead to significant ALT flares and disease progression.

The course of HBeAg-negative CHB is highly variable. Some patients have persistently elevated ALT with detectable viral titers; however, others may have only intermittent rises in ALT. Similar to the immune-active phase, almost all flares of ALT are entirely asymptomatic. If increases in ALT are observed but HBV DNA remains below 2000 IU/mL, other causes of liver disease should be investigated (e.g. fatty liver disease, alcohol, HDV). Unlike during the immunotolerant phase, with HBeAg-negative CHB, higher titers of HBV DNA are associated with an increased risk of progression of liver disease and development of HCC. Antiviral therapy reduces the risk of disease progression and likely lowers the risk of HCC in patients.

Management

If there are intermittent or persistent increases in ALT associated with HBV DNA levels above 2000 IU/mL, antiviral therapy should be considered. Antiviral resistance is generally less of a problem than in patients with HBeAg-positive disease because of the lower viral loads at the start of therapy. Prior to starting therapy, a liver biopsy or non-invasive assessment of fibrosis is generally advised. Exclusion of other causes of liver disease is important in the appropriate clinical scenario (alcohol, fatty liver, HCV coinfection, HDV, etc.).

Assessment of liver fibrosis

HBV is a very dynamic disease and, although treatment is very effective, in many patients it is difficult to stop therapy once it has been instituted. A high percentage of patients will also control their infection/disease with no therapy. The presence of fibrosis is a risk factor for further disease progression and, as a result, most guidelines and experts recommend assessing the degree of fibrosis, either with liver biopsy or non-invasive techniques, prior to starting therapy. In patients with no evidence of fibrosis, therapy can usually be delayed but regular (at least annual) follow-up is required.

Liver biopsy remains the gold standard for assessing the degree of liver fibrosis; however, it is an invasive procedure with a small risk of complications and patients do not like having multiple biopsies, as is often required to manage this very dynamic disease. Fortunately, in recent years, non-invasive tests of liver fibrosis—both serum and elastography tests—have been developed. Non-invasive assessments of fibrosis correlate fairly well with liver biopsy but sensitivity and specificity vary by method (see Chapter 2).

Options for non-invasive assessment of liver fibrosis include: serum markers, transient elastography, and radiographic imaging.

Serum markers

Numerous panels of serum markers have been developed to predict liver fibrosis, which correlate relatively well with liver biopsy findings. Most panels were developed for HCV infection and are generally less predictive in HBV, because of the more dynamic nature of the disease. Serum panels are shown in Chapter 2, with performance characteristics in HCV. In addition to formal serological panels, some evidence of advanced fibrosis can often be gleaned from routine laboratory tests.

- Thrombocytopenia (<150000/μl) often indicates cirrhosis with portal hypertension.
- AST/ALT ratio: ALT is typically higher than aspartate aminotransferase (AST) in chronic HBV infection. With advanced fibrosis, the AST is often higher than ALT.
- Hypergammaglobulinemia: polyclonal increases in IgG are suggestive of advanced liver fibrosis caused by gut bacteria bypassing the liver.

Transient elastography

Transient elastography (TE) uses ultrasound or magnetic resonance to estimate the liver stiffness. Increased liver stiffness is associated with advanced fibrosis. Like other non-invasive tools, TE is very good at extremes of fibrosis, thus it is very accurate at identifying no fibrosis or cirrhosis. However, TE is less precise with intermediate levels of fibrosis. TE may be significantly influenced by the presence of hepatic inflammation, making it relatively unreliable during flares of hepatitis, with a tendency to overestimate the degree of liver fibrosis. Similarly, TE may be very high during acute HBV infection due to hepatic inflammation rather than fibrosis.

- Advantages of TE: non-invasive, rapid, performed in office setting, correlates well with liver biopsy, may predict clinical outcome (variceal bleeding, ascites, etc.).
- Disadvantages of TE: poor accuracy during acute flares of hepatitis and in obese patients or those with ascites, no histological information regarding etiology.

Radiographic imaging

Although in certain instances, ultrasound or other imaging of the liver may be useful diagnostically, imaging of all types is neither sensitive nor specific for the presence of progressive liver fibrosis. Many patients with bridging fibrosis or even early, well-compensated cirrhosis will have a normal-appearing liver on imaging tests. The presence of signs of portal hypertension (splenomegaly, varices, ascites) in the setting of HBV infection are indicators of advanced liver disease, but unfortunately the absence of such features is not adequate to exclude significant hepatic fibrosis.

HBV therapy

Therapy for HBV has improved dramatically in the past decade with the development of potent, well-tolerated, oral antivirals. Therapy for HBV may be divided into two overall approaches: direct-acting antivirals (nucleoside/nucleotide analogues) and immune stimulation (interferon).

Nucleoside/nucleotide analogues

Although HBV is a DNA virus, it has an unusual replication cycle involving an RNA intermediate. From the DNA template, viral RNA is transcribed. The viral RNA serves as the template for reverse transcription to make new HBV DNA. Because of the presence of "reverse transcriptase" activity of the HBV polymerase, many of the reverse transcriptase inhibitors developed for HIV have proven effective at inhibiting HBV replication. HBV encodes only one enzymatically active protein (the polymerase) and as a result all HBV inhibitors target the same stage in replication, namely reverse transcription. To date, all HBV antivirals are nucleoside or nucleotide analogues (NAs). NAs mimic the natural nucleoside/nucleotide and compete for incorporation into nascent virions. Incorporation of the NAs leads to chain termination with production of non-functional, incomplete viral DNA.

Although NAs have much greater affinity for the viral polymerase, they can theoretically inhibit host DNA polymerases as well. Inhibition of the γ DNA polymerase of mitochondrial DNA can lead to mitochondrial toxicity with lactic acidosis. Fortunately, mitochondrial toxicity is very rare with all NAs used for HBV monoinfection. The lactic acidosis syndrome has been reported to occur in patients with advanced liver disease with use of entecavir. Fortunately, side effects of any kind are uncommon with the NAs. Patients tolerate all the oral therapies well. Adefovir and tenofovir may cause dose-related renal toxicity and therefore careful follow-up of renal function is important with these agents.

There are three classes of HBV NAs based on differing structures, resistance patterns, and side-effect profiles.

- L-nucleosides: lamivudine, telbivudine, emtricitabine
  - variable potency but identical resistance profile;
  - resistance to one confers resistance to all in this class;

- notably, resistance occurs more frequently with less-potent agents; lamivudine resistance occurs at a rate of approximately 15% per year with 70% resistance by 5 years, while resistance to telbivudine, a more potent agent, occurs at a rate of 7% per year;
- minimal toxicity.
- Acyclic phosphonates: adefovir, tenofovir
  - potency of adefovir limited by dose (10 mg daily) but good resistance profile (29% at 5 years);
  - resistance to adefovir greater if pre-existing lamivudine resistance (22% at 2 years);
  - tenofovir is very potent and no resistance reported to date;
  - adefovir-resistant mutants are sensitive to tenofovir;
  - renal toxicity reported for both agents; ranges from asymptomatic rise in creatinine with or without drop in phosphate to Fanconi-like syndrome with phosphaturia, amino aciduria, and rarely to renal failure;
  - metabolic bone disease (osteomalacia and osteoporosis) has also been reported with prolonged use, presumably due to phosphate wasting.
- Cyclopentane: entecavir
  - very potent;
  - very good resistance profile in NA-naïve patients (1.4% at 4 years);
  - resistance rate much higher if pre-existing lamivudine resistance (15% at 3 years);
  - double dose (1 mg daily) recommended if pre-existing lamivudine resistance;
  - minimal toxicity; rare reports of lactic acidosis syndrome in patients with decompensated cirrhosis.

A comparison of efficacy for HBeAg-positive patients with 1 year of therapy is as follows:
- HBsAg loss: 3% tenofovir, 2% entecavir, less than 1% other NAs;
- HBeAg seroconversion: approximately 15–20% for all NAs;
- HBV DNA suppression: 70–80% for potent agents (tenofovir/entecavir), 42% for lamivudine, 20% for adefovir;
- ALT normalization: 70% for potent agents (tenofovir/entecavir), 60% for lamivudine, 48% for adefovir;

A comparison of efficacy for HBeAg-negative patients with 1 year of therapy is as follows:
- HBsAg loss: rare with all agents;
- HBV DNA suppression: 80–90% for potent agents (tenofovir/entecavir/telbivudine), 60–70% for lamivudine, 50–60% for adefovir;
- ALT normalization: 80–90% for potent agents (tenofovir/entecavir), 60–70% for lamivudine, 60% for adefovir.

Duration of therapy with nucleoside/nucleotide analogues
For patients with HBeAg-positive disease, treatment should be continued until HBeAg seroconversion (loss of HBeAg and development of anti-HBe) occurs

or resistance develops. Even with prolonged HBV DNA suppression to unde-tectable levels, if HBeAg remains positive patients will universally relapse upon stopping therapy. Once HBeAg seroconversion occurs, treatment should be continued for at least 6 months of consolidation. Recent evidence suggests that even with consolidation therapy, rates of HBeAg seroreversion and HBeAg-negative CHB following cessation of NA therapy are high (up to 70%) and therefore some experts suggest continuing therapy until loss of HBsAg is achieved. Unfortunately, because HBsAg loss is an uncommon event, particu-larly with NA therapy (and almost only seen in those infected with genotypes A and D), such an approach may lead to very prolonged therapy with associ-ated increased costs and risks of long-term toxicity.

For patients with HBeAg-negative CHB, duration of NA therapy is less clear. Most data suggest that even after prolonged suppression of HBV DNA to undetectable levels, relapse is very common upon stopping therapy. Continu-ing therapy until HBsAg clearance is reasonable; however, HBsAg loss is very uncommon in patients who start NA for HBeAg-negative CHB, meaning this approach may lead to exceedingly prolonged treatment.

Because of the need for prolonged therapy once therapy is initiated, it is critical to institute therapy only in those who truly need it.

Interferon/peginterferon

As an alternative to the NAs, which are direct HBV antivirals, interferon and peginterferon may also be used to treat HBV. Interferon is an important component of the innate antiviral immune response. Interferon acts by acti-vating a signaling cascade leading to the activation of numerous antiviral genes within infected cells. Interferon also activates the adaptive immune response.

Although standard interferon is effective, pegylated interferon (peginter-feron) is more commonly used because of its more convenient, once-weekly dosing schedule. There have been no trials comparing standard to pegylated interferon for the treatment of HBV infection and as a result either option may be used. Although some patients do not respond to interferon, no true interferon-resistant HBV has been identified.

The major issue with interferon is tolerability. Many side effects are reported with the most common being flu-like symptoms (myalgias, arthralgias, fatigue, low-grade fever), mild bone marrow suppression, and depression. Stimulation of the immune system may worsen or bring out latent autoimmune conditions. For unclear reasons, patients with HBV tend to tolerate interferon better than those with HCV infection with lower rates of depression and other side effects reported.

Interferon or peginterferon are given for 6 to 12 months. Patients with high ALT and low HBV DNA at baseline are more likely to respond to interferon-based therapy. Viral genotype may also be important with patients with geno-types A and B infection responding much better than those with either genotype D or C. HBsAg titer, if available, may be useful for predicting response to peginterferon. Patients without a decline in HBsAg titer by 12 weeks are very unlikely to respond and therapy can likely be discontinued.

HBeAg seroconversion occurs in 25–30% of patients after 1 year of therapy and appears to be very durable (>70%) over long-term follow-up. Because interferon is immune stimulatory, ALT flares are common during therapy. ALT flares often occur immediately prior to HBeAg seroconversion. Treatment should be continued with ALT flares unless there is evidence of hepatic synthetic dysfunction (jaundice, coagulopathy, etc.). Although synthetic dysfunction with peginterferon is rare, it is reported and thus peginterferon should be avoided in patients with cirrhosis with any evidence of even mild synthetic dysfunction. Importantly, interferon leads to HBsAg clearance in 7–10% of patients, even up to 3–4 years after cessation of therapy, higher than reported for any of the NAs.

Combination therapy

Although combination therapy sounds attractive based on data from other diseases (e.g. HIV), there is minimal evidence to support a benefit to combination therapy in HBV among treatment-naïve patients. All NAs have the same viral target (HBV DNA polymerase) and therefore they compete with each other at the active site of the enzyme. There is no additive or synergistic antiviral effect of combination NA therapy. There may be a benefit in terms of delaying the emergence of resistance; however, this has not been clearly demonstrated. Combination NA therapy is preferable to sequential monotherapy for documented HBV resistance (i.e. add a second agent rather than switch to another agent, particularly for lamivudine resistance treated with adefovir). A "switch" approach may be reasonable with the newer, more potent agents. Combination therapy with lamivudine and peginterferon is not superior to either therapy alone. Whether combination with the more potent NAs and peginterferon would be beneficial is unknown.

Management of NA resistance

Viral breakthrough is defined as an increase in HBV DNA titer by 1 log above the nadir achieved on therapy. Prior to modifying therapy or diagnosing resistance, it is critical to check with the patient about compliance. Up to 30% of viral breakthrough is related to non-compliance rather than resistance.

If the patient reports compliance, recheck the HBV DNA in 1 month. If the titer is still rising, resistance is likely present. Ideally, confirmation with resistance testing is helpful, however it is not widely available. Once resistance is suspected/confirmed, therapy should be modified, even if ALT remains normal:

- For L-nucleoside resistance (lamivudine/telbivudine/emtricitabine)
  - add adefovir
  - switch to tenofovir or tenofovir plus emtricitabine (Truvada)
  - switch to entecavir (use 1mg daily, i.e. double dose and cost).

Table 13.3 Advantages and disadvantages of interferon versus nucleosides/ nucleotide analogues

Peginterferon		Nucleosides/nucleotide analogues	
Advantages	**Disadvantages**	**Advantages**	**Disadvantages**
Defined duration of therapy	Injection	Oral	Long-term/indefinite therapy required
Increased HBsAg loss	Side effects	Well tolerated	Low rates of HBsAg loss
Long-term costs	Short-term cost of therapy	Few drug interactions	Resistance
No resistance	Contraindications	Can be used in decompensated cirrhosis and post-transplant	Long-term costs

- For adefovir resistance
  - add L-nucleoside (lamivudine/telbivudine)
  - switch to entecavir
  - switch to tenofovir or tenofovir plus emtricitabine (Truvada).
- For entecavir resistance
  - switch to tenofovir or tenofovir plus emtricitabine (Truvada).
- For tenofovir resistance
  - switch to entecavir.

The advantages and disadvantages of peginterferon therapy and NA therapy are presented in Table 13.3.

Management in resource-limited settings

Specialized testing, including HBV DNA levels, may not be available in resource-limited areas of the world, many of which have a high prevalence of HBV infection. Lack of access to testing complicates therapy somewhat but, in most instances, appropriate decisions can be made with relatively simple tests. In patients with HBeAg-positive disease, ALT and complete blood count (CBC) can be followed every 6 months with institution of therapy if the ALT increases and does not return to normal (i.e. spontaneous HBeAg seroconversion) within 6 months. In those with active, HBeAg-negative disease, recognition that HBV is the cause of elevated liver tests is more difficult. If liver biopsy is available, it can be quite useful, particularly if there are other possible etiologies for liver inflammation such as fatty liver disease. If liver biopsy is not available, but ALT is persistently elevated in a HBsAg-positive, HBeAg-negative patient, institution of therapy would be appropriate, using improvement of ALT as an imperfect assessment of efficacy. In HBsAg-positive, HBeAg-negative patients with clinical or biochemical evidence of advanced disease (impaired liver synthetic function, low platelets, etc.), the threshold for institution of therapy should be very low, even in the absence of availability of HBV DNA testing.

Once on therapy, if HBV DNA testing is unavailable, ALT, CBC, and creatinine should be followed at 3-monthly intervals. Any ALT elevation should be investigated appropriately with a detailed history and physical examination (medication history including herbal remedies, compliance with HBV therapy, exposures to coinfection, etc). If the ALT elevation persists in a compliant patient, drug resistance should be considered and managed as described above. Notably, ALT flares may be associated with HBeAg seroconversion with both interferon and NA therapy. Therefore in HBeAg-positive patients, before resistance is diagnosed, HBeAg serology should be re-evaluated. Creatinine testing is necessary both to diagnose NA toxicity (with adefovir or tenofovir) and to make dosing adjustments in patients with renal impairment.

In patients on NA therapy with normal ALT, HBeAg and HBsAg should be checked annually. If HBsAg clearance occurs, therapy can be discontinued, but patients must be followed as reactivation with re-emergence of HBsAg has been described.

For all patients, HIV testing is mandatory prior to starting any therapy (see below).

HBV reactivation

Liver disease related to HBV infection is immune mediated and thus the immune status of the host has a major impact on the course of disease. Patients with inactive disease may have severe or even fatal reactivation of disease in the setting of immunosuppression. Reactivation is most commonly reported in patients receiving cytotoxic cancer chemotherapy but has also been reported with prolonged courses of corticosteroids and more recently with biologics used for immune-mediated diseases (rheumatoid arthritis, inflammatory bowel disease). Up to 50% of patients with inactive disease (HBeAg negative, normal ALT, low or undetectable HBV DNA, but still HBsAg positive) will have a flare of HBV-related hepatitis with standard chemotherapy. Typically, HBV DNA titers rise during therapy and the flare of hepatitis occurs following immune reconstitution. A high index of suspicion is necessary to identify HBV reactivation because in patients receiving chemotherapy, many other potential causes for ALT elevation exist. If HBV reactivation occurs, antiviral therapy is indicated; however, in severe cases hepatitis may progress despite therapy. Fortunately this scenario can largely be prevented with the use of pre-emptive antiviral therapy with lamivudine (or likely any NA). Small, randomized controlled trials have shown that using pre-emptive antiviral therapy is more effective than starting therapy only if reactivation occurs. Pre-emptive therapy prevents severe reactivations, which may lead to liver failure and will likely interrupt and thus compromise chemotherapy. If treatment is delayed until the ALT begins to rise, therapy may not be effective. Treatment should be continued for 6 months after the end of all immunosuppression but patients should be followed to ensure that a treatment withdrawal flare does not occur.

Prevention of reactivation CHB (induced by immune suppression).

Because of the potential serious consequences of HBV reactivation and the presence of very effective therapy, the CDC recently recommended that all patients scheduled to receive cytotoxic chemotherapy be screened for HBV (at least HBsAg).

Anti-HBc alone

The term "resolved" infection for individuals who are anti-HBc positive but HBsAg-negative is somewhat of a misnomer because of the presence of the low levels of HBV (in the form of cccDNA) remaining in the liver. With severe immune suppression, even patients who are HBsAg-negative can experience HBV reactivation. Reappearance of HBsAg is usually referred to as "reverse seroconversion". The greatest risk for reverse seroconversion is with allogeneic bone-marrow or stem-cell transplant (up to 50% incidence) but it may also occur with advanced HIV disease and it has been reported to occur in up to 25% of patients receiving rituximab-based chemotherapy. Pre-emptive antiviral therapy is indicated for anti-HBc-positive patients undergoing bone marrow or stem-cell transplant. Whether antiviral therapy would be helpful in the other scenarios, particularly with rituximab therapy, is currently unknown. If therapy is not initiated, HBsAg should be followed regularly with institution of therapy if it becomes positive. The risk of reactivation with standard solid tumor chemotherapy is very low and prophylaxis is not indicated.

Indications for therapy in chronic hepatitis B

Even with ongoing viral replication, therapy for CHB is not always indicated. The indications for which treatment is recommended are discussed below.

1 **Immune active:** HBeAg-positive, elevated ALT, HBV DNA more than 20 000 IU/mL. Treatment should be withheld for 3–6 months to allow for spontaneous HBeAg seroconversion. Assessment of liver fibrosis with either liver biopsy or non-invasive method recommended before starting therapy.

2 **HBeAg-negative chronic hepatitis B:** HBeAg-negative, elevated ALT, HBV DNA more than 2000 IU/mL with no other causes to explain ALT elevation.

3 **Preimmunosuppression:** patients who are HBsAg positive have a high risk of activation of HBV with immunosuppression.

   i **Chemotherapy:** antiviral therapy should be started prior to or concomitant with starting chemotherapy and continued for 6 months after the end of chemotherapy.

   ii **Bone marrow transplant:** all patients who are HBsAg–positive should be treated with pre-emptive antiviral therapy. Patients who are HBsAg-negative but anti-HBc-positive (indicating resolved infection) are at risk of HBV reactivation with severe immunosuppression such as bone marrow transplant. Such patients should receive pre-emptive antiviral therapy. For most patients, lamivudine is adequate because of the low viral loads at the time of starting chemotherapy.

iii **Rituximab/biologics:** rituximab and other biologics have been reported to induce HBV reactivation even in patients who have cleared HBsAg (anti-HBc alone). For patients who are HBsAg-positive, antiviral therapy should be instituted as for other chemotherapy. For patients who are anti-HBc-positive alone, it is unknown if antiviral therapy is beneficial. Close monitoring for reappearance of HBsAg is required.

4 **Decompensated cirrhosis:** in patients with HBV with decompensated cirrhosis, HBV therapy with an NA is well tolerated and indicated if there is detectable HBV DNA in the serum. Short-term improvements in hepatic decompensation and avoidance of liver transplantation have been described. Cases of lactic acidosis have been reported with the use of entecavir in patients with decompensated HBV cirrhosis. Peginterferon is contraindicated in this scenario.

5 **Post liver transplant:** all patients should receive hepatitis B immune globulin (HBIG) and antiviral therapy with an NA post liver transplant to reduce the risk of reinfection of the graft. It may be possible to remove HBIG therapy but NA therapy must be continued indefinitely.

Situations in which antiviral therapy may be considered are:

1 **Fulminant acute HBV:** there are very limited data on the use of treatment in acute HBV. Because spontaneous resolution occurs in more than 95% of immunocompetent adults, showing a benefit to therapy will be difficult. In patients with progressive liver synthetic function (rising bilirubin, INR), treatment with an NA may be warranted.

2 **Cirrhosis with high HBV DNA:** patients with cirrhosis are at risk for liver failure with flares of HBV. Viral suppression may be useful for patients with cirrhosis with detectable HBV DNA levels with normal ALT values. Whether treatment will reduce the incidence of HCC is unknown.

3 **Pregnancy:** hepatitis B vaccination and hepatitis B immune globulin (HBIG) are given within 12 hours of birth to infants born to HBsAg-positive mothers. However up to 10% of infants born to mothers with high viral loads (HBV DNA more than 10E7 IU/mL) will become infected despite appropriate vaccination/HBIG. For woman with high viral loads, treatment with an NA from 32 weeks of gestation may reduce the risk of transmission. If treatment is otherwise unnecessary, it may be stopped 4 weeks after delivery and mothers should be followed closely because of the risk of a treatment withdrawal flare.

Investigations prior to and during antiviral therapy

Investigations prior to starting NAs or peginterferon are:

- Liver enzymes (AST/ALT)
- Liver function (bilirubin, albumin, INR)
- Creatinine with calculation of CrCl
- Urine analysis
- Electrolytes with serum phosphate (if starting adefovir/tenofovir)
- CBC + differential

- **HIV test**—this is critical. All NAs for HBV are active against HIV. Monotherapy with NAs for HIV invariably leads to emergence of resistance and may compromise future HIV care.

Investigations during NA therapy are:
- ALT, creatinine every 3 months
- Electrolytes, phosphate and urine analysis every 3 months if on adefovir/tenofovir
- HBV DNA every 3 months until undetectable then every 6 months
- HBeAg and anti-HBe every 6 months (if HBeAg positive at baseline)
- HBsAg every 12 months once HBV DNA undetectable.

Investigations during peginterferon therapy are:
- CBC + differential, creatinine, ALT, AST, bilirubin, INR, albumin every 1 month
- HBsAg titer (if available) at baseline, week 12 and week 24.

HIV/HBV coinfection

In most areas of high HIV prevalence, HBV is also endemic and as a consequence of their common routes of transmission, HIV/HBV coinfection is common in many regions of the world. Rates of HBV chronicity and disease progression are much higher in HIV/HBV coinfection.

The majority of NAs used for HBV also inhibit HIV replication and therefore it is critical to screen for and consider both viruses when starting and changing therapies. In general, treatment of HIV is not limited by the presence of HBV but anti-HIV regimens should include HBV suppressive therapy. Rates of lamivudine resistance with HIV/HBV coinfection are very high and therefore tenofovir-containing HIV regimens are preferable if available.

Options to treat HBV without treating HIV are limited. Monotherapy with any of the NAs, including entecavir, will lead to the emergence of drug-resistant HIV, which will limit future antiretroviral regimens. Peginterferon therapy is a theoretical option; however, response rates in the HIV-infected population are low. Therefore HIV/HBV co-infection should generally be managed by using an HIV regimen including lamivudine or ideally tenofovir. Monitoring during therapy is similar to the HBV-monoinfection setting.

For patients with HIV/HBV who develop drug-resistant HIV, it is imperative to remember the HBV when changing HIV regimens. Even though a patient may have tenofovir-resistant HIV, this does not mean that tenofovir-resistant HBV is also present. Therefore even if the tenofovir is replaced with another HIV-active agent, the tenofovir must be continued to control HBV. Severe withdrawal flares have occurred when lamivudine or tenofovir were stopped for HIV resistance in the setting of HIV/HBV coinfection.

Hepatocellular carcinoma

Hepatocellular carcinoma (HCC) (see also Chapter 7) is the most dreaded complication of chronic HBV infection. Unlike most other liver diseases, HCC may develop in patients with HBV in the absence of cirrhosis; however, cirrhosis is the most important risk factor for HCC.

The major risk factors for the development of HCC are:
- Cirrhosis
- Increasing age
- Male sex
- Family history of HCC
- HBeAg positivity beyond age 40
- Increasing HBV DNA levels (over age 30)
- HBV genotype C.

If HCC is found early, it is often curable. In contrast, symptomatic HCC is usually very advanced with few treatment options. To identify early and curable HCC, screening is advocated. Screening guidelines are based on age, ethnicity, and the presence of cirrhosis. Screening should be performed with ultrasonography every 6–12 months. Ideally, ultrasound screening should be done in the same facility serially to allow for comparison of scans over time. α-fetoprotein (AFP) may add somewhat to ultrasound for screening, however AFP is often elevated with active hepatitis and therefore is not recommended in patients with active HBV. AFP is also very insensitive, as many HCCs do not produce AFP. AFP is of greatest utility when it is elevated in the setting of an identified lesion on imaging.

Ultrasound screening is recommended for:
- All patients with HBV cirrhosis
- Asian men over age 40 who are HBsAg positive
- Asian women over age 50 who are HBsAg positive
- HBsAg-positive patients over age 40 with a family history of HCC
- HBsAg-positive patients over age 40 with intermittent or persistently elevated ALT and HBV DNA more than 2000 IU/mL
- African men over age 20 who are HBsAg positive (risk possibly increased by exposure to aflatoxin in food).

HDV (delta hepatitis)

Background
HDV is a defective RNA virus that requires HBsAg for its replication. As a result, HDV infection only occurs in the presence of pre-existing or concomitantly acquired HBV infection.

Epidemiology
HDV is currently prevalent in particular geographic regions:
- Horn of Africa (Sudan, Somalia)
- Amazon Basin
- Southeastern Europe (Turkey, Romania)
- Some regions of Asia (Mongolia)

HDV is also common among injection drug-using cohorts worldwide.

Natural history

The natural history of HDV infection depends greatly on whether it is acquired with HBV (**coinfection**) or after HBV is already established (**superinfection**). Coinfection typically worsens the course of acute HBV. The rate of fulminant liver failure with acute coinfection is greater than with acute HBV infection alone.

As with acute HBV infection, the majority of immunocompetent adults clear acute HBV/HDV coinfection. Superinfection is the route of acquisition for most patients with chronic HDV infection.

In chronic infection, HDV typically inhibits HBV replication but causes its own severe and aggressive liver disease. Most patients with HBV/HDV coinfection are:

- HBeAg negative
- Low or undetectable HBV DNA
- Elevated ALT—often very high
- Advanced fibrosis—often cirrhotic at diagnosis.

HDV infection should be considered in HBsAg-positive patients who have active hepatitis despite low or undetectable HBV DNA levels. Some patients with HDV remain HBeAg positive with high levels of circulating HBV. As a result, patients from areas of high HDV prevalence and those with a history of injection drug use should be screened for anti-HDV antibodies.

Serology

Serological markers are useful in determining the stage and activity of HDV infection. The different available markers are described below.

- Anti-HDV antibody: indicates past or current HDV infection
- HDV RNA: indicates ongoing HDV infection (not widely available)
- HBsAg: present
- HBeAg: usually absent
- Anti-HBe: usually present
- HBV DNA: usually low level or undetectable.

Management

Because HDV requires only the HBsAg, which is made *prior* to HBV DNA replication, suppression of HBV DNA replication does not inhibit HDV. As a result, NA therapy for HBV is ineffective at controlling HDV and should only be used if HBV is also active. Peginterferon therapy has been shown to have some efficacy against HDV; however, high doses and prolonged therapy are typically required. If HBsAg clearance is achieved either spontaneously or with therapy, HDV typically resolves.

Novel HDV-specific agents are under clinical development. Liver transplant is an option for patients with decompensated HDV cirrhosis with good post-transplant outcomes.

Case study 13.1

A 58-year-old Asian man with diffuse large cell B-cell lymphoma presents for routine follow up after his third cycle of CHOP-R (cyclophosphamide, doxorubicin, prednisone, and rituximab) chemotherapy. He is found to have an ALT of 475 IU/L, AST of 338 IU/L with a bilirubin of 56 μmol/L. He has ongoing fatigue and nausea related to the chemotherapy but has no new complaints. Investigations reveal that he is HBsAg positive, HBeAg positive with an HBV DNA of $5.7 \times 10E6$. Ultrasound shows a slightly echogenic liver with a reduction in splenomegaly from prior to starting chemotherapy.

Comment. This man has severe reactivation of HBV related to chemotherapy. Most likely he was HBsAg positive, HBeAg negative with low or undetectable HBV DNA prior to starting chemotherapy. Reactivation occurs because of a loss of immune control due to chemotherapy-related immune suppression. Typically, the HBV DNA rises during chemotherapy and this is followed by a hepatitis with immune reconstitution. Despite the ALT elevation, most patients will not develop new symptoms. The presence of bilirubin elevation is a concerning feature. This patient should be started on antiviral therapy (with nucleoside/nucleotide analogues) promptly but some patients may progress to liver failure despite treatment when it is started after reactivation has occurred. The Centers for Disease Control (CDC) in the United States recommends screening all patients for HBsAg prior to starting chemotherapy to prevent such occurrences. Pre-emptive antiviral therapy should be given to all patients found to be HBsAg positive, with the choice of agent dependent on the HBV DNA titer. In this particular case, it is also possible that this man was HBsAg negative but anti-HBc positive prior to starting chemotherapy. With severely immunosuppressive regimens, particularly those containing rituximab, there is a risk of reverse seroconversion with reappearance of HBsAg in patients who are HBsAg negative but anti-HBc positive at the start of therapy. Whether pre-emptive therapy is warranted for such patients is unknown but HBsAg should be checked regularly with the addition of antiviral therapy if it becomes positive.

Case study 13.2

A 23-year-old Somali man is found to have an asymptomatic elevation of ALT (186 IU/L) and AST (223 IU/L). Other laboratory investigations reveal a bilirubin of 13 g/dL, albumin of 39 g/L, INR of 1.1, hemoglobin of 142 g/L, WBC of 3.8, and platelet count of 107 000/μL. He left Somalia as a teenager and believes that he has always been very healthy. He is HIV negative and takes no medications. Serology reveals that he is HBsAg positive, HBeAg negative, anti-HBe positive with an HBV DNA of 1232 IU/mL.

Comment. This man has high liver enzymes despite being HBeAg negative with a low HBV DNA titer. It is very unlikely that an HBV DNA titer of 3 logs is likely to

(Continued)

cause this degree of enzyme elevation and other causes of liver disease should be investigated. HDV coinfection should be a strong consideration, particularly given his country of origin in the Horn of Africa where HDV is endemic. HDV usually suppresses HBV replication and hence HBV DNA titers are often low or even undetectable despite high enzymes and marked hepatitis on liver biopsy. HDV often has a very aggressive course and despite his young age it is likely that this man has already progressed to cirrhosis. The low platelet count and AST/ALT ratio of greater than 1 are both suggestive of advanced fibrosis. Treatment options are limited but long-term peginterferon therapy may have some benefit. Other etiologies that should be considered would include autoimmune hepatitis, Wilson disease, and fatty liver, all of which can coexist with HBV infection.

Multiple choice questions

1. A 25-year-old Asian woman who is HBsAg positive, HBeAg positive with an HBV DNA titer of 9.2 log IU/mL and ALT of 17 IU/L should:
   A. Begin HCC surveillance with ultrasounds every 6 months because her high viral load puts her at increased risk of HCC
   B. Start treatment with peginterferon
   C. Should be observed with no intervention
   D. Should undergo a liver biopsy to assess her degree of liver inflammation and fibrosis
   E. Is in the immune clearance phase of HBV infection

2. The most important risk factor for HCC in patients with HBV is:
   A. Male sex
   B. Cirrhosis
   C. HBV DNA titer
   D. Elevated ALT
   E. HBV genotype

Answers

1. C
2. B

Further reading

Chen CJ, Yang HI, Su J, et al.; REVEAL- HBV Study Group. Risk of hepatocellular carcinoma across a biological gradient of serum hepatitis B virus DNA level. JAMA 2006; 295: 65–73.

Feld JJ, Heathcote EJ. Hepatitis B e antigen-positive chronic hepatitis B: natural history and treatment. Semin Liver Dis 2006; 26: 116–29.

Hsu C, Hsiung CA, Su IJ, et al. A revisit of prophylactic lamivudine for chemotherapy-associated hepatitis B reactivation in non-Hodgkin's lymphoma: a randomized trial. Hepatology 2008; 47: 844–53.

Liaw YF, Sung JJ, Chow WC, et al. Lamivudine for patients with chronic hepatitis B and advanced liver disease. N Engl J Med 2004; 351: 1521–31.

Loomba R, Rowley A, Wesley R, et al. Systematic review: the effect of preventive lamivudine on hepatitis B reactivation during chemotherapy. Ann Intern Med 2008; 148: 519–28.

McMahon BJ. Natural history of chronic hepatitis B. Clin Liver Dis 2010; 14: 381–96.

Patterson SJ, George J, Strasser SI, et al. Tenofovir disoproxil fumarate rescue therapy following failure of both lamivudine and adefovir dipivoxil in chronic hepatitis B. Gut 2011; 60: 247–54.

Zoulim F, Locarnini S. Management of treatment failure in chronic hepatitis B. J Hepatol 2012; 56 (Suppl.): S112–22.

Chronic viral hepatitis in adults and children: hepatitis C

CHAPTER 14

Eberhard L. Renner[1] and Eve A. Roberts[2]

[1]GI Transplantation, Toronto General Hospital, University Health Network, and University of Toronto, Toronto, Ontario, Canada

[2]Departments of Paediatrics, Medicine, and Pharmacology, University of Toronto, and Division of Gastroenterology, Hepatology and Nutrition, The Hospital for Sick Children, Toronto, Ontario, Canada

Key points

- The hepatitis C virus (HCV) is a small, parenterally transmitted RNA virus; today it is acquired almost exclusively by the use of unsterile needles.
- It occurs in six distinct genotypes, genotype 1 being the most prevalent in North America, Europe and Japan.
- HCV causes an acute hepatitis that is clinically silent in most cases and persists in the majority (80%) of patients, leading to chronic hepatitis.
- Chronic hepatitis C remains clinically silent and progresses to cirrhosis in about 10% of patients within 20 years. Once cirrhosis is established, it causes significant morbidity and mortality from hepatic decompensation and hepatocellular carcinoma.
- Non-hepatic manifestations of chronic hepatitis C infection are relatively common, especially asymptomatic or symptomatic mixed cryoglobulinemia, which may cause renal failure.
- Concomitant alcohol consumption, male gender, coinfection with HIV or HBV, and older age at time of infection accelerate the progression to cirrhosis.
- Every new patient should be asked for risk factors of HCV infection including: a history of transfusion of blood and blood products prior to the early 1990s, a history of past or present i.v. drug use (or snorting cocaine with a straw), a history of piercings and tattoos and medical procedures performed without appropriate sterile techniques, coming from a high prevalence region of the world, or being born to a mother with HCV infection.

Hepatology: Diagnosis and Clinical Management, First Edition. Edited by E. Jenny Heathcote.
© 2012 John Wiley & Sons, Ltd. Published 2012 by John Wiley & Sons, Ltd.

- Patients with any of the above risk factors should be screened by anti-HCV antibody testing; positive test results need to be confirmed by direct detection of circulating virus using an HCV RNA PCR assay.
- Antiviral therapy should be considered in every patient with confirmed HCV infection. Patients with HCV infection should be referred for consideration/conduct of antiviral treatment to physicians with expertise and up-to-date knowledge in the field.
- Therapy of hepatitis C virus infection is rapidly evolving; the current standards consist of pegylated interferon-α and ribavirin. The addition of new, directly acting antiviral agents improve cure rates, but not without cost (both in terms of side effects and financial).
- Efficacy of therapy depends on genotype, with cure rates (i.e. sustained virological response (SVR)) being achieved with current standard therapy in 50% of genotype 1 and 4, and 80% of genotype 2 and 3 infected patients. Side effects of therapy are common and can be severe.
- Infants of mothers who have chronic hepatitis C should be tested for hepatitis C infection by checking anti-HCV antibodies—but only after 18 months old when a positive test signifies actual infection. Since many parents are unwilling to be uncertain about HCV transmission for such a long time, testing for serum HCV RNA plus ALT can also be performed when the infant is 2–6 months old. If the test result is negative, this indicates that HCV infection of the infant has not occurred.

Introduction

Chronic hepatitis due to hepatitis C virus (HCV) infection is the single most important infectious cause of death in Ontario, the most populous province of Canada.[1] It is also the most frequent indication for liver transplantation worldwide. HCV was first identified in 1989 using molecular cloning techniques and the serum of patients with post-transfusion non-A/non-B hepatitis.[2] A diagnostic test allowing detection of circulating anti-HCV antibodies in the serum of HCV infected patients was reported simultaneously.[3] It has since become clear that HCV was responsible for almost all cases of post-transfusion non-A/non-B hepatitis, which has all but vanished since mandatory testing of all blood products was introduced in the early 90s. During the last 20 years, much has been learned about the virus, such as its epidemiology, diagnosis, natural history, and its ability to avoid immune clearance by the host and cause chronic hepatitis in the majority of infected patients. Last but not least, effective therapies have been developed and continue to be improved at the time of this writing.[4] This chapter reviews aspects of chronic hepatitis that are relevant for the clinician not trained in hepatology.

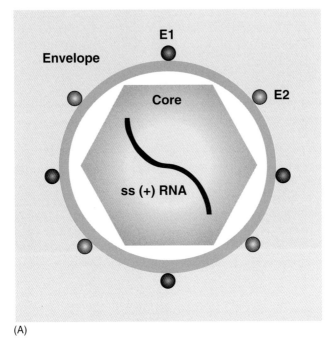

(A)

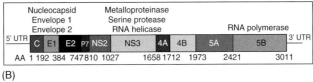

(B)

Fig. 14.1 Schematic of the hepatitis C virus. (A) Schematic depiction of the hepatitis C virus (HCV). The envelope contains the E1 and E2 viral proteins. The core is the viral core protein and harbors the viral genome, a 9.6-kD positive-sense (+), single stranded (ss) RNA. (B) Schematic depiction of the genomic organization of HCV. The genome is translated into a single precursor protein that is post-translationally processed and cleaved into the individual viral proteins. This process is initiated by host cell enzymes and, upon its liberation, completed by the HCV protease. HCV RNA polymerase and protease are essential for viral replication and therefore form prime targets for the new directly acting antiviral drugs.

The virus

HCV is a small (around 50 nm), enveloped, positive sense, single-stranded RNA virus that belongs to the Flaviviridae family (Fig. 14.1). Its genome consists of 9600 base pairs and encodes for three structural and seven non-structural proteins. The former consist of the nucleocapsid (core) and two envelope proteins (E1 and E2); the latter includes a protease/helicase (NS3-4A) and an

RNA-dependent RNA polymerase (NS5B). The life cycle of the virus proceeds from viral attachment and entry into the host cell, to viral RNA translation into a single polyprotein and its post-translational processing into specific structural and non-structural viral proteins, to viral RNA replication, and, finally, virion assembly and release (for review see reference 4). Processes involved in all of these steps are currently under investigation as potential targets for new antiviral drugs. Prime targets are the viral protease and RNA polymerase, since they are indispensable for HCV replication. Thus, several HCV protease and HCV polymerase inhibitors are currently in late clinical development.

HCV exists in six major, genetically distinct subtypes (genotypes 1–6) with distinct geographical distribution. Genotype 1 is the predominant genotype in North America and Europe (50–80%) with genotypes 2 and 3 accounting almost entirely for the remainder cases, whereas in Egypt almost 100% of cases are genotype 4 infections, and genotype 3 predominates in Pakistan.

Unlike DNA polymerases, RNA polymerases do not have a proof-reading mechanism and are therefore prone to mistakes. HCV's RNA-dependent RNA polymerase is no exception and numerous mutations occur during HCV replication. Based on HCV's small size (9600 base pairs) and its very high replications rate—it has been estimated that each day 10^{12} new virions are produced in an infected individual—every possible mutation likely occurs daily in a patient with chronic HCV infection. HCV therefore never occurs as a single genotype entity, but rather as a family of closely related, slightly different variants, so called quasispecies, which still belong to the same genotype. It is thought that HCV's high replication rate paired with its high mutation rate facilitates viral escape from host defenses. It is intuitively understandable that this also facilitates appearance and selection of resistant HCV species during antiviral therapies and forms a major obstacle to vaccine development.

Epidemiology

HCV infection has been reported from all over the world and is a major global health problem. The WHO estimates that about 3% of the world's population or worldwide approximately 170 million people are chronically infected with HCV. The prevalence of chronic HCV infection varies in different regions of the world and, according to WHO estimates, ranges from less than 1% in Northern Europe and Canada to 10% or above in some countries such as Egypt (Table 14.1). In Canada, an estimated 250 000 people are infected with HCV.[5]

HCV is a classic parenterally transmitted virus. Thus, HCV infection worldwide is highly prevalent in hemophiliacs (50 to >90%) and i.v. drug users. HCV was responsible for more than 90% of transfusion-associated non-A/non-B hepatitis; since introduction of mandatory screening of all blood products in the early 1990s, this route of transmission has virtually disappeared. Today, new infections occur almost exclusively through illicit drug use (sharing needles or snorting of cocaine with a straw) and medical procedures performed without adequate sterile precautions taken. In the absence of appropriate sterile

Table 14.1 Global prevalence of hepatitis C virus infection according to WHO[6]

Prevalence	Geographic regions/countries
<1%	Canada, Mexico, Argentina, Chile, Germany, Scandinavia, UK, Australia
1–2.4%	USA, France, Italy, Russia, Middle East, South Africa, India, Pakistan, Japan
2.5–4.9%	Brazil, Central Africa, China
5–9.9%	Tunisia, parts of Central Africa, South East Asia
≥10%	Peru, Egypt, Mongolia

technique, HCV can be transmitted through piercing and tattooing. Sexual transmission is possible in patients with high-risk behavior such that mucosal membranes are damaged, but rare without and can be virtually eliminated by safe sex practices (use of condoms). However, no health authority worldwide feels that the low risk (in the absence of high-risk behavior) would justify recommending safe sex practices in all monogamous relationships involving an HCV infected partner. HCV is not transmitted by breast feeding, kissing, sneezing/coughing, sharing eating utensils or drinking glasses, or other normal social contact, including hand shaking or hugging, food, or water. Vertical transmission from mother to child during pregnancy or perinatally is well documented and has become the main route of infection for HCV in children. Unfortunately, there is no "protective" antibody to HCV, that is, no effective postexposure prophylaxis.

In 1995, there were 2600 hospitalizations for HCV-related complications in the USA, leading to charges of US$514 million. Costs related to in-patient and out-patient care of HCV-infected patients were estimated to amount to almost US$5.5 billion.[6] Modeling studies from several Western countries using local epidemiological information and natural history data (see below) predict that the disease burden and the costs related to complications of chronic hepatitis C, that is, the morbidity and the need for liver transplantation due to decompensated cirrhosis and hepatocellular carcinoma, will continue to increase at least until around 2020, while the incidence of cirrhosis will start to decline around 2005–2010.[7]

Natural history

Once transmitted, HCV infects and replicates in liver cells, causing an acute hepatitis that only infrequently becomes clinically manifest (Fig. 14.2). While HCV has also been shown to be able to infect selected cell types outside the liver, including some white blood cells, the clinical significance of such

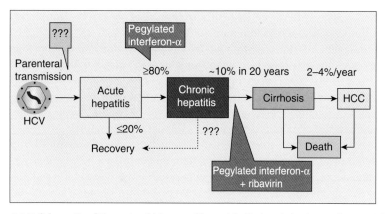

Fig. 14.2 Schematic of the natural history of hepatitis C virus infection and potential interventions. Upon (parenteral) transmission, the hepatitis C virus (HCV) homes to the liver and leads to an acute hepatitis, which rarely becomes clinically manifest. Currently, there is no vaccination available to protect against HCV infection. The ensuing innate and adaptive host immune response is able to clear the virus in a minority of patients (around 20%). If detected in the acute phase, HCV infection can be effectively treated and cured in more than 90% of patients with interferon-α-based monotherapy. In the majority of patients (about 80%), HCV is able to persist and leads to chronic hepatitis, which remains asymptomatic until late in its course. The inflammatory reaction associated with chronic hepatitis C triggers a wound-healing response leading to fibrosis and progression to cirrhosis over decades. Thus, 10% of patients with chronic hepatitis C develop established cirrhosis within 20 years. Treatment of chronic hepatitis C with pegylated interferon-α and ribavirin can cure the infection and prevent progression to cirrhosis in 50% of genotype 1 and 4, and 80% of genotype 2 and 3 infected patients, respectively. Once cirrhosis is established, chronic HCV infection leads to morbidity and mortality secondary to decompensation and hepatocellular carcinoma (the latter develops in 2–4% of patients per year). Factors accelerating fibrosis progression and development of cirrhosis include older age at time of infection, any concomitant alcohol consumption, male gender, and coinfection with HIV or HBV.

potential extrahepatic infections remains unclear. HCV is not cytopathic; that is, it does not kill its host cell during replication. Instead it stimulates a host reaction that attempts to clear the virus and causes inflammation and collateral liver damage. Both innate and adaptive immune mechanisms are involved; however, innate immunity, in particular the type I interferon system (interferon-α and interferon-β), plays a pivotal role. This is illustrated by the facts that (1) HCV has evolved to undercut the type of interferon response at several levels, which is thought to facilitate its persistence and (2) high-dose exogenous interferon-α is effective in treating clinical HCV infection (see below). During infection, the host mounts an antibody response against HCV. Although these anti-HCV antibodies are useful for diagnosis (see below), clinically they have little relevance as they neither neutralize the virus nor convey immunity and thus if re-exposed, reinfection may occur.

Upon acute infection, only about 20% of patients are able to eliminate the virus spontaneously (Fig. 14.2). In the remaining 80%, HCV will escape the host defenses, persist, and cause chronic infection with ongoing liver inflammation. Chronic hepatitis C does not cause symptoms and remains undetected if not specifically sought. If spontaneous clearance of HCV in a *chronically* infected individual is at all possible, it is a rare event, at least in adults.

As with any chronic inflammation, chronic hepatitis (of any cause) triggers a wound-healing response with activation of hepatic stellate cells that synthesize and deposit collagen, thus leading to progressive liver fibrosis and, finally, cirrhosis. In chronic hepatitis C, this process takes decades; about 10% of chronically infected patients develop cirrhosis within 20 years (Fig. 14.2). Only once cirrhosis is established, morbidity and mortality ensue. Patients decompensate with ascites, portal hypertensive bleeding, jaundice (due to liver dysfunction), and/or hepatic encephalopathy. Per year, about 2–4% of HCV-infected cirrhotic patients develop hepatocellular carcinoma. The life expectancy of patients with HCV infection is shorter than that of a normal population, and the difference is attributable solely to an increased mortality from cirrhosis and its complications, including HCC. Fibrosis progression and cirrhosis formation is accelerated by any amount of concomitant alcohol consumption, concomitant HIV or HBV infection (or other chronic liver disease), male gender, and older age at the time of infection.

Extrahepatic complications of hepatitis C

It is not unusual for individuals infected with hepatitis C to present not with symptoms of liver disease but rather with an extrahepatic manifestation. Perhaps the most common is cryoglobulinemia, which often goes undiagnosed as a non-organ-specific complication of an undiagnosed hepatitis C. Lesions typically associated with cryoglobulinemia may be asymptomatic or cause variably sized red skin blotches due to a small vessel vasculitis, which may affect internal organs such as kidneys. This can affect any part of the body but most often lower legs and arms. Another common non-hepatic complication is lymphoproliferative disease (B-cell lymphoma).[8]

Diagnosis

Since HCV infection typically remains clinically silent in the acute hepatitis phase and through most of the chronic hepatitis phase, that is until complications of cirrhosis occur, it is of prime importance to ask about risk factors for acquiring hepatitis C in any patient with a "hepatitis" (Table 14.2). In addition, patients with known risk factors should be tested for HCV infection.

A highly sensitive and specific, commercially available enzyme linked immunoassay (EIA) is the screening test of choice. This test becomes positive

Table 14.2 Risk factors for hepatitis C virus infection that mandate screening, including pregnant women

History of or current illicit drug use (i.v. or cocaine snorting sharing a straw)

Transfusion of blood or blood products before mandatory testing for HCV was introduced (1992 in Canada)

Immigration from a country with high HCV prevalence

History of tattoos, piercings, or medical procedures performed without adequate sterile precautions

Traumatic sexual behavior, including current or previous sexual partners known to have used illicit i.v. drugs and *in vitro* fertilization from anonymous donors

History of incarceration

Known HIV positivity

Children of HCV infected mothers

as short as 2 weeks after acquiring HCV infection, but this may take longer, especially in immunocompromised individuals. Of note, IgG antibodies can cross the placenta. In babies born to HCV-infected mothers, such passive mother-to-child antibody transfer may lead to a positive anti-HCV antibody test in the absence of true infection of the baby. Thus, children should not be tested for anti-HCV antibodies prior to age 18 months. In an immunocompetent individual, a negative HCV antibody rules out chronic HCV infection. A positive antibody test indicates that the patient has had contact with the virus, but it does not prove current infection; as with many antibodies, anti-HCV can persist for years beyond clearance of the virus. Thus, the presence of ongoing infection needs to be confirmed in all anti-HCV-positive individuals by direct detection of the viral genome using a sensitive RNA assay, usually a commercially available RT-PCR assay. HCV RNA in serum becomes detectable by RT-PCR as early as 1 week after infection.

Determination of HCV genotype and HCV viremia level using a commercially available line-probe assay and quantitative RT-PCR test is only required prior to initiating therapy. Genotype and level of pretreatment viremia are important prognostic markers to predict outcome and treatment duration in adults (see below).

Therapy

All patients with HCV infection should be considered for antiviral therapy. Hence all individuals with risk factors for HCV infection should be considered for screening. Treatment of chronic hepatitis C remains a rapidly evolving field and should therefore be undertaken only by physicians with appropriate up-to-date knowledge and expertise. Referring patients for an expert opinion regarding indication for and conduct of treatment is often the best plan. Therefore, the following focuses on the overarching principles of current antiviral therapy, rather than providing detailed treatment schemes that will be outdated almost as fast as they are written down.

As with any treatment, the decision to treat has to balance a number of factors, including the likelihood of chronic hepatitis C reaching a stage associated with significant morbidity and mortality during the lifetime of the patient (e.g. age, comorbidities, severity of HCV-related liver disease), the chance of being cured by the therapy (efficacy), and the risk of experiencing side effects during treatment (safety and tolerability). If treatment were highly effective, safe, and well tolerated, HCV infection per se would likely be an indication for treatment in all patients with chronic hepatitis C. It should be emphasized that the extent of aminotransferase elevation correlates poorly with the hepatic inflammatory activity and fibrosis stage in hepatitis C; in fact, patients may have completely normal aminotransferases at the time of liver biopsy despite a chronic hepatitis being present. Other laboratory tests and technologies to assess fibrosis stage, such as FibroTest and FibroScan, may be able to discriminate the extremes, namely cirrhosis from minimal fibrosis. However, the overlap of test results in the mild to moderate fibrosis stages is too large to make these tests clinically useful in decision making regarding antiviral therapy. A liver biopsy therefore continues to play an important role in assessing the immediate need for antiviral therapy, especially in patients with genotype 1 (and 4) infection that respond suboptimally to current treatment regimens (see below).

The current standard antiviral therapy for hepatitis C consists of a combination of pegylated interferon-α and ribavirin. While interferon-α has numerous direct and indirect antiviral effects, the mechanism(s) of action of ribavirin are less clear, but includes immunomodulation.[9] Treatment aims at durable elimination of HCV, that is a sustained virological response (SVR), defined as undetectable HCV RNA in serum 24 weeks after cessation of therapy. Patients who reach an SVR almost never relapse later on and are regarded as cured. However, they do not have a protective immunity and HCV re-infection can occur with repeat risk behavior.

The standard of care for treatment of chronic hepatitis C is a combination of pegylated recombinant interferon-α plus ribavirin. Genotypes 2 and 3 respond much better to therapy (SVR 80% after 24 weeks of therapy) than genotypes 1 and 4 (SVR 50% after 48 weeks of therapy).[10,11] High baseline levels of HCV viremia, a slow decline of viremia during therapy, advanced fibrosis/cirrhosis, inability to adhere to full dose therapy (tolerability/side effects), and African American ethnicity are associated with impaired SVR rates. While the latter has recently been linked to a genetic polymorphism (IL-28B) upstream of the interferon-λ gene,[12] the role of interferon-λ and of the polymorphism in HCV infection and response to interferon-based antiviral therapy remains to be elucidated. If viremia levels decline very rapidly leading to undetectable HCV in serum after 4 weeks of treatment, there is a very high (90%) chance of reaching an SVR with continuing treatment, irrespective of genotype. Conversely, adult patients who do not respond with a decline in viremia levels of at least 2 logs at week 12 of treatment have a very low (<5%) probability of reaching an SVR with continuing therapy, but remain at risk for side effects; in this situation, continuing treatment does not carry a favorable risk–benefit ratio and so it should be stopped.

Side effects of pegylated interferon-α include flu-like symptoms lasting 1–2 months in the vast majority of patients, mood changes ranging from a frequent mild irritability to rare severe depression (including suicidal ideation), a decrease in neutrophil (and platelet) counts requiring dose reduction (and/or treatment with granulocyte colony stimulation factor [GCSF] in up to one-third of patients), and, last but not least, triggering of autoimmune diseases including autoimmune thyroiditis. While most side effects are reversible upon cessation of treatment, generally within 2–4 weeks, autoimmune diseases may persist and require lifelong therapy (e.g. thyroid hormone replacement). Pre-existing autoimmune conditions such as psoriasis are frequently aggravated during therapy. Ribavirin is concentrated in red blood cells and leads to a hemolytic anemia and in combination with pegylated interferon-α the hemo-globin levels typically drop by 30–40 g/L during the first 4–8 weeks of treatment. This may require dose reductions and/or treatment with erythropoietin in some patients. Ribavirin is excreted by the kidneys and is not dialyzable. Patients with impaired renal function are therefore at risk of accumulating ribavirin and require dose adjustments from the start. Ribavirin is fetotoxic and has a risk for teratogenicity when either the mother *or father* is taking ribavirin at the time of conception/pregnancy. In some age groups this hazard imposes special problems for managing treatment.

Populations that are difficult to treat because of decreased efficacy and/or increased risk for side effects includes patients with decompensated cirrhosis, renal failure, HIV coinfection, transplant recipients, and other patients who are immunocompromised/on immunosuppressive drugs, and i.v. drug users. Treating such patients requires special experience and caution.

Several new antiviral drugs designed to act directly on viral (but also host) targets essential for HCV replication are currently in clinical development. The HCV protease inhibitors telaprevir and boceprevir are the first of these compounds to be licensed in 2011. These drugs will be used in conjunction with the standard pegylated interferon-α plus ribavirin regimen to avoid resistance selection that rapidly occurs with monotherapy. Based on currently available data from the phase III studies,[13–16] these drugs will permit shorter duration of treatment and also increase SVR rates in genotype 1 infection (by 20%). Their side effects may be severe, particularly in those with cirrhosis. The most effective and tolerable treatment regimens are currently still being determined. There is a possibility of IFN and ribavirin-free treatments becoming available in the future![17,18]

For patients with HCV-related cirrhosis, especially if decompensated or complicated by HCC, a liver transplant offers the only chance for long-term survival although, once transplanted, the graft is universally reinfected by HCV, antiviral therapy tolerance is suboptimal, and is less likely to result in cure. Thus it is best to treat all those with cirrhosis before they develop liver failure—as an SVR pretransplant means no recurrence post transplant. Should an SVR be achieved, liver failure is unlikely to ensue although the risk of HCC is not entirely eliminated.

Special considerations in pediatric patients

Any discussion of hepatitis C infection in children has to include aspects of maternal infection because nowadays almost all chronic hepatitis C occurring in children is due to infection by mother-to-infant transmission (also known as vertical transmission). In North America, children who developed transfusion-associated hepatitis C are now young adults. Among an immigrant population, however, from countries where hepatitis C is endemic and standards of blood unit screening for transfusion and sometimes even medical procedures are suboptimal, some children or teenagers with transfusion-associated chronic hepatitis C will still be found. Often they have some other important medical problem such as a congenital anemia. In general, chronic hepatitis C in children is slowly progressive and seemingly mild. The therapeutic approach used in adult patients cannot be transferred uncritically to the pediatric age bracket, and early treatment of children with chronic hepatitis C is often appropriate and justified. Extended natural history studies suggest that most patients with chronic HCV infection from childhood onwards will develop hepatic fibrosis and possible cirrhosis over the first 2–4 decades of life and thus are at risk for developing clinically important chronic liver disease at a age which most would regard as the "prime of life". Cirrhosis has been reported in children with chronic hepatitis C and more than 100 children have already been transplanted in North America for end-stage liver disease related to chronic hepatitis C; however, hepatocellular carcinoma is rare, though reported in early adolescence.

In general, mother-to-infant transmission of HCV infection occurs with mothers who are viremic. In order to get a handle on the scope of this problem, studies need to be very large; a review of those involving more than 15 000 pregnant women, indicated that the percent of viremic women in such cohorts is approximately 0.8%. Universal screening of pregnant women for HCV infection may not be cost effective; however, risk factors (Table 14.2) should be sought by direct questioning. With respect to the risk of transmission of HCV from mother to child, an exhaustive analysis of the literature up to 2001 showed that the risk was 1.7% if the mother was only known to be positive for anti-HCV antibodies but 4.3% if the HCV RNA testing was positive once. If the HCV RNA was detected twice, then the risk was 7.1%. Further experience reporting transmission rates with viremic mothers suggests that this latter rate is most relevant, and the overall risk for the HCV-monoinfected woman appears to be 5–7% per pregnancy. Transmission risk is increased if the mother is coinfected with HCV and HIV, probably two- to threefold overall. High viral load ($>10^5$–10^6 viral copies/mL) also seems to be associated with increased rates of transmission of infection; however, viral load fluctuates during pregnancy and thus is not a reliable predictor. The use of fetal internal ("scalp-vein") monitoring and prolonged rupture of membranes also appear associated with increased risk of transmission. The data regarding amniocentesis are so incomplete that its risk cannot be assessed. There is no advantage to elective caesarean section in mothers with chronic hepatitis C in terms of reducing risk of transmission of HCV. With vaginal delivery, major tears should be avoided. Breast feeding is generally recognized as permissible, although care must be taken to ensure that the nipples do not get cracked and bleed (e.g. mastitis) and the mother does not have a clinical flare of hepatitis postpartum. Even with the best precautions some transmission of HCV to the infant may take place because approximately 30% of this infection may occur *in utero* instead of around the time of birth.

Determining whether or not the infant gets HCV infection by mother-to-infant transmission is unfortunately less straightforward. The transplacental transfer of anti-HCV antibodies makes it impossible to test the infant for anti-HCV antibodies before 18 months of age. Testing cord blood is useless as the results are impossible to interpret; direct testing for viral RNA is not sufficiently informative when the infant is 1 month-old to warrant testing so early. It is also quite obvious that some infants get an acute infection and clear it in the first year of life. The current standard recommendation is not to test for anti-HCV before the child is 18 months old. If it is negative at 18 months, then the child does not have chronic hepatitis C. In situations where diagnostic information is needed earlier, testing for HCV RNA at 2 months is reasonable. If it is negative, then this is highly reassuring. If it is positive, it should be tested again when the infant is 6 months old, when it may be negative with spontaneously resolved infection. Serum alanine aminotransferase (ALT) should be checked each time (recognizing that the upper limit of normal for ALT is higher in the first year of life than in adults).

The natural history of chronic hepatitis C in childhood is somewhat different from that in adults. In addition to resolution of acute infection in very early infancy, there is a tendency for young children to attain a spontaneous resolution of chronic HCV infection in the first few years of life. Studies have shown that this tendency to spontaneous resolution is the same whether the infection is acquired by mother-to-infant transmission or through some sort of transfusion. A large Canadian natural history study showed that 25% of the cohort achieved spontaneous resolution of chronic HCV infection at approximately 7 years old for those infected at or around birth, and at approximately 12 years old for those where the infective episode was identified.[19] Several recent European retrospective studies indicate that the general rate of spontaneous resolution is rather low in children, on the order of 6–15%. Most children with chronic hepatitis C are asymptomatic; extrahepatic manifestations of chronic hepatitis C appear rare in children. Nevertheless, it is clear that chronic hepatitis C in children is a progressive disease, even if it is indolent. Some children have no distinct abnormality on liver biopsy; most have mild inflammation and comparatively little fibrosis. Cirrhosis is uncommon, occurring in approximately 1% of children. Fatty liver, either due to the HCV infection or associated with childhood obesity, may increase the rate of disease progression.[20,21] An important but under-recognized aspect of chronic hepatitis C in childhood is that it entails significant social stigmatization for the child and family, and thus it can have a broad negative impact on the child's social growth and development. Practical issues like going to day-care, playing sports, participating in school trips, dating, and other routine aspects of adolescence loom large for parents; restrictions are problematic for their HCV-infected children.

Accordingly, the threshold for treating children is somewhat more relaxed than for treating adults. There is quite a lot of available research data regarding treatment in children. Two recent pediatric randomized controlled trials have established that combination therapy with pegylated interferon-α plus ribavirin is currently the best standard treatment.[22] No child should be treated before the age of 3 years because of the potential for severe neurotoxicity associated with interferon-α. Ribavirin is given using a weight-based regimen, as is customary with most drug treatment regimens in the pediatric age bracket. Children tolerate this regimen very well, although the usual side effects of anemia, neutropenia, transient flu-like syndrome, and weight loss because of anorexia may occur. SVR is on the same order as with adults. Optimal length of treatment in relation to HCV genotype is still being determined. Teenage sexual behavior may be problematic when ribavirin is used, and pregnancy tests must be done frequently. Likewise depression and suicidal ideation, impulsive behaviors, or change in general emotional outlook all need to be monitored closely. Suicidal ideation is an indication for stopping treatment. Practitioners need to be aware that the use of complementary and alternative medicine is highly prevalent in families where a child has chronic hepatitis C.[23]

The decision to treat a child with chronic hepatitis C is complex, but in principle any child over 3 years old might be at least considered for treatment. For the child with chronic hepatitis C due to mother-to-infant transmission, it may make sense to monitor the disease for another 3–4 years in case later spontaneous resolution occurs. For the child with genotype 2–3 infection, pre-emptive treatment may make sense even with relatively mild liver disease, especially if the family is not coping well or if the child has other chronic health problems whose treatment will be hampered in the face of chronic hepatitis C. For children with chronic hepatitis C due to genotype 1 or 4–6, waiting for even better therapeutic regimens while the child has trivial disease may be the better choice. These issues are important for the generalist who is providing continuity of care to the family or teenager because the decision about treatment and the treatment itself are stressful and require increased medical support.

Likewise it is not really clear how to manage the child who has had spontaneous remission of chronic HCV infection. Most will not have cirrhosis, and the prevailing inclination is to regard them as cured. However, giving in to this definite sense of relief is not necessarily the best plan. They probably need some ongoing surveillance and counseling about lifestyle choices, notably about alcohol use and maintenance of healthy body weight. They may have questions about child bearing. As we accumulate more children who have been treated successfully and achieved SVR, similar considerations will apply to them. Finally, displaced homeless "street kids" are children/teenagers who are at high risk for chronic hepatitis C and may not have the opportunity for adequate treatment; they pose an important challenge for ongoing management of pediatric chronic hepatitis C.

Case study 14.1

A 55-year-old male business analyst of Pakistani descent presents with new-onset ascites. He was completely asymptomatic until 4 weeks ago when he noticed increasing abdominal girth and ankle edema. In the past he had been noted at the time of a routine check to have abnormal liver enzymes and at that time was asked to stop his usual one to three beers a day. He has moderate ascites and ankle edema, a few spider nevi on the chest, and palmar erythema.

Upon advice he stops all alcohol consumption and his fluid retention improved. Routine laboratory tests ordered show: ALT of 75 IU/L, ALP within normal limits, total bilirubin mildly elevated (35 μmol/L), INR 1.4, albumin 33 g/L, creatinine, electrolytes, and glucose within normal limits, CBC was normal except for a decreased platelet count of $84 \times 10^6/\mu L$. The ultrasound shows a small nodular liver but without any circumscribed nodule suggestive of HCC, ascites, and an enlarged (15 cm) spleen. The blood tests for potential etiologies show the following: HBsAg negative, anti-HBs and anti-HBc positive, anti-HCV positive, all markers for both hereditary and autoimmune liver diseases are negative. The patient is surprised to hear that he likely has cirrhosis and states that he never used i.v. drugs but he had required surgery as a young man when he was living in Pakistan. Ongoing hepatitis C is confirmed with a positive HCV RNA test, the viral load being 2.4×10^5 IU/L. In view of the clinical evidence of cirrhosis, a gastroscopy is recommended to check for the presence of esophageal varices.

Consultation by a gastroenterologist/hepatologist states as diagnosis "HCV-related cirrhosis (genotype 3)". His MELD score is calculated to be 11 on the basis of cirrhosis with well-controlled fluid retention and grade 1 esophageal varices (i.e. too small to recommend prophylactic beta-blockers therapy). It is thought too early to consider liver transplantation (a survival benefit is seen only if the MELD score is 15 or higher). Given that treatment of genotype 3 HCV has a greater than 50% likelihood of cure with just 24 weeks of pegylated interferon-α/ribavirin, antiviral therapy is recommended despite the higher risk due to the established cirrhosis with a history

(Continued)

of past liver failure as antiviral therapy with elimination of the virus (SVR) will prevent further liver failure and less chance of the need for a transplant as HCC risk is reduced. Antiviral therapy is started and his treatment course although fraught with problems does lead to an SVR. However, because he has obvious cirrhosis, regular 6-monthly ultrasounds to screen for HCC should continue. Despite his reduced rate of risk of HCC, the risk is not zero (at least within the first 5 years of being virus free). He remains abstinent from alcohol and has no evidence of hepatic failure in follow up.

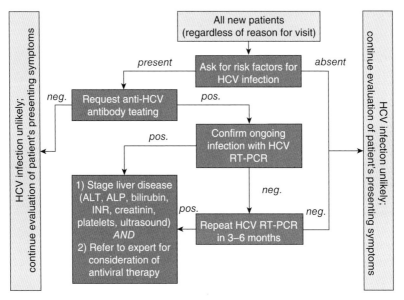

Fig. 14.3 Practice points/management algorithm: approach to the patient with possible HCV infection.

Case study 14.2

As a busy general practitioner, you are pleased to see your patient, a 32-year-old physicist, who is thrilled to be pregnant with her first child. The pregnancy is going well, totally uncomplicated, as she enters the third trimester. This woman had required extensive surgery in 1986, following a horrendous automobile accident. The blood bank had to go to extreme lengths to meet her intraoperative transfusion needs because she has a rare blood type. Given this transfusion history, which she had forgotten about, you test her anti-HCV and it is positive; you test her serum HCV RNA and it also positive with a high viral load (Fig. 14.3). You discuss the options with her. You tell her not to worry because the mother-to-infant transmission rate is low.

A couple of months later, you see your patient on the obstetrics ward. She has a beautiful new daughter. The vaginal delivery went well, except that membranes were ruptured for 12 hours; they avoided using any internal fetal monitoring. Your patient wants to know about breast feeding and you tell her to go ahead and breast feed. The next day you see your patient before her discharge home and she is obviously distraught. She is terrified of breast feeding because it is another risk for transmitting HCV to her child, though one she can control. You remind her of the benefits of breast feeding for both child and mother, and you cite the consensus of current textbooks and practice guidelines in favor of breast feeding in this situation. In the end you recognize that her extreme risk-intolerance outweighs any benefits breast feeding might have. You recommend an infant formula.

It is the first well baby visit at 1 month, and the infant girl is doing fine. She is gaining weight and has no visible jaundice, but she is still not sleeping through the night. Her mother wants to know whether the baby has "caught hepatitis C". You tell her that the anti-HCV test cannot be done until the baby is 18 months old. The mother goes almost berserk: she cannot go a year and half without knowing whether her child has this disease. You know that she is going through a lot postpartum, coping with the new baby and the new reality of her own medical diagnosis. However, you also know that testing for HCV RNA at 1 month is useless because the test is not sensitive enough then. Therefore you make an appointment for bringing the baby back for the test after she is 2 months old. The baby turns out to be negative then; under some continuing duress, you recheck her at 6 months old and the HCV RNA is still undetectable. At 18 months old the baby proves to be anti-HCV negative.

Multiple choice questions

1. Which of the following statements is correct?
   A. HCV is a small, enveloped DNA virus.
   B. HCV infection is still spread almost exclusively by transfusion of blood or blood products.
   C. Chronic hepatitis C is a rare disease. While chronic hepatitis C usually does not cause symptoms until cirrhosis is established, acute hepatitis C is almost always symptomatic.
   D. Screening for HCV infection is based on anti-HCV antibody testing, positive results requiring confirmation by detection of circulating virus using an HCV RNA RT-PCR assay.
   E. Because current standard therapy (pegylated interferon-α and ribavirin) has limited efficacy and serious side effects, it is not considered in most patients.

2. The regimen of pegylated interferon-α plus ribavirin cannot be used to treat children with chronic hepatitis C in which of the following situations?
   A. A 16-year-old girl is under detention (for the next 2 years, per court order) in a supervised facility where personnel will monitor treatment.
   B. The child has chronic infection with genotype 1 HCV.
   C. The child is less than 3 years old.
   D. Liver biopsy shows that the child has only mild fibrosis.
   E. The child is dyslexic.

Answers

1. D
2. C

References

1. Kwong JC, Crowcroft NS, Campitelli MA, et al. Ontario Burden of Infectious Disease Study Advisory Group; Ontario Burden of Infectious Disease Study (ONBOIDS): An OAHPP/ICES Report. Toronto: Ontario Agency for Health Protection and Promotion, Institute for Clinical Evaluative Sciences, 2010. http://www.ices.on.ca/file/ONBOIDS_FullReport_intra.pdf.
2. Choo QL, Kuo G, Weiner AJ, et al. Isolation of a cDNA clone derived from a blood-borne non-A, non-B viral hepatitis genome. Science 1989; 244: 359–62.
3. Kuo G, Choo QL, Alter HJ, Gitnick GL, et al. An assay for circulating antibodies to a major etiologic virus of human non-A, non-B hepatitis. Science 1989; 244: 362–4.
4. Pawlotsky JM, Chevaliez S, McHutchison JG. The hepatitis C virus life cycle as a target for new antiviral therapies. Gastroenterology 2007; 132: 1979–98.
5. Public Health Agency of Canada. Hepatitis C: Get the facts. You can have it and not know it, 2010. http://www.phac-aspc.gc.ca/hepc/pubs/getfacts-informezvous/index-eng.php.
6. Leigh JP, Bowlus CL, Leistikow BN, et al. Costs of hepatitis C. Arch Intern Med 2001; 161: 2231–7.
7. Remis RS. Modelling the incidence and prevalence of hepatitis C infection and its sequelae in Canada, 2007, final report. Public Health Agency of Canada, 2007. http://www.phac-aspc.gc.ca/sti-its-surv-epi/model/pdf/model07-eng.pdf.
8. Blackard JT, Kemmer N, Sherman KE. Extrahepatic replication of HCV: insights into clinical manifestations and biological consequences. Hepatology 2006; 44: 15–22.
9. Feld JJ, Hoofnagle JH. Mechanisms of action of interferon and ribavirin in treatment of hepatitis C. Nature 2005; 436: 967–72.
10. Manns MP, McHutchison JG, Gordon SC, et al. Peginterferon alfa-2b plus ribavirin compared with interferon alfa-2b plus ribavirin for initial treatment of chronic hepatitis C: a randomised trial. Lancet 2001; 358: 958–65.
11. Fried MW, Shiffman ML, Reddy KR, et al. Peginterferon alfa-2a plus ribavirin for chronic hepatitis C virus infection. N Engl J Med 2002; 347: 975–82.
12. Ge D, Fellay J, Thompson AJ, et al. Genetic variation in IL28B predicts hepatitis C treatment-induced viral clearance. Nature 2009; 461: 399–401.

13. Jacobson IM, McHutchison JG, Dusheiko G, et al. ADVANCE Study Team. Telaprevir for previously untreated chronic hepatitis C virus infection. N Engl J Med 2011; 364: 2405–16.

14. Poordad F, McCone J, Bacon BR, et al. SPRINT-2 Investigators. Boceprevir for untreated chronic HCV genotype 1 infection. N Engl J Med 2011; 364: 1195–206.

15. McHutchison JG, Manns MP, Muir AJ, et al. PROVE3 Study Team. Telaprevir for previously treated chronic HCV infection. N Engl J Med 2010; 362: 1292–303.

16. Bacon BR, Gordon SC, Lawitz E, et al. HCV RESPOND-2 Investigators. Boceprevir for previously treated chronic HCV genotype 1 infection. N Engl J Med 2011; 364: 1207–17.

17. Zeuzem S, Buggisch P, Agarwal K, et al. Dual, triple, and quadruple combination treatment with ribavirin or PegIFN/RBV for up to 28 days in treatment naïve G1 HCV subjects. 61st Annual Meeting of the American Association for the Study of Liver Diseases (AASLD 2010), Oral presentation LB#1.

18. Gane EJ, Stedman CA, Hyland RH, et al. Once daily PSI-7977 plus RBV: Pegylated interferon alpha not required for complete rapid viral response in treatment-naïve patients with HCV GT2 or GT3. 62nd Annual Meeting of the American Association for the Study of Liver Diseases (AASLD 2011), Abstract 34.

19. Yeung LT, To T, King SM, et al. Spontaneous clearance of childhood hepatitis C virus infection. J Viral Hepat 2007; 14: 797–805.

20. Bortolotti F, Verucchi G, Camma C, et al. Long-term course of chronic hepatitis C in children: from viral clearance to end-stage liver disease. Gastroenterology 2008; 134: 1900–7.

21. Delgado-Borrego A, Healey D, Negre B, et al. Influence of body mass index on outcome of pediatric chronic hepatitis C virus infection. J Pediatr Gastroenterol Nutr 2010; 51: 191–7.

22. Schwarz KB, Gonzalez-Peralta RP, Murray KF, et al. The combination of ribavirin and peginterferon is superior to peginterferon and placebo for children and adolescents with chronic hepatitis C. Gastroenterology 2011; 140: 450–8.

23. Erlichman J, Salam A, Haber BA. Use of complementary and alternative medicine in pediatric chronic viral hepatitis. J Pediatr Gastroenterol Nutr 2010; 50: 417–21.

Liver disease due to alcohol

CHAPTER 15

Nazia Selzner

Multi Organ Transplant Program and Division of Gastroenterology, Toronto General Hospital, University Health Network, Toronto, Ontario, Canada

---

Key points

- Alcoholic liver disease (ALD) encompasses a spectrum of injury, ranging from fatty liver to frank cirrhosis.
- Although alcoholic fatty liver secondary to excessive alcohol ingestion resolves with abstinence, in those who continue to drink steatosis predisposes to hepatic fibrosis and cirrhosis.
- The risk of liver disease increases with the quantity and duration of alcohol intake. The prevalence of alcoholic liver disease is influenced by many factors, including genetic factors (e.g. predilection to alcohol abuse, sex) and environmental factors (e.g. availability of alcohol, social acceptability of alcohol use, concomitant hepatotoxic insults).
- The diagnosis of ALD is based on a combination of features, which include a history of significant alcohol intake, clinical evidence of liver disease, and supporting laboratory abnormalities.
- A variety of scoring systems have been used to assess the severity of alcoholic hepatitis and to guide treatment; Maddrey's discriminant function, the Glasgow score, and the Model for End-Stage Liver Disease (MELD) score help the clinician decide whether corticosteroids should be initiated, whereas the Lille score is designed to help the clinician decide whether to stop corticosteroids after 1 week of administration.
- Treatment of ALD can be divided into three components: treatment of alcoholism, nutritional support, and specific drug treatments.

Hepatology: Diagnosis and Clinical Management, First Edition. Edited by E. Jenny Heathcote.
© 2012 John Wiley & Sons, Ltd. Published 2012 by John Wiley & Sons, Ltd.

Alcoholic liver disease (ALD) is a general term describing a spectrum of conditions ranging from fatty liver to alcoholic hepatitis to cirrhosis, all of which can be present simultaneously and are potentially reversible with abstinence (with time even remodeling of hepatic fibrosis takes place). Regular alcohol use, even for just a few days, can result in a fatty liver (also called steatosis), a disorder in which hepatocytes contain macrovesicular droplets of triglycerides. Fatty liver develops in about 90% of individuals who drink more than 60 g/day of alcohol, but may also occur in individuals who drink less. Fatty liver is generally reversible with abstinence and is not believed to progress to a chronic form of liver disease if abstinence or moderation is maintained. Alcoholic hepatitis (AH) is an acute form of alcohol-induced liver injury that occurs with the consumption of a large quantity of alcohol over a prolonged period of time; it encompasses a spectrum of severity ranging from asymptomatic derangement of blood tests to fulminant liver failure and death. Cirrhosis involves replacement of the normal hepatic parenchyma with extensive thick bands of fibrous tissue and regenerative nodules, which may result in the clinical manifestations of portal hypertension and liver failure. Hepatic fibrosis occurs in 40–60% of the patients who ingest more than 40–80 g/day for an average of 25 years. This chapter reviews the epidemiology, clinical manifestation, and management of patients with alcohol-induced liver disease.

Epidemiology and risk factors

The risk of liver disease increases with the quantity and duration of alcohol intake. Although necessary, excessive alcohol use is not sufficient to promote ALD. Only one in five heavy drinkers develops AH, and one in four develops cirrhosis.[1]

The typical age at presentation of AH is between 40 and 50 years, with the majority occurring before 60. The reasons why only a minority of alcoholics develops hepatitis are incompletely understood. Environmental and host factors that increase the risk of alcoholic cirrhosis are presented in Table 15.1.

Although women are at increased risk of developing ALD when they drink alcohol, the majority of patients with AH are males because men are twice as likely as women to abuse alcohol.

Different alcoholic beverages contain varying quantities of alcohol (Table 15.2). The risk for developing cirrhosis increases with the ingestion of more than 60–80 g/day of alcohol for 10 or more years in men, and more than 20 g/day in women.[2] The amount of alcohol consumption that places an individual at risk of developing AH is not known. However, in practice, most individuals with AH drink more than 100 g/day. The typical patient has drunk heavily for two or more decades, although an occasional patient has abused alcohol for less than 10 years.

However, clinical presentation after abstinence for more than 3 months should raise concern for underlying advanced alcoholic cirrhosis or other causes of chronic liver disease. Occasional patients deny alcohol abuse and

Table 15.1 Risk factors associated with alcoholic cirrhosis

Being female
Amount of alcohol ingested
Drinking multiple types of alcohol (e.g. beer plus wine, etc.)
Alcohol consumption between meals
Social acceptability of alcohol use
Availability of alcohol
Concomitant chronic hepatitis C viral infection
Poor nutrition
Genetic polymorphisms of genes involved in the metabolism of alcohol (including alcohol dehydrogenase, acetaldehyde dehydrogenase, and the cytochrome P450 system)

Table 15.2 Alcohol contents of beverages

Type of alcohol	Alcohol content
1 beer (Canadian)	15 g
4 oz wine	10 g
1 oz liquor	10 g

discreet discussions with family members are required to obtain the true history of the patient's alcohol use.

Clinical presentation and diagnosis

The diagnosis of ALD is based on a combination of features, including a history of significant alcohol intake, clinical evidence of liver disease, and supporting laboratory abnormalities. **Fatty liver** is usually diagnosed in the asymptomatic patient who is undergoing evaluation for elevated serum aminotransferase levels; typically, aspartate aminotransferase (AST) levels are less than twice the upper limit of normal and the AST value is greater than that for the alanine aminotransferase (ALT). No laboratory test is diagnostic of fatty liver. Ultrasonographic findings include a hyperechogenic, enlarged liver. Typical histologic findings of fatty liver include fat accumulation in hepatocytes, which is often macrovesicular but it is occasionally microvesicular. The centrilobular region of the hepatic acinus is most commonly affected. In severe fatty liver, however, fat is distributed throughout the acinus. Fatty liver is not specific to alcohol ingestion; it is associated with obesity, insulin resistance, hyperlipidemia, malnutrition, and various medications. Attribution of fatty liver to alcohol use therefore requires a detailed and accurate patient history.

Table 15.3 Manifestations of alcoholic hepatitis

Clinical manifestations
  Rapid onset of jaundice
  Fever
  Anorexia
  Ascites
  Proximal muscle loss
  Encephalopathy
  Enlarged and tender liver

Biochemical signs
  Elevated serum levels of aspartate aminotransferase < 300 IU/mL
  Ratio aspartate aminotransferase alanine aminotransferase > 2:1
  Elevated white blood cell count (neutrophilia)
  Elevated total serum bilirubin level (conjugated)
  Elevated INR

Histologic findings
  Ballooned hepatocytes
  Mallory bodies
  Large fat droplets
  Sinusoidal fibrosis
  Foamy degeneration of hepatocytes

Alcoholic hepatitis (AH) is a clinical syndrome of jaundice and liver failure. The typical age at presentation is 40 to 60 years. The clinical and biochemical sign of AH are presented in Table 15.3.

The diagnosis of **alcoholic cirrhosis** rests on finding the classic signs and symptoms of end-stage liver disease in a patient with a history of significant alcohol intake. Patients can present with any or all the complications of portal hypertension, including ascites, variceal bleeding, and hepatic encephalopathy. The histology of end-stage alcoholic cirrhosis, in the absence of acute AH, resembles that of advanced liver disease from many other causes, without any distinct pathologic findings.

Prognosis

The severity of AH can be assessed by calculating Maddrey's discriminant function,[3] the MELD score,[4] the Glasgow score,[5] and the Lille score[6] (Table 15.4). In clinical practice, any of these scoring systems can be used to select patients suitable for pharmacologic therapy. Of note, the Lille score, which is based on pretreatment data plus the response of the serum bilirubin level to a 7-day course of corticosteroid therapy, can be used to determine whether corticosteroids should be discontinued due to the lack of response.[6]

These various scoring systems are presented in the Table 15.4.

Table 15.4 Various prognosis scoring systems and their components

Name	Components				Prognosis value
Maddrey's discriminant function (DF)	4.6 (patient's PT – control PT) + total bilirubin (mg/dL)				Poor prognosis if score ≥ 32
Model for end-stage liver disease (MELD score)	$3.8 \times \log_e$(bilirubin in mg/dL) + $11.2 \times \log_e$(INR) + $9.6 \times \log_e$(creatinine mg/dL) + 6.4				Poor prognosis if > 21
Lille score	$3.19 - 0.101 \times$ age, + $0.147 \times$ albumin on day 0 + $0.0165 \times$ the change in bilirubin, – $0.206 \times$ renal insufficiency, rated as 0 if absent and 1 if present, – $0.0065 \times$ bilirubin level – $0.0096 \times$ prothrombin time				If > 0.45 indicates lack of response to corticosteroids
Glasgow alcoholic hepatitis score	**Score:**	**1**	**2**	**3**	Poor prognosis if score > 9
	Age	<50	≥50	—	
	WCC (10^9/L)	<15	≥15	—	
	Urea (mm/L)	<5	≥5	—	
	PT ratio	<1.5	1.5–2.0	≥2	
	Bilirubin (μmol/L)	<7.3	7.3–14.6	>14.6	

PT, prothrombin time; WCC, white cell count.

Treatment

Treatment of ALD can be divided into three components: treatment of alcoholism, nutritional support, and specific drug treatments (Fig. 15.1).

Treatment of alcoholism

Abstinence from alcohol is essential to prevent the progression of liver disease. However, the majority of the patients are often unable to achieve complete and durable alcohol abstinence and therefore referral to an addiction specialist and follow-up with a support group is appropriate. Among the medications intended to reduce craving for alcohol, naltrexone and acamprosate have some proven efficacy for short-term abstinence in alcoholic patients. Baclofen, a γ-aminobutyric acid beta-receptor agonist, reduces craving among alcohol-dependent subjects without liver disease and is also safe and effective at maintaining abstinence among alcohol-dependent subjects with alcoholic cirrhosis.

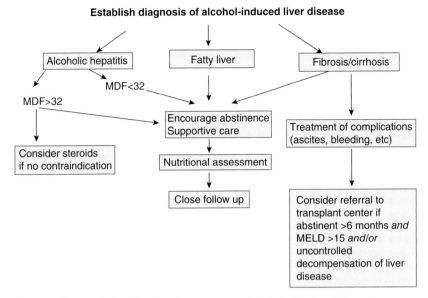

Fig. 15.1 Proposed algorithm for the management of alcohol-induced liver disease. MDF, Maddrey's discriminant function.

Nutritional support

Almost all patients with AH have some degree of malnutrition, but estimating the severity of malnutrition remains a challenge because sensitive and specific clinical or laboratory parameters are lacking. Assessment of the degree of malnutrition can be performed using urinary creatinine excretion and mid-arm muscle area for subjects without ascites or edema, while creatinine height index is preferable for patients with ascites. Other methods of assessment have included assessment of muscle mass, grip strength, response to skin tests (frequently anergic), and serum levels of prealbumin, vitamins (e.g. vitamin A, folic acid, B_{12}), and minerals (e.g. phosphorus, zinc).[7] The degree of malnutrition correlates directly with short and long-term mortality of patients with alcoholic hepatitis. Patients with mild malnutrition have a 14% mortality rate at 1 year post diagnosis of AH, compared to 76% mortality rate in those with severe malnutrition. Nutritional supplementation is generally associated with an improvement in liver test results, but only rarely with a survival benefit.

Medical therapy

The use of corticosteroids as specific therapy for AH has been controversial.[8] Prednisolone, 40 mg/day for 28 days (with or without a 2-week taper), is the most widely recommended drug to treat AH. The mechanism of action is believed to be its effect on decreasing the transcription of proinflammatory cytokines such as tumor necrosis factor-alpha (TNF-α). Indication and contraindications for treatment are presented in Table 15.5.

Table 15.5 Indication and contraindications for corticosteroid therapy

Indications: any of the following
Maddrey's discriminant function of ≥32
MELD > 21
Glasgow alcoholic hepatitis scale > 9
Hepatic encephalopathy

Contraindications
Uncontrolled sepsis
Recent upper gastrointestinal bleeding
Renal insufficiency
Chronic hepatitis B infection

Corticosteroid treatment of AH has been evaluated in 13 randomized controlled trials and in at least three meta-analyses. The results of the meta-analyses are conflicting but it appears that in a selected group of patients with severe liver dysfunction, as manifested by hepatic encephalopathy or a markedly abnormal discriminant function, that is above 32 (see Table 15.4 for formula), corticosteroids may have a survival benefit. Some studies suggest that the decision to stop corticosteroids because of lack of efficacy can be determined by calculating the Lille score after 7 days of treatment. A Lille score greater than 0.45 indicates a lack of response to corticosteroids and predicts a 6-month survival rate of less than 25%. All patients need to be screened for hepatitis B prior to the introduction of corticosteroid (or other immunosuppressive therapy).

Another therapeutic approach is the use of pentoxifylline, an inhibitor of TNF synthesis. Elevated TNF levels have been associated with higher mortality from AH. A randomized, double-blind, controlled trial demonstrated a survival benefit of treatment with pentoxifylline in patients with severe alcoholic hepatitis. The survival advantage was primarily due to a decrease in the development of the hepatorenal syndrome in pentoxifylline-treated patients. Although promising, these findings have yet to be validated by independent investigation.

Other therapies that have been investigated in the treatment of AH but not found to be beneficial include propylthiouracil, infliximab, insulin and glucagon, calcium channel blockers, and antioxidants such as vitamin E.

Liver transplantation
Treatment of the patient with alcoholic cirrhosis is similar to any other type of cirrhosis, and includes prevention and management of ascites, spontaneous bacterial peritonitis, variceal bleeding, encephalopathy, malnutrition, and hepatocellular carcinoma. Patients with evidence of hepatic decompensation (ascites with or without spontaneous bacterial peritonitis, hepatic encephalopathy, variceal bleeding) should be referred to a transplantation center.

Acute AH (see Table 15.3 for definition) is an absolute contraindication for liver transplantation. Most transplantation centers currently require patients with a history of alcohol abuse to have documented abstinence of at least 6 months before undergoing transplantation.[9] This requirement theoretically has a dual advantage of predicting long-term abstinence and allowing recovery of liver function from acute alcoholic hepatitis.

Case study 15.1

A 55-year-old woman is admitted to the hospital for abdominal pain, fever, and jaundice. She had been drinking one bottle of wine every evening with her meals since she lost her husband 5 years ago until a week prior to her admission. She continued to work as a secretary until 3 weeks prior to her admission, when she became increasingly weak but stated that she was "feeling well". She had lost 8 pounds over the last 6 months. Two years ago she was told she had an "enlarged liver" during her yearly physical check up. Unfortunately, she refused the ultrasound and the liver biopsy that was recommended by her physician at that time.

On physical examination she appeared cachectic. Her temperature was 38°C. She was jaundiced, had bilateral finger clubbing, and palmar erythema. The liver was 20 cm in span and tender. The spleen was not enlarged. The abdomen was not distended.

Laboratory tests showed WBC $20\,000 \times 10^9$/L, hematocrit 40%, and platelets $150\,000 \times 10^9$/L platelets. Liver biochemical and function tests shows AST of 250 IU/L, ALT of 99 IU/L, bilirubin of 245 μ/mol/L, and INR of 1.3. All viral serologies (HBV, HCV) and autoimmune markers were negative. α_1-antitrypsin and ceruloplasmin blood levels were normal.

Comments

This case history is a typical presentation of an acute alcoholic hepatitis in a patient with chronic history of alcohol consumption. Note the typical presentation of the patient with the combination of fever, jaundice, abdominal pain, and enlarged tender liver. Despite signs and symptoms of liver disease, patients usually state that they are "feeling fine". She had most probably had simple steatosis 2 years earlier and should have been questioned about her alcohol history and abstinence should have been recommended. Her Maddrey's discriminant function is more than 32 and she would be a candidate for corticosteroids treatment.

Multiple choice questions

1. Which of the following is incorrect regarding alcoholic liver disease?
   A. Fatty liver due to excess consumption of alcohol is irreversible.
   B. Alcoholic hepatitis is defined by the presence of inflammation in the liver.
   C. Severe alcoholic hepatitis may lead to acute hepatic failure.
   D. Fatty liver can predispose to cirrhosis in those individuals who continue to drink.

2. Which of the following is correct regarding treatment of alcoholic hepatitis?

   A. Treatment of ALD can be divided into three components: treatment of alcoholism, nutritional support, and specific drug treatments.

   B. Steroids should be recommended in patients with Maddrey's discriminant function less than 32.

   C. Liver transplantation is an option for all patients with severe acute alcoholic hepatitis.

   D. Hepatic encephalopathy is a contraindication for steroid therapy.

Answers

1. A
2. A

References

1. Grant BF, Dufour MC, Harford TC. Epidemiology of alcoholic liver disease. Semin Liver Dis 1988; 8: 12–25.
2. O'Shea RS, Dasarathy S, McCullough AJ. Alcoholic liver disease. Am J Gastroenterol 2010; 105: 14–32.
3. Maddrey WC, Boitnott JK, Bedine MS, et al. Corticosteroid therapy of alcoholic hepatitis. Gastroenterology 1978; 75: 193–9.
4. Dunn W, Jamil LH, Brown LS, et al. MELD accurately predicts mortality in patients with alcoholic hepatitis. Hepatology 2005; 41: 353–8.
5. Forrest EH, Evans CD, Stewart S, et al. Analysis of factors predictive of mortality in alcoholic hepatitis and derivation and validation of the Glasgow alcoholic hepatitis score. Gut 2005; 54: 1174–9.
6. Louvet A, Naveau S, Abdelnour M, et al. The Lille model: a new tool for therapeutic strategy in patients with severe alcoholic hepatitis treated with steroids. Hepatology 2007; 45: 1348–54.
7. Nielsen K, Kondrup J, Martinsen L, et al. Nutritional assessment and adequacy of dietary intake in hospitalized patients with alcoholic liver cirrhosis. Br J Nutr 1993; 69: 665–79.
8. Lucey MR, Mathurin P, Morgan TR. Alcoholic hepatitis. N Engl J Med 2009; 360: 2758–69.
9. Lucey MR, Brown KA, Everson GT, et al. Minimal criteria for placement of adults on the liver transplant waiting list: a report of a national conference organized by the American Society of Transplant Physicians and the American Association for the Study of Liver Diseases. Transplantation 1998; 66: 956–62.

Drug-induced liver disease

CHAPTER 16

Leslie B. Lilly

Multi Organ Transplant Program, Toronto General Hospital, University Health Network, Toronto, Ontario, Canada

Key points

- Virtually any drug can be a source of hepatotoxicity.
- Drugs are the commonest identified cause of fulminant hepatic failure in most Western centers.
- Recognition of the pattern of drug injury may aid in identification of the agent; in some case, characteristic histology on liver biopsy may be invaluable in deciding which drug is implicated, especially in ill patients receiving numerous medications.

Introduction

Drug-induced liver disease (DILD) is clearly common, although the exact incidence and prevalence are difficult to ascertain due to under-reporting. It is worth noting that hepatotoxicity is one of the most common reasons for termination of drug development programs or clinical trials. In addition, there are clearly genetic predispositions to some types of DILD, as well as gender and age effects. Pre-existing medical conditions may predispose to drug injury and the severity of that injury; studies have implicated diabetes mellitus and alcohol use. While most drug reactions are considered idiosyncratic, and therefore unpredictable and dose-independent, there may be a dose dependency for the most severe cases of DILD.

In a recent review, antimicrobials were reported to be the most common class of agents implicated in DILD, accounting for almost half of reported cases. Central nervous system agents were second; immunomodulatory drugs, analgesics, antineoplastic agents, antihypertensives, and lipid-lowering agents were among the other classes of drugs reported.

Hepatology: Diagnosis and Clinical Management, First Edition. Edited by E. Jenny Heathcote.
© 2012 John Wiley & Sons, Ltd. Published 2012 by John Wiley & Sons, Ltd.

Acute liver injury is the typical pattern in DILD; however, a small proportion of patients may develop chronic disease.

Mechanisms of drug-induced liver injury

It is not surprising, given the wide variety of classes of drugs that can cause liver injury, that a variety of mechanisms leads to hepatotoxicity. One involves cell membrane disruption with subsequent cell death, due to covalent binding of drug to cell proteins, which triggers an immunologic response to newly created adducts. Another pathway of injury leads to cholestasis through interruption of bile transport pumps or alterations in actin microfilaments. A direct toxic effect on mitochondrial function, with subsequent lipid accumulation and steatosis/steatohepatitis, represents yet another mechanism of drug injury. These pathways and others are discussed in detail elsewhere.

Patterns of drug injury

It is often a help to look at DILD according to the pattern of injury produced, in an effort to narrow down the potential agents in patients who may be exposed to multiple medications with hepatotoxic potential. An hepatocellular pattern, reflecting hepatocyte necrosis, is characterized by much higher elevation in aminotransaminases (AST, ALT) when compared with cholestatic markers (bilirubin, ALP). The former is typical of acetaminophen toxicity, as well as antituberculous medications, valproic acid, ketoconazole, and non-steroidal anti-inflammatory drugs (Box 16.1). A cholestatic picture is more commonly seen with many antibiotic-related DILD (penicillin derivatives and erythromycin) as well as estrogen-based hormones (Box 16.2). There are many compounds, however, that produce a mixed picture, including sulfa drugs, phenytoin, angiotensin-converting enzyme (ACE)-inhibitors, and others (Box 16.3). Other DILD may be complicated by the cholestatic effect of the oral contraceptive pill. Drugs that induce fatty liver (amiodarone, tamoxifen, tetracycline) typically present with signs of more hepatocellular injury than cholestasis. Immunologically mediated injury, such as that seen with phenytoin, nitrofurantoin, or halothane, tends to present with the mixed pattern of abnormal liver biochemistry.

The timing of abnormal biochemistry with drug exposure may be helpful. Although there is some controversy regarding the true incidence of statin-induced hepatotoxicity, is it generally considered that a rise in aminotransaminases within a few weeks of use may be attributed to these agents. Extremely rapid onset of idiosyncratic DILD is rare, although seen with drugs in the erythromycin class and among the fluoroquinolones.

In contrast, methotrexate-induced hepatic injury is thought to be related to the cumulative dose of the medication, which means that it may take several years to appreciate the development of drug-related fibrosis and often simultaneous chronic alcohol consumption may have an additive effect.

Box 16.1 Drugs associated with hepatocellular pattern of liver injury*

- Acetaminophen
- Amiodarone
- Anticonvulsants
  - Valproic acid
- Antihypertensives
  - Lisinopril, losartan
- Antimicrobials
  - Isoniazid, ketoconazole, pyrazinamide, rifampin, tetracycline
- Antipsychotics/antidepressants
  - Fluoxetine, paroxetine, risperidone, sertraline, trazodone
- Highly active antiretroviral treatment (HAART) drugs
- Non-steroidal anti-inflammatory drugs
- Statins
- Miscellaneous
  - Methotrexate, omeprazole, acarbose

*NB: May appear to have cholestatic features if the individual is taking oral contraceptives.

Box 16.2 Drugs associated with cholestatic pattern of liver injury

- Antimicrobials
  - Amoxicillin–clavulanic acid, erythromycin and its derivatives, terbinafine
- Steroids
  - Anabolic steroids, estrogens, oral contraceptives
- Antidepressants/antipsychotics
  - Chlorpromazine, mirtazapine, phenothiazines, tricyclics
- Miscellaneous
  - Clopidogrel, irbesartan

Box 16.3 Drugs associated with mixed pattern of liver injury

- Anticonvulsants
  - Carbamazepine, phenobarbital, phenytoin
- Antihypertensives
  - Captopril, enalapril, verapamil
- Antimicrobials
  - Clindamycin, nitrofurantoin, sulfonamides, trimethoprim–sulfamethoxazole
- Miscellaneous
  - Amitriptyline, azathioprine, trazodone

> ## Box 16.4 Patterns of drug-mediated liver injury (with examples)
>
> - Acute liver failure (see Table 16.1)
>   - extensive macrovesicular steatosis (e.g. tetracycline)
>   - necrosis with inflammation (most idiosyncratic drug reactions, including isoniazid, antibiotics, anticonvulsants)
>   - necrosis without inflammation (acetaminophen, cocaine, ecstasy)
> - Acute hepatitis (see Box 16.5)
> - Chronic hepatitis
>   - no autoimmune markers (sulfonamides, lisinopril, tamoxifen)
>   - with autoimmune markers (minocycline, nitrofurantoin, methyldopa, hydralazine)
>   - methotrexate
> - Acute cholestasis
>   - bland cholestasis (no inflammation; anabolic steroids, oral contraceptives)
>   - cholestasis with hepatitis (macrolide antibiotics, chlorpromazine)
> - Chronic cholestasis (and ductopenia)
>   - penicillins (amoxicillin–clavulanic acid, clindamycin, sulfonamides)
> - Granulomatous hepatitis
>   - antimicrobials (isoniazid, sulfonamides, dapsone, penicillin)
>   - anticonvulsants, antipsychotics (phenytoin, chlorpromazine)
>   - others (nitrofurantoin, diltiazem, allopurinol, methyldopa, amiodarone)
> - Steatosis/steatohepatitis
>   - microvesicular (tetracycline, cocaine, valproic acid, Reye syndrome)
>   - macrovesicular (steroids, non-steroidal anti-inflammatory drugs, tamoxifen, alcohol)
>   - steatohepatitis (amiodarone)
> - Vascular injury (veno-occlusive disease)
>   - chemotherapeutic agents
>
> Adapted from Ramachandran and Kakar, 2009.

It is also possible to classify DILD by the histologic findings seen on liver biopsy (Box 16.4), although it is usually unnecessary to obtain liver tissue in this situation. However, a patient may be receiving more than a single drug that can cause DILD, for example, and stopping the drugs to determine etiology may not be an option. Alternatively, underlying liver disease may make determination of the role of DILD in new biochemical abnormalities difficult, and biopsy may be helpful. Patients may be critically ill, with sepsis or hemodynamic disturbances that can affect liver biochemistry or liver function, and biopsy is more often required to determine the relative contributions of these various hepatotoxic possibilities.

Table 16.1 Drugs implicated in acute liver failure

Drug	Biochemical/histological pattern
Acetaminophen Antituberculous drugs (rifampin, isoniazid) Ketoconazole Valproic acid Phenytoin	Hepatitis (hepatocellular necrosis)
Amoxicillin–clavulanic acid ACE inhibitors Erythromycin	Cholestasis
Amiodarone Tamoxifen	Non-alcoholic steatohepatitis
Sulfa compounds Phenytoin Nitrofurantoin	Mixed hepatocellular/cholestatic

---

Box 16.5 Drugs associated with acute hepatitis type of injury

- Non-steroidal anti-inflammatory drugs
- Anticonvulsants (phenytoin, valproic acid, carbamazepine, chlorpromazine)
- Antimicrobial agents
  - Antibacterials (penicillins, amoxicillin–clavulanic acid, cephalosporins, tetracycline, sulfonamides, erythromycin)
  - Antifungals (fluconazole, ketoconazole, griseofulvin)
  - Antivirals (zidovudine, nevirapine, efavirenz)
  - Antiparasitics (albendazole, thiabendazole)
- Antihypertensives (methyldopa, hydralazine, ACE inhibitors, labetalol)
- Antiarrhythmics (quinidine, procainamide)
- Hypolipidemics (statins, clofibrate, nicotinic acid)
- Hypoglycemics (rosiglitazone)
- Others (sulfonylureas, allopurinol)

Approach to the patient with suspected drug-induced liver disease (Box 6.6)

Patients who have developed liver injury related to medications may present with very non-specific symptoms, including nausea, fatigue, or a vague right upper quadrant discomfort. Anorexia may be present. More specific symptoms such as pruritus or jaundice may of course occur. Liver biochemistry should

Box 16.6 Approach to the patient with suspected drug-induced liver disease

A Hepatocellular pattern
  1 Exclude other causes of predominant transaminase elevation
    (a) Viral hepatitis
      (i) HAV-IgM, HBsAg, anti-HBc IgM, HCV-Ab, others
    (b) Ischemic hepatopathy ("shock liver")
      (i) Review of recent hemodynamic profile
      (ii) Doppler assessment hepatic veins, portal veins
    (c) Autoimmune hepatitis
      (i) ANA, immunoglobulins
    (d) Alcohol
  2 If above non-contributory, discontinue, if possible, suspect agents (Boxes 16.1 and 16.5, and Table 16.1)
Consider liver biopsy if liver profile fails to improve or no clear etiology has been identified (Box 16.4)
B Cholestatic pattern
  1 Exclude other common potential causes of cholestasis
    (a) Biliary tract obstruction
      (i) Ultrasound or CT/MRI to assess biliary tree
      (ii) MRCP to further clarify biliary anatomy if necessary
      (iii) ERCP for therapeutic intervention
    (b) Intrinsic cholestatic liver disease
      (i) Serology for PBC, MRCP for PSC
    (c) Sepsis
    (d) TPN
  2 If above non-contributory, discontinue, if possible suspect agents (Box 16.2 and Table 16.1)
  3 Consider liver biopsy if liver profile fails to improve or no clear etiology has been identified (Box 16.4)
C Mixed pattern
  1 Exclude other common potential causes of a mixed enzyme pattern
    (a) Infiltrative disorders (malignancy, steatosis)
    (b) Some viral hepatitides (e.g. persistent hepatitis A)
    (c) Sepsis with hemodynamic compromise
  2 If above non-contributory, discontinue, if possible, suspect agents (Box 16.3 and Table 16.1)
  3 Consider liver biopsy if liver profile fails to improve or no clear etiology has been identified (Box 16.4)

ANA, antinuclear antibodies; CT, computed tomography; ERCP, endoscopic retrograde cholangiopancreatography; MRCP, magnetic resonance cholangiopancreatography; MRI, magnetic resonance imaging; PBC, primary biliary cirrhosis; PSC, primary sclerosing cholangitis; TPN, total parenteral nutrition.

be obtained. A careful drug history is an essential part of the assessment of patients with abnormal liver biochemistry. This includes not only prescription drugs, but over the counter and herbal or naturopathic medications as well. Alcohol use should be specifically explored. Patients are often unaware of the wide variety of over the counter drugs that contain acetaminophen, and may be inadvertently ingesting higher than recommended dosages, resulting in disturbed liver biochemistry or liver failure. As drug-related hepatotoxicity is relatively rare, even very large-scale clinical trials may fail to identify an important idiosyncratic drug reaction; only when compounds go into wide clinical use in millions of patients do such reactions sometimes become evident. Further, mechanisms for reporting drug reactions are not uniformly used, resulting in under-reporting of adverse outcomes. Liver injury due to a drug may not become overt until the drug is stopped and may take 6 weeks to develop; thus, past as well as present drug intake needs to be questioned.

There are some patient populations that appear to be at increased risk of DILD. Adults appear more susceptible than children, and men tend to be affected less often than women. Pregnancy may increase susceptibility, along with obesity and malnutrition. Depletion of glutathione stores, often the case in alcoholic liver disease, seems to predispose to acetaminophen-induced liver injury and possibly plays a role in many other individuals with DILD.

The most important factor determining susceptibility to DILD is likely genetic variability, although the field of pharmacogenomics remains in its infancy.

While pre-existing liver disease may not increase the likelihood of a drug causing liver injury (unless due to alcohol), it may limit the capacity of the organ to recover from any injury that has taken place.

The management of suspected DILD must include identification and exclusion of other potential causes of the abnormal liver profile; non-alcoholic fatty liver disease is becoming an important cause of persistently abnormal liver biochemistry, and should be suspected in patients with or at risk for the metabolic syndrome. Viral serology should be performed, and imaging (usually ultrasonography initially) may be appropriate. It may sometimes be necessary to investigate for autoimmune liver disease or metabolic conditions that involve the liver (hemochromatosis, for example) before arriving at the conclusion that the abnormalities in liver tests are potentially drug induced.

Prompt discontinuation of the suspected drug should follow, and usually results in improvement in liver biochemistry, although this can take up to several months (even years with cholestatic drug injury), depending on the agent involved. In those rare cases where fulminant hepatic failure has been precipitated, liver transplantation may be required. Indeed, in many series it is a drug (acetaminophen) that is the leading cause of fulminant hepatic failure. According to Hy's rule, the combination of hepatocellular injury and jaundice induced by a drug is associated with a particularly poor prognosis, with a fatality rate of 10–50%.

> **Case study 16.1**
>
> Consultation is requested on a 71-year-old man in the CCU with abnormal liver enzymes. The laboratory values are: total bilirubin 27 mol/L, AST 184 IU/L, ALT 140 IU/L, ALP 260 IU/L. They had all been normal 1 week earlier when the patient was admitted for chest pain, an abnormal ECG, and elevated troponins. He had a history of atrial fibrillation managed with digoxin and coumadin, and type 2 diabetes mellitus managed with diet only. A diagnosis of myocardial infarction was made.
>
> Within 24 h the patient had experienced a number of ventricular arrhythmias associated with hypotension, and was treated with dopamine and amiodarone, in addition to coumadin and nitrates. Further, on the third day following admission he had become febrile, and right lower lobe pneumonia was diagnosed on chest radiography. He was started on tazosin, but developed a rash, and was switched to levofloxacin per os.
>
> Elevated liver enzymes were noted on the fifth day of admission, and when they did not resolve after 48 h a hepatology consultation was requested.

Multiple choice questions

1. A 57-year-old female patient is referred for abnormal liver biochemistry. There is no history of underlying liver disease, and imaging (ultrasound, magnetic resonance cholangiopancreatography) is unremarkable. The liver biochemistry is as follows: total bilirubin 21 μmol/L, AST 60 IU/L, ALT 80 IU/L, ALP 360 IU/L. You suspect DILD, and she is on several potentially hepatotoxic drugs. Which of the following is the most likely to account for this pattern?
   A. Acetaminophen
   B. Estrogens
   C. Trimethoprim–sulfamethoxazole
   D. Losartan
   E. None of the above

2. A 24-year-old man is referred for abnormal liver biochemistry and altered mental status. He has no known history of liver disease, and viral serology (hepatitis A, B, and C) is all negative. There is no history of mental illness or suicidal ideation. He drinks, on average, four to six beers per day. A week ago, he suffered a knee injury while playing hockey and has been taking 3.5 g of acetaminophen daily, recommended by his family physician, and according to the package insert. He takes no other medications, either by prescription or over the counter. On examination he is drowsy and has asterixis. Ultrasound of the liver and vessels is unremarkable. The liver biochemistry is as follows: total bilirubin 34 μmol/L, AST 6700 IU/L,

ALT 8100 IU/L, ALP 123 IU/L, INR 3.7. Serum acetaminophen level is *unde-tectable*. Which is the most appropriate course of action?

A. Stop the acetaminophen and discharge the patient home
B. Stop the acetaminophen and admit to hospital for observation
C. B *plus* initiation of *N*-acetylcysteine
D. B *plus* consult with local transplant center for possible transfer and assessment
E. C *plus* D

Answers

1. C
2. E

Further reading

Bader T. The myth of statin-induced hepatotoxicity. Am J Gastroenterol 2010; 105: 978–80.

Björnsson E. Drug-induced liver injury: Hy's rule revisited. Clin Pharmacol Ther 2006; 79: 521–8.

Ghabril M, Chalasani N, Bjornsson E. Drug-induced liver injury: a clinical update. Curr Opin Gastroenterol 2010; 26: 222–6.

Lat I, Foster DR, Erstad B. Drug-induced acute liver failure and gastrointestinal complications. Crit Care Med 2010; 38: S175–87.

Lee WM. Drug-induced hepatotoxicity. N Engl J Med 2003; 349: 474–85.

Navarro VJ, Senior JR. Drug-related hepatotoxicity. N Engl J Med 2006; 354: 731–9.

Ramachandran R, Kakar S. Histological patterns in drug-induced liver disease. J Clin Pathol 2009; 62: 481–92.

Obesity and its hepatic complications in adults and children

CHAPTER 17

E. Jenny Heathcote[1] and Eve A. Roberts[2]

[1]Division of Gastroenterology, Toronto Western Hospital, University Health Network, University of Toronto, Toronto, Ontario, Canada

[2]Departments of Paediatrics, Medicine, and Pharmacology, University of Toronto, and Division of Gastroenterology, Hepatology and Nutrition, The Hospital for Sick Children, Toronto, Ontario, Canada

---

Key points: adults

- Obesity rates are increasing worldwide. Adults with a body mass index (BMI) of more than 30 (Caucasian) or more than 27 (Asian) are classified as obese and have a 10-fold increased risk of cirrhosis over the general population. Waist size may be even more relevant.

- Liver disease secondary to obesity accounts for one-third of all chronic liver disease in adults in North America.

- Non-alcoholic fatty liver disease (NAFLD) is a spectrum of liver disorders, in order of severity: simple steatosis (fat only), non-alcoholic steatohepatitis (NASH: fat + inflammation ± fibrosis), and cirrhosis.

- The prevalence of NAFLD varies according to ethnicity (greater in Asians than Caucasians) and may cluster in families, which suggests a genetic disposition.

- NAFLD is present in 70% of people who are obese but may also affect lean individuals.

- NAFLD may be associated with obesity, insulin resistance, and hyperlipidemia (in the absence of regular alcohol consumption). These three components are the main elements of the "metabolic syndrome".

- Non-alcoholic steatohepatitis (NASH), which requires liver biopsy for diagnosis, is present in 18.5% of those who are obese. In severely obese individuals (BMI >40), the rate of NASH is 30%, with 2–3% having cirrhosis (if diabetic, 10–25% have cirrhosis).

- NASH is progressive: approximately 30% develop severe fibrosis after 10 years of follow-up. Regression of cirrhosis may occur with sustained weight loss.

- Nevertheless, patients with NASH more often die from coronary heart disease (10%) or extrahepatic malignancy (5%) than from a complication of cirrhosis (2%).

Hepatology: Diagnosis and Clinical Management, First Edition. Edited by E. Jenny Heathcote.
© 2012 John Wiley & Sons, Ltd. Published 2012 by John Wiley & Sons, Ltd.

> **Key points: children**
>
> - NAFLD is the most common chronic liver disease in children in North America.
> - Cirrhosis associated with NAFLD may occur in childhood.
> - The "insulin resistance syndrome" characterizes children with NAFLD. Insulin resistance is probably acquired through an interaction of genetic make-up and environmental factors (diet, lack of exercise, poor sleep habits). The "metabolic syndrome" has not been defined in children.
> - Waist circumference is highly informative for diagnosing NAFLD in children. Most, but not all, children with NAFLD have a BMI in the overweight or obese range for their age/sex.
> - NAFLD must be distinguished from all other causes of fatty liver not associated with hyperinsulinemia/insulin resistance. Wilson disease is an important consideration.
> - Liver biopsy is required for complete diagnosis and helps to eliminate competing diagnoses.
> - No effective pharmacological treatment has been established for children. Dietary intervention with a low-glycemic-index diet and lifestyle changes to incorporate regular exercise are effective in improving the liver disease as weight loss is achieved.

Definition

Non-alcoholic fatty liver disease (NAFLD) denotes a spectrum of liver disorders associated with abnormal insulin action. The spectrum is comprised of simple steatosis (accumulation of large droplets of fat in hepatocytes without inflammation), non-alcoholic steatohepatitis (NASH; accumulation of large droplet fat along with inflammation and/or fibrosis), and the resulting cirrhosis in which steatosis may no longer be obvious. Most people who have NAFLD are overweight or obese.

Liver test abnormalities as a consequence of obesity in the absence of excess alcohol intake are most often due to simple hepatic steatosis, which is usually not associated with advanced liver disease. NASH is a more severe liver disease associated with infiltration of the liver with inflammatory cells and progressive fibrosis. In adults, NASH is more likely to be present in older individuals (>50 years old) with a high body mass index (BMI), type 2 diabetes and elevated aspartate aminotransferase (AST) and/or alanine aminotransferase (ALT) values, although the latter may fall to normal with disease progression.

Pathogenesis

Hyperinsulinemia is essential to the disease mechanism. Insulin resistance is the main feature, which may be a response to sustained hyperinsulinemia. Varying degrees of insulin resistance between the liver and extrahepatic tissues may account for some of the abnormalities in NAFLD. The hepatic response to insulin appears to be more disordered for lipid metabolism than for glucose metabolism. Hyperinsulinemia leads to mobilization of stored lipid (and adipocytokines) from adipose tissue and promotes hepatic steatosis. Free fatty acids (FFA) contribute to the development of hepatic steatosis and liver damage. FFA are highly toxic; they damage intracellular membranes through lipid peroxidation. FFA-mediated damage to mitochondria inhibits α-oxidation of hepatic FFA. Since insulin inhibits oxidation of FFA, hyperinsulinemia may enhance FFA damage to hepatocytes. FFA also activate hepatocellular signaling pathways related to inflammation and apoptosis. Insulin up-regulates hepatocellular SREBP-1c (sterol response element binding protein-1c). With the excess of FFA available, up-regulating SREBP-1c probably generates increased hepatocellular production of triglycerides and very-low-density lipoproteins, and thus the hypertriglyceridemia characteristic of NAFLD. Finally, insulin up-regulates a hepatocellular protein known as suppressor of cytokine signaling (SOCS)-3, which down-regulates hepatocellular insulin receptors. Thus, the hyperinsulinemia itself is capable of promoting acquired insulin resistance in the liver and sustaining a vicious cycle.

The transition from simple steatosis to NASH suggests contribution of additional types of hepatic injury. Possibly, FFA toxicity to hepatocellular organelles accumulates and, additionally, FFA activate various inflammatory or fibrogenic pathways. It is unclear why most obese individuals have simple hepatic steatosis rather than NASH. Oxidant stress, inflammatory cytokines, and low-grade systemic inflammation may play a role. Some inflammatory cytokines may exacerbate hepatocellular insulin resistance and mitochondrial dysfunction. In individuals with NASH the cell injury in the lipid-laden hepatocytes promotes oxidative stress and lipid peroxidation. It has been suggested that the abnormal disposal of hepatic fat in obese individuals is a result of impaired autophagy. Accumulation of fatty acids in hepatocytes promotes endoplasmic reticulum stress, which induces proinflammatory cytokines, which promote the deposition of collagen in the liver causing progression of hepatic fibrosis associated with impaired generation of new hepatocytes.

In children, an important question is how this disease process gets started. It is most likely that over-nutrition and lack of physical exercise lead to critical metabolic changes, which involve sustained hyperinsulinemia and consequently hepatic steatosis. The prevalent "junk-food diet" of developed countries is delicious and fun to eat, and it is high in calories from sugars (notably sucrose and fructose) and saturated fats, and low in antioxidants and fiber. Studies in rodents have demonstrated repeatedly that this kind of diet creates hyperinsulinemia and hepatic steatosis. Children who spend much of their time in front of screens (television, computer, or hand-held games), who are chauffeured from one place to another, or who have no opportunities for sports and safe playgrounds are at risk. Likewise, for reasons not yet clear, children who do not get enough sleep are likely to be overweight/obese with attendant metabolic abnormalities.

Table 17.1 Epidemiology of liver disease related to obesity in adults

Ethnicity	Greatest in Asians, least in African Americans
Prevalence	Responsible for 1/3 of all chronic liver disease in the non-alcoholic in North America
Obesity (BMI > 30 in Caucasians, >27 in Asians)	70% hepatic steatosis, 20% steatohepatitis, rate of cirrhosis unknown
Severe obesity (BMI > 40)	90% steatosis, 30% steatohepatitis (2–3% cirrhosis)
Diabetes (type 2)	75% have hepatic steatosis
Hyperlipidemia	↑ Triglycerides, 60% NAFLD ↑ Cholesterol, 30% NAFLD
Familial	Genetic, also related to common eating habits and exercise pattern

BMI, body mass index; NAFLD, non-alcoholic fatty liver disease.

Genetic predispositions clearly exist, although identification of relevant genes is incomplete. Some of these genes regulate metabolic processes. Some genes may relate to inflammatory injury.

Non-alcoholic fatty liver disease in adults

Epidemiology
The risk of NAFLD in adults correlates with BMI. In those who are obese, simple steatosis can be found in 70% (whereas hepatic steatosis is reported present in liver tissue in 3.5% of individuals with a normal BMI) (Table 17.1). NASH is present in 18.5% of those who are obese, but 2.7% of cases are lean individuals who may have been obese when younger. In those with severe obesity (BMI > 40), typically 60% have simple steatosis, 30% have NASH, and 1% cirrhosis, but the percentage with cirrhosis increases if diabetes is present.

Individuals of Asian origin are at the highest risk of NAFLD whereas African Americans are at least risk. For Hispanics the risk is between that for Asians and African Americans. It is unclear whether familial disease is genetic or related to common eating and exercise habits, but it is obvious that NAFLD is highly influenced by an imbalance between overall calorie consumption and systemic calorie utilization.

Clinical features
As in most with a chronic liver disease, the affected individual remains free of symptoms or signs, although some may have acanthosis nigricans and/or a

> ### Box 17.1 Liver disease in obese adults—tips for history and physical
>
> History
> - Eating pattern (including soft drinks/fruit juice)
> - Exercise pattern
> - Alcohol intake
> - Body weight, current *and* past
> - Family history of liver disease and metabolic syndrome (diabetes)
> - Hirsutism (polycystic ovary syndrome)
>
> Physical examination
> - Body mass index and waist circumference
> - Buffalo hump
> - Acanthosis nigricans
> - Skin stigmata of cirrhosis (unusual)
> - Systemic blood pressure
> - Evidence of peripheral vascular disease
> - Hepatomegaly—texture
> - Splenomegaly (if present check for varices)
> - Ascites, hepatic encephalopathy

buffalo hump (Box 17.1). Thus physicians need to have a high index of suspicion in obese subjects (particularly in those with abdominal obesity), who are physically inactive with or without elevation of serum aminotransferase levels.

Individuals with NAFLD may not be obese at the time of diagnosis; thus it is important to establish prior body weight in all individuals with abnormal liver tests.

Sometimes the individual gives a history of non-specific abdominal pain (often in the right upper quadrant). Associated disorders include systemic hypertension, hyperlipidemia, and type 2 diabetes.

A frequent misunderstanding is that the degree of elevation of the serum aminotransferase values is a guide to the severity of the underlying liver disease. In the setting of probable NAFLD, this misunderstanding compromises diagnosis of this disease. Thus any individual who is overweight, particularly with central obesity, should be a "suspect" for NAFLD and worked up appropriately. Liver enzyme levels may be within the normal range, especially in those with advanced disease.

Before the diagnosis of NAFLD can be made, it is essential to make an in-depth evaluation of both current and past alcohol intake (see Chapter 15). Women are more susceptible to alcohol-mediated liver disease than men. In women, more than 20 g alcohol/day and men more than 30–40 g alcohol/

> **Box 17.2 Disease associations with non-alcoholic fatty liver disease in adults**
>
> - Metabolic syndrome ($\uparrow$ uric acid, $\uparrow$ BP, $\uparrow$ lipids, $\uparrow$ cholesterol)
> - Polycystic ovarian syndrome
> - Sleep apnea

> **Box 17.3 Causes of hepatic steatosis in adults not due to obesity or alcohol use**
>
> - Total parenteral nutrition
> - Drugs: methotrexate, stavudine, didanosine, amiodarone, prednisone, L-asparaginase
> - Toxins (industrial)
> - Kwashiokor
> - Small bowel bacterial overgrowth
> - Genetic diseases: Wilson disease

day may be hepatotoxic regardless of the type of alcohol consumed (see Chapter 8).

Associated disorders in adults

Individuals found to have a fatty liver may also have type 2 diabetes, and 75% of those with type 2 diabetes have a fatty liver. In individuals with elevated serum triglycerides, 60% have a fatty liver whereas only 30% of those with an isolated elevation of serum cholesterol have a fatty liver.

Fatty liver is often associated with systemic hypertension, less often with hyperuricemia, polycystic ovary syndrome, sleep apnea, and small bowel bacterial overgrowth (Box 17.2). Most individuals with a fatty liver will have impaired exercise tolerance, as measured by oxygen consumption during exercise.

Those who have had chemotherapy for blood dyscrasias or other tumors and those who undergo surgery on the pituitary gland may be at an increased risk for developing NAFLD. Whether women with hypothyroidism are at increased risk for NAFLD remains unknown.

Differential diagnosis

The major disease entity in adults is *alcoholic* fatty liver disease. Other causes of hepatic steatosis are intake of specific hepatotoxins, certain medications such as methotrexate, total parenteral nutrition, kwashiokor, and some genetic disorders (Box 17.3).

Reye syndrome and fatty liver of pregnancy are very different; their clinical presentation is highly specific and liver histology shows only microvesicular fat.

Evaluation of liver disease

Severity of liver disease in adults with NAFLD is in part age dependent, cirrhosis being unusual before the age of 50. Not uncommonly, cirrhosis is a chance finding at the time of abdominal surgery. In this situation, volume and/or salt overload postoperatively is a frequent complication, which may precipitate the onset of ascites. Other manifestations of portal hypertension, such as bleeding varices, may be problematic. As is the case with all cirrhotic patients, there is an increased chance of hepatocellular carcinoma (HCC). As both the early detection of HCC using 6-monthly liver ultrasound examinations and its treatment markedly improve survival, it is most important to evaluate the severity of liver disease in everyone suspected of having fatty liver disease.

NASH cannot be diagnosed accurately without a liver biopsy and those at greatest risk of NASH are the elderly and those with very high BMI, type 2 diabetes, or abnormal AST:ALT (ratio > 1).

Laboratory features

Most individuals with NAFLD will have an elevation (often very minimal) in AST and/or ALT values (Box 17.4). Simultaneous measurement of fasting glucose and insulin is used to estimate insulin resistance by employing the HOMA-IR formula, a well-validated surrogate for direct testing of insulin resistance.

HOMA-IR = Fasting insulin (IU/ml)
$\times$ Fasting glucose (mmol/L) divided by 22.5

The HOMA-IR is abnormal in adults if it is greater than 2. Other possible laboratory abnormalities include hypertriglyceridemia, hypercholesterolemia, hyperuricemia, elevated IgA levels, and detectable antinuclear antibody (ANA) in 25–30% of those with NASH.

Box 17.4 Standard laboratory work up in all obese adults

- CBC (low platelet count is a marker of cirrhosis)
- Liver biochemistry AST:ALT ratio; and electrolytes
- Liver function tests: INR, serum albumin, and bilirubin
- Fasting glucose and insulin (to compute HOMA-IR)
- Fasting (12 h) cholesterol and triglycerides
- Serum uric acid
- Ultrasound of the liver (regardless of above results)

Investigations

Although examination of liver tissue is the gold standard, it is clearly not feasible to perform this in everyone thought to have NAFLD! However, in those who are most at risk of progressive liver disease, such as type 2 diabetic patients who are obese, liver biopsy is the preferred test for correct diagnosis if NAFLD is suspected. The new non-invasive tests used to measure degree of hepatic fibrosis are not reliable in obese individuals and do not allow evaluation of the degree of hepatic inflammation.

Any patient with suspected NAFLD and at high risk for cirrhosis requires a thorough preoperative work-up prior to any surgery. It is important to know preoperatively whether cirrhosis is present or not. Numerous precautions are necessary in any patient with cirrhosis of any etiology before, during, and following any surgical intervention so as to prevent postoperative hepatic decompensation with ascites, variceal hemorrhage, and/or hepatic coma (see Chapters 4 and 6).

Natural history

The outcome of patients identified as having a fatty liver obviously depends on the severity of their background liver disease, but even in those with cirrhosis death is more likely to be a consequence of concurrent vascular disease, that is coronary artery disease. Those with simple steatosis have been thought to normally run a benign course. However, these figures are from patients diagnosed with NAFLD 20–30 years ago and may not represent the outcome of those diagnosed with NAFLD in the 21st century simply because the management of coronary artery disease has improved greatly.

Of those found to have NASH without prominent fibrosis on their first liver biopsy, one-third will progress to severe fibrosis, or even cirrhosis, over 5–10 years, particularly those who also have inflammation in the portal tracts. Hepatic failure in those with cirrhosis due to NASH occurs in 17% at 1 year, 23% at 3 years, and 52% at 10 years. Liver failure is frequently precipitated by surgery (see Chapters 5, 6, and 8), particularly if this is abdominal or cardiac. However, bariatric surgery for gross obesity is not necessarily contraindicated as the consequent weight loss can lead to reduction of insulin resistance and diabetes. An additional 10–12% will die (often of other causes) over a 10 to 15-year follow-up. Hepatocellular carcinoma is confined to patients with NASH, usually those with cirrhosis.

Management

The most effective therapy is to institute dietary changes, as well as promote a regular exercise program (Box 17.5). In those who make these changes in lifestyle, a 10–15% weight reduction promotes loss of fat within the liver and will also reduce inflammation and liver cell injury. This is accompanied by a reduction in insulin resistance. Success with this relatively simple intervention lowers both liver and cardiac risk. Most important among the dietary changes

> **Box 17.5 Management of probable non-alcoholic fatty liver disease in the obese adult**
>
> 1 Education regarding food intake (quality and quantity)
> 2 Promote daily exercise of any form (e.g. walking ≥ 10 000 steps/day, although vigorous exercises may be more effective)
> 3 Treat associated metabolic complications
> 4 Refer for sleep study if sleep apnea suspected
> 5 Consider referral for liver biopsy if there is a clinical suspicion of cirrhosis—especially in patients > 50 years old and/or with a low platelet count or prior to anticipated surgical procedure
> 6 Bariatric surgery—only if no cirrhosis present and all other measures fail to reduce weight
> 7 Liver transplantation for hepatic failure and/or HCC (young patients)

is the need to eliminate the intake of concentrated fructose syrup (present in most soft drinks and in many other foods) which increases triglycerides. It remains unproven as to whether increasing the intake of omega-3 fatty acids improves fatty liver. Regular exercise improves glucose disposal in skeletal muscle mitochondria regardless of whether or not the exercise is accompanied by weight loss, hence the term "fit–fat".

Many different drug therapies have been evaluated, none of which has been shown to improve liver histology to the degree seen with dietary changes and regular exercise. Ursodeoxycholic acid is ineffective. Insulin sensitizers, that is thiozolidinediones (pioglitazone), actually promote weight gain and appear to be of little benefit unless accompanied by appropriate dietary changes and increased exercise. Vitamin E may have some benefit. Lipid modulatory drugs, for example fibrates, are promising, whereas the statins have no beneficial effect on liver fat. The only treatment that reliably has an effect of reducing weight and hepatic fat is bariatric surgery, which itself is fraught with complications and thus is infrequently recommended in those with a BMI greater than 40 or those with cirrhosis (only if Child's A). Sleeve gastrectomy rather than Roux-en-y gastric bypass is recommended.

In cirrhotic individuals with liver failure and/or HCC, liver transplantation remains the treatment of choice; however, particularly in those older than 60 years the 1-year survival without liver replacement surgery is only 50%. Rapid recurrence of NAFLD in the graft is usual.

Non-alcoholic fatty liver disease in children

Epidemiology

Since its first description in the early 1980s, NAFLD has become the leading cause of chronic liver disease in children in North America. Childhood obesity is a major worldwide problem. Although there are some issues relating to how to define obesity in children, in general the incidence of childhood obesity has doubled or tripled in the past 20 years in most developed countries, such that approximately one-quarter of all children are either overweight or obese. Similar trends are beginning to be found in countries with rapidly growing economies in Asia and South America.

Children from certain ethnic backgrounds appear to be predisposed to NAFLD. Ethnicities with increased risk include: Hispanics, mainly non-Cuban; Asians, specifically from China, the Philippines, and Japan; and indigenous peoples of North and South America. African Americans seem to have a decreased risk.

Clinical features

Children are usually diagnosed in the preteen years or early adolescence, but toddlers have been found to have NAFLD. NAFLD is usually asymptomatic. Some children complain of non-specific abdominal pain. Children with NAFLD may have asymptomatic elevations of serum aminotransferases. Jaundice is extremely rare.

The vast majority of children with NAFLD are overweight or obese, but a few, in the order of 10–15%, have a normal BMI for their age/gender. It is critically important to use pediatric BMI reference values, which have been adjusted for age/gender, since the adult thresholds for overweight and obesity per BMI do not apply to children. In fact, through childhood the BMI curve is biphasic. BMI does not evaluate visceral adiposity. Waist circumference (WC) provides useful additional diagnostic information. Children with NAFLD almost universally have an abnormally large WC. Again, reference values for age/gender need to be consulted. Alternatively, the waist/height ratio (should be <0.5 for all ages and genders) can be used.

Physical examination may reveal acanthosis nigricans affecting the neck, axillae, or knuckles. Hepatomegaly may be mildly tender. Splenomegaly is rare.

Though asymptomatic, most children with NAFLD have hepatic steatosis severe enough to be detected by imaging. Indeed many children are referred for assessment because of a "bright liver" detected when abdominal sonography has been performed for some other indication.

Associated disorders

Some children with NAFLD have type 2 diabetes mellitus, which is becoming highly prevalent in the pediatric age bracket. The typical child with NAFLD has hyperinsulinemia with insulin resistance but is euglycemic. Hepatic steatosis with glycogenosis has also been described in some children with type 1 diabetes mellitus (Mauriac syndrome), but whether this is the same as NAFLD is debatable.

Children with congenital disorders of hypothalamic function or acquired hypothalamic dysfunction after surgery (most commonly craniopharyngioma resection) are hyperphagic and at risk for NAFLD with rapid development of cirrhosis.

Any child who is a survivor of childhood neoplasia, for example acute lymphoblastic leukemia, appears to be at increased risk of obesity and the metabolic derangements associated with NAFLD. Chemotherapy may play a role in the development of this hepatic complication.

Various rare genetic disorders involve dysregulation of insulin action. Details of disease mechanism distinguish these disorders from typical childhood NAFLD, but clinically they are very similar. These diseases include: Bardet–Biedl syndrome, Alström syndrome, polycystic ovary syndrome (PCOS), the various lipodystrophy syndromes despite absence of obesity, Turner syndrome, and Dorfman–Chanarin syndrome.

Differential diagnosis

NAFLD must be distinguished from hepatic disorders characterized by hepatic steatosis (with or without inflammation, fibrosis, or actual cirrhosis) but not due to dysregulated insulin action (Box 17.6). Simply having hepatic steatosis is not the same as having NAFLD. Unlike adults, where the major differentiation is from alcohol-associated liver disease, in children most of these disorders are metabolic. Drug-induced liver injury may be present, and some children abuse alcohol. A secondary issue is to identify other causes of liver disease in children who happen to be overweight or obese; this is an emerging problem and usually arises when a child is found to have elevated serum aminotransferases.

In terms of genetic diseases that may present with fatty liver, cystic fibrosis and Wilson disease are at the top of the list in terms of urgency for diagnosis. Hepatic steatosis is extremely common with both cystic fibrosis and Wilson disease; treatment is entirely different from that for NAFLD. It is essential to make these diagnoses as soon as possible for best clinical outcome. In East Asians, type 2 citrullinemia is important because treatment involves specific dietary restrictions.

Box 17.6 Differential diagnosis of fatty liver (macrovesicular steatosis) in children

Acquired dysregulated insulin action: non-alcoholic fatty liver disease
Inherited metabolic disorders with dysregulated insulin action:
  Bardet–Biedl syndrome
  Alström syndrome
  Polycystic ovary syndrome
  Lipodystrophy syndromes

Inherited metabolic disorders:
  Cystic fibrosis
  Wilson disease
  α_1-antitrypsin deficiency
  Hereditary tyrosinemia, type I
  Homocystinuria
  Galactosemia
  Hereditary fructose intolerance
  Glycogen storage diseases (mainly types I, VI)
  Sialidosis, mannosidosis, fucosidosis
  Refsum disease
  Abeta- or hypobetalipoproteinemia
  Neutral lipid storage disease
  Cholesterol ester storage disease
  Dorfman–Chanarin syndrome
  Tangier disease
  Familial hyperlipoproteinemias
  Citrullinemia type 2
  Systemic carnitine deficiency (usually microvesicular fat)
  Weber–Christian disease
  Chronic granulomatous disease
  Porphyria cutanea tarda
  Schwachman syndrome (pancreatic insufficiency)
Systemic disease:
  Chronic hepatitis C
  Celiac disease
  Inflammatory bowel disease
  Diabetes mellitus
  Nephrotic syndrome
Nutritional:
  Hyperphagic disorders (congenital or acquired disorders of hypothalamus)
  Jejunoileal bypass; gastric reduction operations
  Dehydration, severe infection
  Acute starvation
  Protein–calorie malnutrition (kwashiorkor)
  Total parenteral nutrition
Drugs:
  Amiodarone
  Methotrexate
  Prednisone/glucocorticoids
  L-asparaginase
  Vitamin A (in excess)
  Ethanol

Some patients with chronic hepatitis C, particularly those infected with genotype 3, develop insulin resistance and thus may have a fatty liver disorder, which is closely related to NAFLD. Chronic hepatitis B needs to be excluded as a cause of abnormal serum aminotransferases, but it may coincide with NAFLD.

Evaluation of liver disease

The vast majority of children with NAFLD have only simple steatosis. A few already have cirrhosis and portal hypertension. Clearly, these children are at risk for the major complications of severe chronic liver disease. Approximately 10% of children with NASH will develop cirrhosis; thus, evaluation of liver disease is aimed toward identifying those at the severe end of the disease spectrum. Simple indices have been proposed to identify those children with more advanced disease (Box 17.7). Children with NASH are candidates for drug treatment; those with NAFLD-related cirrhosis require close medical supervision.

Particularly in the pediatric age bracket, it is not acceptable to dismiss simple steatosis as benign. Studies in children suggest that 1–2% of these children will

---

Box 17.7 Criteria for prompt liver biopsy in children with fatty liver

Inconclusive diagnostic process:

Features highly consistent with autoimmune hepatitis (↑IgG; specific autoantibodies associated with type 2 AIH; high-titer ANA or SMA in type 1 AIH)

Non-diagnostic results from biochemical tests relating to Wilson disease

Absence of pathophysiological profile (↑WC; ↑HOMA-IR; dyslipidemia) of NAFLD

Features of potentially severe NAFLD:

Young age (<10 years old)

Hepatosplenomegaly

Thrombocytopenia

Extremely elevated serum AST or ALT (10–20 × ULN)

Very severe insulin resistance (by HOMA-IR) (>6.3)

Hypothalamic disorder

Family history of severe NAFLD

Other:

Comorbid liver diseases such as chronic viral hepatitis B or C, or α_1-antitrypsin deficiency

Planned pharmacological intervention for NAFLD

AIH, autoimmune hepatitis; ALT, alanine aminotransferase; ANA, antinuclear antibody; AST, aspartate aminotransferase; NAFLD, non-alcoholic fatty liver disease; SMA, smooth muscle antibody; ULN, upper limit of normal; WC, waist circumference.

eventually develop cirrhosis. Children with fatty liver severe enough to be evident on liver sonography require evaluation for diseases besides NAFLD. If they have NAFLD, they require early intervention (with dietary/lifestyle treatments) to reverse the liver disorder.

Laboratory features

Mild elevations of serum aminotransferases are often present. There is no reliable correspondence between AST/ALT abnormalities and the presence or absence of inflammation. As in adults, most children have dyslipidemia, more often hypertriglyceridemia than hypercholesterolemia. Insulin resistance should be established by the HOMA-IR test, which requires simultaneous measurement of fasting glucose and fasting insulin. The HOMA-IR has been validated in children but the cut-off for children is 3.15, somewhat higher than that for adults. Most children with NAFLD are euglycemic.

The definition of the "metabolic syndrome" has not been standardized for children, and thus it cannot be used as part of the laboratory evaluation of NAFLD in children. Finding evidence for an "insulin resistance syndrome" has the same physiological impact as diagnosing the metabolic syndrome in an adult.

Investigations

Hepatic steatosis must be identified through imaging. Sonography is the usual modality, although it is somewhat insensitive. Approximately 40% of hepatocytes must contain appreciable fat for the liver to look fatty by ultrasound examination. CT scan can be used but it requires too much radiation to be practical. MR imaging is highly sensitive; it avoids the radiation problem but it can be quite unpleasant for a child to undergo the test. Magnetic resonance spectroscopy (MRS) testing is a new technique for measuring hepatic fat; it is relatively easy to perform, well-tolerated, and suitable for sequential studies. Unfortunately, it remains a research tool at the current time.

The complete diagnosis of NAFLD requires a liver biopsy. Imaging methods do not assess fibrosis. Elastography, a non-invasive procedure for measuring liver stiffness, is not validated for childhood NAFLD. Liver biopsy stages the severity of fibrosis and permits assessment of inflammation; it provides data to eliminate some of the competing diagnoses. Liver biopsy involves risk and discomfort for the patient. Consequently, expert opinion is divided as to whether it must be performed in every child who appears to have NAFLD. Patients whose diagnosis of NAFLD is not secure and those who are at risk for severe disease require early liver biopsy. Criteria for triaging a child with fatty liver disease to prompt liver biopsy are given in Box 17.7.

Children with NASH typically have a different histological picture than adults with NASH. Instead of findings that closely resemble alcoholic hepatitis, childhood NASH displays little ballooning of hepatocytes, Mallory–Denk bodies, or polymorphonuclear leukocytes in the inflammatory infiltrate. Macrovesicular steatosis may be severe. The inflammatory infiltrate is mostly with chronic inflammatory cells, and it may be subtle. Fibrosis is often present but tends to be periportal. The reason for this different histological pattern remains uncertain.

Natural history

Obese children tend to remain obese as adults. Children with severe disease in the NAFLD spectrum appear to progress: NASH may progress to cirrhosis and NAFLD-related cirrhosis can progress to end-stage liver disease. Liver transplantation is problematic because NAFLD recurs in the graft, and the rate of progression in the liver graft may be more rapid than it had been in the native liver. NAFLD predisposes to hepatocellular carcinoma.

If 1–2% of children with simple steatosis eventually develop cirrhosis, then statistically we may expect up to 20000 new cirrhotic patients, probably as adults, for every 1 million children with NAFLD as simple steatosis in childhood.

Studies are already showing that children with NAFLD are at increased risk for cardiovascular disease. Primary systemic hypertension is becoming more prevalent in childhood due to obesity. Obese children also are at increased risk for sleep apnea and its complications, degenerative joint disease, and suffer a social disadvantage (notably, bullying).

Therapy

Studies in pediatric clinics have shown that treatment is most effective when it is provided by a multidisciplinary management team to deal with the diverse aspects of this disorder (medical, endocrinological, dietary, psychosocial). Treatment is directed towards management of obesity, insulin resistance, or reducing oxidative stress. For those with more advanced disease, treatment is also aimed at hepatic complications.

The only treatment that has been demonstrated as effective in childhood NAFLD is the treatment of obesity by weight loss. Reduction in body weight was associated with normalization of serum aminotransferases in several clinical series; substantial improvement in liver histology has been reported. Although caloric restriction is generally used, redesigning the diet so that it has a low glycemic index may be more effective. The point of this diet is to avoid postprandial hyperinsulinemia. It involves inclusion of fruits, vegetables, legumes, whole-grain or high fiber, or traditionally processed grains and pasta, and exclusion or limited consumption of white potatoes, sugar (sucrose) including all soft drinks, and highly refined white flour, as well as avoidance of foods high in saturated or trans fats. Regular physical exercise is important for reducing postprandial hyperinsulinemia and for giving the child a further measure of control. Family-based behavioral intervention may also enhance overall success.

At the present time, no drug treatment has been shown conclusively to be effective for children with NAFLD. Metformin showed efficacy in a small study of adolescents, and it is used routinely in children with type 2 diabetes mellitus or polycystic ovary syndrome. A multicenter, randomized, controlled trial in pediatric NAFLD is underway. Vitamin E (800 IU/day of natural vitamin) may be effective although studies to date in children are mainly unconvincing. For children with morbid obesity and NAFLD, bariatric surgery may be effective; however, the long-term complications of bariatric surgery performed in childhood are unknown.

It is evident that primary prevention through education and early intervention are important in dealing with NAFLD in children, and effective public health measures need to be developed urgently.

Case study 17.1

A 55-year-old woman, at the time of her annual check up with her family physician, is found to have mild elevation of her serum aminotransferase values (ALT ranging from 55–85 IU/L (ULN 30 IU/L) which persisted over the next few months. She was asked to abstain from all alcoholic beverages (she used to have a glass of wine with dinner most nights). She was referred to a gastroenterologist who saw her and noted a waist circumference of 99 cm, firm hepatomegaly, no splenomegaly, BMI above 30. She stated she had been abstinent from all alcohol for the last 6 months. However, her ALT values remained elevated. Testing for hepatitis B and C was negative. Other blood tests showed a normal CBC, elevated triglycerides, normal fasting glucose but elevated HbA1C. Both her mother and older sister are diabetics treated with oral agents. Her iron studies were normal.

In view of her obesity, the patient was advised to increase her exercise by walking or cycling on a daily basis and reducing her fat and carbohydrate intake (including cessation of all soft drinks). However, no change in weight could be achieved. Rather, she became heavier and in 2 years time was given a diagnosis of diabetes, which required treatment with oral agents. She began to complain of vague RUQ pain and an ultrasound of her abdomen showed her to have gallstones and a fatty liver. She underwent surgical removal of her gallstones and at the time of surgery the surgeon noted cirrhosis—no liver biopsy was taken! The RUQ pain did not resolve following cholecystectomy. She returned to her family physician who, because of the finding of cirrhosis, arranged a screening ultrasound 6-monthly due to the increased risk of HCC in all cirrhotic patients. However, after a few years the ultrasound screening was "forgotten" until she presented to the Emergency Room with an UGI hemorrhage, shown to be due to bleeding varices—the latter were banded successfully. Ultrasound done at the time showed a probable HCC invading the main portal vein. This tumor was not thought amenable to surgery and she was considered an unsuitable liver transplant candidate as her tumor had spread outside her liver. She died a month later following a massive UGI hemorrhage.

Case study 17.2

Mike is a 12-year-old boy who is referred for evaluation of abnormal liver biochemistries. His GP checked these tests because Mike's mother had just been found to have chronic hepatitis B. Mike was negative for HBsAg and anti-HBc but his AST was 110 IU/L and ALT 98 IU/L. Mike feels well. He gets teased about being chubby and does not play sports. He is really good at computer games and likes to chat with his friends on Facebook after school. His medical history is notable for lactose intolerance; both parents and one aunt have type 2 diabetes mellitus. His mother says that Mike's diet is just the normal one for his age but she does mention that he drinks two to three cans of soft drink daily since he cannot drink milk. On examination Mike is a healthy looking East Asian male who appears obese. BMI is 26 (obese range for age/gender); waist circumference is 99 cm (39 inches). Acanthosis nigricans is evident around the neck. Abdominal exam reveals obesity but neither liver nor spleen is palpable. Fasting blood work reveals a normal blood glucose, elevated serum triglycerides (1.9 mmol/L), elevated fasting insulin with HOMA-IR = 4.4.

Hepatic sonogram shows a bright liver with focal fatty sparing. Liver biopsy shows extensive macrovesicular steatosis with delicate periportal fibrosis and focal chronic inflammatory infiltrates.

You discuss the diagnosis of NAFLD with Mike and his parents. Your first task is to convince them that this is an actual medical problem and that he will not simply outgrow it. Then you give Mike very simple instructions relating to a low-glycemic index diet (but you do not call it a "diet") and ask him to keep an exercise calendar to record 30–60 minutes of exercise each day. Over the next few months of regular follow-up, Mike's weight is lower and he feels better. He is proud of his achievement, and you congratulate him liberally on his healthy lifestyle. With continued surveillance and support, he maintains this improvement. Serum aminotransferases normalize and follow-up liver sonogram is no longer diagnostic of fatty liver.

Multiple choice questions

1. Which statement is correct?
   A. All those with fatty liver disease are either overweight or obese.
   B. "Inactive" cirrhosis may have been due to prior fatty liver disease.
   C. Specific therapies have been shown to be effective in fatty liver disease.
   D. Fatty liver disease is highest in African Americans.

2. Non-alcoholic fatty liver disease in children is:
   A. A "non-problem" because few children are cirrhotic
   B. Uncommon in childhood
   C. Limited to a few ethnic groups
   D. Associated with insulin resistance and various complications of obesity such as cardiovascular disease and sleep apnea
   E. Likely to exacerbate psychological disorders associated with disturbed body image

Answers

1. B
2. D

Further reading

Adams LA, Lymp JF, St Sauver J, et al. The natural history of nonalcoholic fatty liver disease: a population-based cohort study. Gastroenterology 2005; 129: 113–21.

Aithal GP, Thomas JA, Kaye PV, et al. Randomized, placebo-controlled trial of pioglitazone in nondiabetic subjects with nonalcoholic steatohepatitis. Gastroenterology 2008; 135: 1176–84.

Brunt EM, Janney CG, Di Bisceglie AM, et al. Nonalcoholic steatohepatitis: A proposal for grading and staging the histologic lesions. Am J Gastroenterol 1999; 94: 2467–74.

Dixon JB, Bhathal PS, O'Brien PE. Nonalcoholic fatty liver disease: predictors of nonalcoholic steatohepatitis and liver fibrosis in the severely obese. Gastroenterology 2001; 121: 91–100.

Harrison SA, Fecht W, Brunt EM, et al. Orlistat for overweight subjects with nonalcoholic steatohepatitis: A randomized, prospective trial. Hepatology 2009; 49: 80–6.

Harrison SA, Torgerson S, Hayashi P, et al. Vitamin E and vitamin C treatment improves fibrosis in patients with nonalcoholic steatohepatitis. Am J Gastroenterol 2003; 98: 2485–90.

Harrison SA, Torgerson S, Hayashi PH. The natural history of nonalcoholic fatty liver disease. A clinical histopathological study. Am J Gastroenterol 2003; 98: 2042–7.

Johnson NA, Sachinwalla T, Walton DW, et al. Aerobic exercise training reduces hepatic and visceral lipids in obese individuals without weight loss. Hepatology 2009; 50: 1105–12.

Keskin M, Kurtoglu S, Kendirci M, et al. Homeostasis model assessment is more reliable than the fasting glucose/insulin ratio and quantitative insulin sensitivity check index for assessing insulin resistance among obese children and adolescents. Pediatrics 2005; 115: e500–3.

Lindor KD, Kowdley KV, Heathcote EJ, et al. Ursodeoxycholic acid for treatment of nonalcoholic steatohepatitis: results of a randomized trial. Hepatology 2004; 39: 770–8.

Loomba R, Sirlin CB, Schwimmer JB, et al. Advances in pediatric nonalcoholic fatty liver disease. Hepatology 2009; 50: 1282–93.

Mager DR, Patterson C, So S, et al. A prospective study of metabolic and dietary characteristics in children with NAFLD. Eur J Clin Nutr 2010; 64: 628–35.

Maheshwari A, Thuluvath JP. Cryptogenic cirrhosis and NAFLD: Are they related? Am J Gastroenterol 2006; 101: 664–8.

Malik SM, deVera ME, Fontes P, et al. Outcome after liver transplantation for NASH cirrhosis. Am J Transplant 2009; 9: 782–93.

Manchesini G, Bugianesi E, Forlani G, et al. Nonalcoholic fatty liver, steatohepatitis and the metabolic syndrome. Hepatology 2003; 37: 917–23.

Manco M, Bedogni G, Marcellini M, et al. Waist circumference correlates with liver fibrosis in children with non-alcoholic steatohepatitis. Gut 2008; 57: 1283–7.

Nelson A, Torres DM, Morgan AE, et al. A pilot study using simvastatin in the treatment of nonalcoholic steatohepatitis: a randomized placebo-controlled trial. J Clin Gastroenterol 2009; 43: 990–4.

Roberts EA. Pediatric nonalcoholic fatty liver disease (NAFLD): a "growing" problem? J Hepatol 2007; 46: 1133–42.

Sacks FM, Bray GA, Carey VJ, et al. Comparison of weight-loss diets with different compositions of fat, protein, and carbohydrates. N Engl J Med 2009; 360: 859–73.

Sanyal AJ, Campbell-Sargent C, Mirshahi F, et al. Nonalcoholic steatohepatitis: association of insulin resistance and mitochondrial abnormalities. Gastroenterology 2001; 120: 1183–92.

Schwimmer JB, Behling C, Newbury R, et al. Histopathology of pediatric nonalcoholic fatty liver disease. Hepatology 2005; 42: 641–9.

Schwimmer JB, Celedon MA, Lavine JE, et al. Heritability of nonalcoholic fatty liver disease. Gastroenterology 2009; 136: 1585–92.

Schwimmer JB, Deutsch R, Rauch JB, et al. Obesity, insulin resistance, and other clinico-pathological correlates of pediatric nonalcoholic fatty liver disease. J Pediatr 2003; 143: 500–5.

Schwimmer JB, Pardee PE, Lavine JE, et al. Cardiovascular risk factors and the metabolic syndrome in pediatric nonalcoholic fatty liver disease. Circulation 2008; 118: 277–83.

St George A, Bauman A, Johnston A, et al. Steatohepatitis and metabolic liver disease. The independent effects of physical activity in patients with non-alcoholic fatty liver disease. Hepatology 2009; 50: 68–76.

van der Poorten D, Milner KL, Hui J, et al. Visceral fat: a key mediator of steatohepatitis in metabolic liver disease. Hepatology 2008; 48: 449–57.

Vanni E, Bugianesi E. The gut-liver axis in nonalcoholic fatty liver disease: Another pathway to insulin resistance? Hepatology 2009; 49: 1790–2.

HIV-associated liver diseases

CHAPTER 18

David K.H. Wong

University of Toronto, and Division of Gastroenterology, Toronto Western Hospital, University Health Network, Toronto, Ontario, Canada

Key points

- Everyone infected with human immunodeficiency virus (HIV) should be screened for hepatitis B and hepatitis C as all three viruses share routes of infection.
- Anyone with liver disease should be assessed (at least annually) for both activity of the liver disease and severity of underlying liver fibrosis, ideally using non-invasive methods to determine the presence of cirrhosis.
- Individuals with HIV and liver disease should ideally be cared for in settings with expertise in both HIV and liver disease.

Introduction

The natural history of HIV/AIDS has evolved rapidly from the inevitable death sentence of the 1980s and early 1990s to a chronic infection that can be controlled through the use of combination antiretroviral therapy (cART). In the late 1990s, combination therapy was chosen from the drug classes of nucleoside/nucleotide reverse transcriptase inhibitors (NRTI), non-nucleoside reverse transcriptase inhibitors (NNRTI), and protease inhibitors (PI). In 2011, additional classes of drugs became available, such as fusion inhibitors, entry inhibitors, and integrase inhibitors.[1] The ability to target the HIV virus at so many sites of replication means that it is possible to completely suppress HIV replication in the large majority of infected individuals. The challenge of medication adherence remains. Fortunately, this is less problematic as the pill burden has decreased with the development of new drug formulations, allowing single-pill combination therapy and once-daily dosing regimens, as well as development of medications that minimize side effects. With HIV controlled, the major cause of mortality in those with HIV infection is now liver disease.[2]

Hepatology: Diagnosis and Clinical Management, First Edition. Edited by E. Jenny Heathcote.
© 2012 John Wiley & Sons, Ltd. Published 2012 by John Wiley & Sons, Ltd.

The evaluation of liver disease in HIV is difficult as the cause is frequently multifactorial even if the injuring agent was stopped many years in the past. There are many theories about mechanisms of liver injury in HIV but there is rarely the accompanying proof of the mechanism in the published literature. For example, a thorough history of alcohol consumption is almost never available in publications about other causes of liver disease. Everyone with HIV infection should be screened for hepatitis B and hepatitis C infection as all three viruses share common routes of infection (Fig. 18.1a and b). Everyone with risk

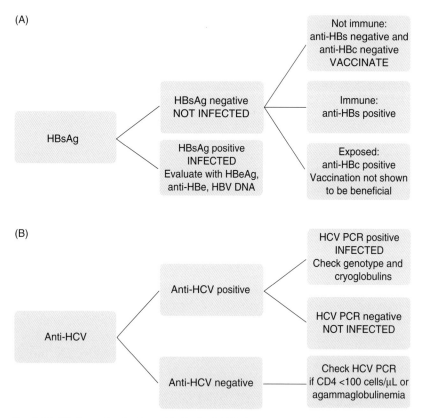

Fig. 18.1 (A) Screening for hepatitis B: check HBsAg, anti-HBs, IgG anti-HBc. (B) Screening for hepatitis C: check anti-HCV, confirm with HCV PCR. Everyone with HIV should be screened for hepatitis B (HBsAg, anti-HBs, anti-HBc) and hepatitis C (anti-HCV). Those who remain susceptible to HBV infection (HBsAg negative, anti-HBs negative, and anti-HBc negative) should be vaccinated. Many with HIV have been previously exposed to hepatitis B (anti-HBc positive) and it is unclear if they will benefit from vaccination. In those not currently infected and yet have behaviors associated with high risk of infection (multiple sexual partners, injection drug use), HBsAg and anti-HCV should be checked annually and whenever new ALT/AST elevation is observed.

behaviors that put them at risk for hepatitis B virus (HBV) infection should be vaccinated. Arguably, screening should be done annually in those with ongoing high-risk behaviors for acquiring viral hepatitis. Hepatitis B testing and characterization for HBV activity with HBeAg (hepatitis B e antigen) status and HBV DNA viral load is rarely done in most centers as part of routine HIV care. Mitochondrial toxicity is postulated as a cause of liver disease in those with HIV on antiretroviral therapy but tests of mitochondrial function or electron microscopic studies of liver tissue for mitochondrial morphology are almost never done. Immune reconstitution inflammatory syndrome (IRIS) is postulated but other factors such as rebounding hepatitis B, C, or D viremia suggesting viral reactivation are not routinely excluded. Thus, the approach to evaluating the liver of the individual must be a systematic approach with good communication between the hepatologist and the HIV specialist.

Evaluation of HIV

Components of the evaluation of HIV infection are:
- year of HIV diagnosis and route of acquisition;
- CD4 nadir (lowest count) and current CD4;
- HIV viral load;
- medication history, noting especially:
  ○ years of exposure to the D drugs: ddC (dideoxycytidine (Zalcitabine), an HIV-specific NRTI, FDA approved in 1992, no longer marketed), ddI (dideoxyinosine, an HIV-specific NRTI, FDA approved in 1991), d4T (stavudine (Zerit) an HIV-specific NRTI, FDA approved in 1994), as well as AZT (zidovudine, an HIV-specific NRTI, FDA approved in 1987)
  ○ prior exposure to 3TC (lamivudine (Epivir), an HBV- and HIV-specific NRTI, FDA approved for HIV in 1995 and for HBV in 1998) when HBV infection may have been present, and so probability of 3TC-resistant HBV is high
  ○ ATV (atazanavir (Reyataz) an HIV-specific PI) can dramatically raise the indirect (unconjugated) bilirubin without liver injury

The HIV history is important to the overall evaluation of an individual infected with HIV who has liver disease. The year of HIV diagnosis and route of acquisition is not only informative for assessment of risk behaviors, which may put them at ongoing risk for viral hepatitis, but it may give insight into how these individuals may react to any proposed therapy. For example, those with ongoing injection drug use may not place a high priority to antiviral therapies that may have a lot of side effects. Those who survived HIV infection in the 1990s and were exposed to many of the early HIV medications may be skeptical about unproven therapies. The CD4 count for HIV is similar to the degree of liver fibrosis for liver disease—both are measures of disease severity and markers for increased risk of complications once certain CD4 count thresholds are reached. Uncontrolled HIV infection leads to falling CD4 counts that are associated with increased risk of death once they fall below a certain threshold. The threshold for initiating HIV therapy has been a moving target but once below 200 cells/μL, the risk of opportunistic infections rises to the point that prophylactic antibiotics (sulfamethoxazole plus trimethoprim) are indicated. It is important to record the nadir CD4 count (the lowest recorded CD4) since the CD4 will rise with HIV suppressive therapy but if therapy is interrupted, the CD4 will rapidly fall to the nadir within a few months. The HIV viral load should be negative in the majority who are on effective cART. A detectable viral load suggests treatment failure due to poor adherence and/or drug resistance. The complete HIV medication history is important in several ways. The duration of exposure to "D drugs" (ddC, ddI, d4T) and perhaps long-term use of AZT may have led to mitochondrial injury and predispose patients to nodular regenerative hyperplasia, a form of non-cirrhotic portal hypertension. Atazanavir raises the indirect (unconjugated) fraction of bilirubin, which does not seem to be associated with liver injury. Any medication started within the last 12 months should be noted as it may be responsible for an idiosyncratic liver injury.

Assessing and managing liver disease

Liver disease in those with HIV is a broad field. Although this chapter touches on the common liver diseases in those with HIV, the reader is referred to other chapters in this book for more detailed information if required. The approach to the assessment of liver disease can be summarized in the following five steps:
1 Establish the diagnosis (Box 18.1)
2 Determine the activity or pace of liver injury (Box 18.2)
3 Determine the severity of liver fibrosis (Box 18.3). If cirrhosis is present, determine the severity of cirrhosis.
4 Treat the underlying cause of liver disease to prevent ongoing liver injury (Box 18.4)
5 Manage the complications of cirrhosis (Box 18.5)

Viral hepatitis—hepatitis C

Hepatitis C virus (HCV) coinfection is a major cause of morbidity and mortality in those with HIV infection. HCV is a curable infection but the cure is imperfect, both in terms of efficacy and side effects. Although it is ideal to cure HCV infection in those with the most severe liver disease, it is not feasible to treat the sickest patients with the currently available therapies. Hepatitis C treatment is risky in those with cirrhosis and mild liver dysfunction, as frank liver failure can develop during therapy. Early studies showed that though therapy with the current standard of pegylated interferon-α_{2a} 180μg or pegylated interferon-α_{2b} 1.5μg/kg in combination with lower-dose ribavirin 800mg/day × 48 weeks could cure HCV infection, the sustained virological response (SVR) was lower than that observed in those with HCV without HIV infection: 14–29% for HCV genotype 1 and 43–62% for HCV genotype 2 and 3. When

Box 18.1 Differential diagnosis of hepatitis

1 Viral hepatitis
  a. Hepatitis A (IgM anti-HAV)
  b. Hepatitis B (HBsAg)
    (i) IgM anti-HBc is positive in acute HBV infection but can also be positive in chronic HBV infection during a severe ALT flare
  c. Hepatitis C (anti-HCV, HCV PCR if anti-HCV may be falsely negative, such as in acute HCV infection <12 weeks after infection, CD4 very low <100 cells/μL, agammaglobulinemia)
  d. Hepatitis D (IgG anti-HDV)
2 Fatty liver
  a. Alcohol history (Did you ever, in your life, drink alcohol on a daily basis? When was the last time you had an alcoholic beverage?—many people "quit" a few days before seeing a doctor)
  b. Metabolic syndrome (diabetes, dyslipidemia, central obesity, rapid weight changes)
    (i) Recognize that a simple prescription of diet and exercise almost always fails in the long run
    (ii) Assess for factors that contribute to weight gain
      (1) Medications (glitazones for diabetes, antidepressants, antipsychotics, steroids, etc.)
      (2) Musculoskeletal injuries that may limit mobility
      (3) Medical conditions (hypothyroid, depression)
      (4) Behavioral (what social situations lead to over-eating)
  c. Medications (ddC > ddI > d4T > AZT, estrogens, androgens)
3 Drug induced liver injury (DILI)
  a. Careful medication history, paying particular attention to when medications were started
    (i) Drugs used for HIV
    (ii) Drugs used for non-HIV conditions
    (iii) Complementary and alternative medicines, other non-prescribed medicines

Box 18.2 How active is the hepatitis?

1 The height of the ALT/AST is an imperfect reflection of the pace of liver injury. However, it is probably true that if the ALT/AST <100, the pace of injury is not rapid whereas if ALT/AST >>200, the pace of injury is probably faster.
2 Viral load testing
  a. Hepatitis B is unlikely to be active if the HBV DNA viral load <1000 IU/mL. However, it may still be inactive if the viral load is very high >100 000 000 IU/mL

(Continued)

(>1E8 IU/mL). To date, the only definitive test to determine if HBV is active is if ALT normalizes when HBV viral load is fully suppressed. Conversely, if HBV viral load is fully suppressed and yet ALT remains abnormal, HBV is unlikely to be the cause of the ongoing hepatitis.

b. Hepatitis C has resolved (not active) if HCV RNA viral load is undetectable when not on any HCV-active therapy. Anti-HCV usually remains detectable after resolution of infection and cannot be used to diagnosis reinfection with hepatitis C. If ALT becomes persistently elevated again in the future, a positive HCV PCR test confirms reinfection.

c. Hepatitis D is similar to hepatitis C in that infection is resolved if HDV viral load is negative when not on HDV-active therapy.

Box 18.3 How severe is the liver damage: is there cirrhosis?

1 How severe is the degree of fibrosis—is there cirrhosis?
   a. Liver biopsy
   b. Non-invasive markers of liver fibrosis (see Chapter 2)
      (i) Serum markers
      (ii) Elastography (stiffness) based tests
   c. Imaging characteristics (see Chapter 26)
      (i) Surface of the liver is nodular
      (ii) Lobar redistribution: left lobe enlarges while right lobe shrinks
2 How severe is the cirrhosis?
   a. Portal hypertension
      (i) Hypersplenism (platelets <150 × 10^9/L, leukopenia), splenomegaly
      (ii) Distended portal vein, patent umbilical vein
      (iii) Esophageal/gastric/rectal varices
      (iv) Ascites (usually if albumin <30 g/L)
   b. Impaired liver synthesis
      (i) INR elevated (all factors low except factor VIII)
      (ii) Albumin low <35 g/L
   c. Impaired excretion
      (i) Jaundice (elevated direct/conjugated bilirubin)
   d. Encephalopathy
   e. Common tools for assessing severity of cirrhosis
      (i) Model for End-stage Liver Disease (MELD): uses INR, bilirubin, creatinine
      (ii) Child–Pugh–Turcotte: uses INR, albumin, bilirubin, ascites, encephalopathy

---

Box 18.4 Management of hepatitis

Establish a diagnosis for cause(s) of ongoing active liver injury
1 Hepatitis B:
  a. First line = 3TC/FTC–tenofovir backbone for HIV therapy
  b. Alternatives are generally suboptimal
    (i) Entecavir: high risk of resistance and treatment failure if pre-existing M204V/I from prior 3TC. Entecavir monotherapy has been reported to cause M184V mutation in HIV
    (ii) Adefovir: less potent than tenofovir and so HBV may not be fully suppressed, leading to long-term risk for resistance. There is concern that adefovir monotherapy may result in tenofovir resistance for HIV but, to date, this has not been reported
    (iii) Interferon: poor efficacy in HIV coinfection
2 Hepatitis C:
  a. Therapy to 2011: pegylated interferon-α_{2a} 180 µg weekly or pegylated interferon-α_{2b} 1.5 µg/kg in combination with ribavirin 13–15 mg/kg daily
    (i) Efficacy in HCV genotype 1: 14–29%
    (ii) Efficacy in HCV genotype 2: 43–62%
    (iii) HIV drugs to avoid during HCV therapy
      (1) DDI, D4T: risk of liver failure in those with cirrhosis
      (2) AZT: severe anemia during treatment
  b. Future: likely addition of HCV-specific protease inhibitor by 2012, many other classes of antiviral agents by 2014
3 Fatty liver:
  a. Stop alcohol
  b. Stop drugs that may be contributing to fatty liver
    (i) ddC, ddI, d4T
    (ii) AZT
  c. Treatment of metabolic syndrome
    (i) Weight loss program
    (ii) Lipid lowering agents are *not* contraindicated and are generally safe
4 DILI:
  a. Stop the offending drug

---

weight-based ribavirin dosing (800 mg–1200 mg) was used, SVR improved to 36–39% for HCV genotype 1 and 53–73% for HCV genotype 2 and 3.[3]

Given the importance of dosing, the main focus of treating HCV in HIV has become management of interferon–ribavirin associated side effects. The most prominent side effect is anemia, due to ribavirin-induced hemolysis and interferon-induced marrow suppression. Concomitant use of AZT during HCV therapy can lead to profound anemia and so AZT (also found in Combivir

---

Box 18.5 Management of cirrhosis

1 Gastroscopy to look for esophageal varices
   a. Repeat every 2–3 years if no varices
   b. Repeat every 1–2 years if small varices
   c. Prophylaxis with non-selective beta-blockers, such as propranolol or nadolol, if large varices (see Chapters 4 and 5)
2 Ultrasound for hepatoma screening
   a. Repeat every 6 months
   b. Contrast-enhanced imaging (CT, MRI, ultrasound) if nodule >1 cm detected and not previously characterized (see Chapter 5)
3 Signs of liver failure
   a. INR, bilirubin, and creatinine are required to calculate the MELD score. High MELD scores >12–14 should prompt a discussion about liver transplant (see Chapters 2 and 4)
   b. Dietary sodium restriction <2 g/day if albumin falling, peripheral edema, or ascites develops
      (i) If hyponatremia develops, fluid restriction should be implemented in addition to the dietary sodium restriction, i.e. saline should not be given!
   c. Avoid precipitating renal failure (hepatorenal syndrome)
      (i) Avoid nephrotoxic agents in liver failure, particularly non-steroidal anti-inflammatory drugs (acetaminophen remains safe in doses <3–4 g/day), aminoglycosides, drugs that can cause hypotension
   d. Encephalopathy/confusion
      (i) Carefully review medications that can cause confusion. Adjust dosing or stop offending medications (see Chapter 5)
         (1) Narcotics, sedatives, antipsychotics
      (ii) Lactulose, rifaximin

---

and Trizivir) should be switched to another agent where possible. Neuropsychiatric side effects can also be problematic and so familiarity with the use of antidepressants and antipsychotics is helpful. Altered taste and anorexia can lead to profound weight loss, particularly if ddI or d4T are part of the cART regimen. ddI and probably d4T are contraindicated during hepatitis C therapy, particularly if cirrhosis is present, as acute onset of liver failure has been reported.

Treatment of HCV genotype 1 will change from 2012 onwards with the availability of HCV genotype 1-specific protease inhibitors. Many other newer agents, such as polymerase inhibitors, NS5A inhibitors, and cyclophilin inhibitors, all with activity against all HCV genotypes, are anticipated by 2015. The initial challenge will be to determine how they can be used in conjunction with the other HIV medications as many of the HIV medications and the newer HCV medications affect drug metabolism through the hepatic cytochrome P450 system. However, the issue of drug–drug interaction is a familiar and ongoing issue with HIV treatment and, currently, very few (if any) medications cannot be used in the setting of HIV therapy.[4]

There is no single test that is useful to estimate the duration of HCV infection. The gold standard for timing the infection is if there was a prior HCV test that was negative. A history of blood donation is useful as blood has been routinely screened for HCV in the developed world since 1992. Since most people have never had prior HCV testing, most HCV coinfected individuals are presumed to have chronic HCV infection. Acute HCV infection has been reported in the cohort of HIV positive men who have sex with men (MSM). These individuals may or may not have had prior HCV testing but they do get regular monitoring of liver enzymes during cART therapy for HIV. Transmission is thought to be predominantly through sexual practices that break the mucosal barrier and result in bleeding, between men who are HIV positive but who may not know the partner's HCV status.

Who to treat. Everyone with HCV infection (defined as a positive HCV PCR (polymerase chain reaction) test result) should be assessed for treatment as HCV is a potentially curable infection that can otherwise lead to severe liver injury. Those with signs of liver failure (elevated INR) should be assessed for liver transplantation. Those with compensated cirrhosis or advanced liver fibrosis should be offered treatment with currently available agents. Those with acute HCV infection, within a year of exposure to HCV, should be offered therapy since the probability of eradicating acute HCV infection is so high (see Chapter 12).[5] Those with mild chronic HCV-related liver disease who do not seem to have advanced liver fibrosis or evidence of rapid fibrosis progression may opt to wait for newer therapies that have higher efficacy and lesser side effects. Those with vasculitis affecting the skin, kidneys (membranoproliferative glomerulonephritis), or nerves should be evaluated for type II (essential mixed) cryoglobulinemia complicating HCV infection. Symptomatic cryoglobulinemia is an indication for HCV treatment even in the absence of significant liver disease.

Viral hepatitis—hepatitis B

An effective hepatitis B virus (HBV) vaccine has been available since 1981. HBV vaccination is recommended in those with HIV infection as well as those at risk for HIV infection, as the two viruses share many routes of infection. Nevertheless, there are several potential limitations to the HBV vaccine. The full course of vaccination may not have been administered in those with a history of HBV vaccination. Furthermore, the HBV vaccine may not have elicited a protective anti-HBs titer. Although many feel that a history of vaccination should induce memory T-cell responses that would provide protection even if anti-HBs titers fall over time, this has not been proven with direct virus exposure and it is unclear if this is true in those with HIV infection. As such, any individual with an acute hepatitis should be assessed for current HBV infection even if there was a past history of HBV vaccination.

The natural history of hepatitis B is complicated largely because there are so many different serological tests for HBV. Furthermore, HBV is not a cytopathic virus. Rather, liver injury is thought to be immune mediated. The degree of immune control versus immune liver injury is variable from person to person. HIV infection makes immune control of HBV less likely and those with previously inactive HBV infection may experience reactivation of HBV following the acquisition of HIV infection. Fortunately, some of the NRTIs used for HIV are even more active against hepatitis B, namely 3TC (lamivudine), TDF (tenofovir (Viread), an HBV- and HIV-specific NRTI, FDA approved for HIV in 2001, for HBV in 2008), and ADV (adefovir (Hepsera) an HBV-specific NRTI, FDA approved in 2002). The following observations should be borne in mind when evaluating the individual with HBV–HIV coinfection:

1 HBsAg (hepatitis B surface antigen) is much more sensitive than HBV DNA viral load testing. It is common to see someone who remains HBsAg positive even if HBV DNA has been undetectable by sensitive PCR for many years.

2 HBV DNA viral load can be extremely high, over 12 logs, compared to HIV, which is typically no higher than 4–6 logs. As such, even highly potent therapies may not fully suppress HBV viremia. After a year of potent HBV antiviral therapy, it is expected that 30–40% of those who are HBeAg positive and 10% of those who are HBeAg negative to remain viremic. These responses are no different from those with HBV monoinfection when treated with entecavir monotherapy, tenofovir monotherapy, or even entecavir–tenofovir combination therapy.

3 For every rule in HBV, there is an exception that is not so uncommon. For example, it is possible for hepatitis B to persist (HBV DNA >12 IU/mL) despite testing HBsAg negative (occult hepatitis B). Although being anti-HBs positive usually means immunity to hepatitis B, individuals can be chronically infected and yet test both HBsAg positive and anti-HBs positive. Similarly, every combination of HBeAg and anti-HBe has been observed (the common two: HBeAg positive/anti-HBe negative, HBeAg negative/anti-HBe positive and the uncommon two: HBeAg positive/anti-HBe positive and HBeAg negative/anti-HBe negative). The natural history of the less common variants is not well reported but occult hepatitis B is thought to be an inactive form of HBV infection.

4 HBV viral load (HBV DNA) does not correlate with the degree of liver injury as HBV is not a cytopathic virus. Those with extremely high viral loads may have no immune-mediated injury, but some might. However, those with very low HBV viral loads are unlikely to have ongoing HBV-mediated liver injury: alanine aminotransferase (ALT) levels are usually normal once the HBV DNA goes below 1000 IU/mL.

5 There is no obvious synergy in potency of antiviral effect for HBV combination therapy—the maximum degree of HBV viral suppression is what you

would expect from the most potent agent. Combination therapy for hepatitis B likely decreases the risk of developing drug-resistant mutations compared to monotherapy with less potent agents like 3TC and ADV (see below).

6 Lamivudine (3TC) 150 mg is a moderately potent inhibitor of HBV but its potency is lost with mutations at rtM204. 3TC has been used for HIV infection since the mid 1990s and the probability of rtM204 mutation in HBV is over 80% after 3–4 years of 3TC exposure.

7 Tenofovir (TDF) 300 mg is a very potent inhibitor of HBV. To date, HBV resistance to TDF has not been described. FTC (emtricitabine, an HBV- and HIV-specific NRTI, FDA approved for HIV 2003 but not approved for HBV) 200 mg is similar to 3TC and is available in combination with TDF (Truvada).

8 Adefovir (ADV) is probably a potent inhibitor of HBV but dose-dependent nephrotoxicity limits its use at potent doses. At the low dose of 10 mg, ADV is less potent. If HBV DNA viral load is not fully suppressed after a year of ADV monotherapy, ongoing treatment is associated with an increased risk of mutations at N236 and/or A181 leading to treatment failure of HBV. Although such a low dose of ADV has no demonstrated activity against HIV, it is theoretically possible to generate HIV-resistant mutations with cross-resistance to TDF though this has not yet been reported.

9 Entecavir (ETV (Baraclude), an HBV-specific NRTI, FDA approved in 2005) 0.5 mg is very potent against HBV but not very potent against HIV. Although it was initially thought that it could be used as monotherapy for HBV without treating HIV, this is not optimal as it can result in HIV resistance mutations at M184 that will make HIV cross-resistant to 3TC.

10 Treatment failure due to resistance is defined as a confirmed 1 log rise in HBV DNA from nadir, after confirming adherence. While on treatment, HBV DNA should be tested every 3 months until the HBV DNA becomes negative. Once negative, HBV DNA testing every 6 months should be sufficient, assuming that patient adherence is good.

11 HBV treatment failure, due to resistance, poor adherence, or switch in HIV therapy such that HBV is no longer adequately covered, can lead to virological rebound that can be followed by clinical hepatitis, which in turn can rapidly progress to liver failure.

Who to treat. Everyone with HBV infection (defined as HBsAg positive test) should be assessed for treatment. Even if untreated, HBV must be monitored every 6–12 months by HBV DNA viral load testing. If HBV is treated, the goal is to achieve undetectable HBV DNA viral load to minimize the subsequent risk of treatment failure due to resistance. Suppression of HBV DNA to below the threshold of 1000 IU/mL, under which ALT should normalize, may take from 3–6 months, depending on the pretreatment viral load. It is expected that with tenofovir or entecavir-based therapy, just over 60% of those who are HBeAg positive and about 90% of those who are HBeAg negative should have undetectable HBV DNA levels after 1 year of therapy.[6] For those who remain HBV DNA positive, HBV viremia may persist for years (personal observation) but viral load tends to fall slowly (<1 log IU/mL) over time. HBV DNA should be monitored every 3 months while on therapy to look for virological rebound, which would suggest treatment failure, either due to poor adherence or drug resistance.

If HIV currently does not yet need treatment whereas HBV does require treatment, ADV monotherapy can be considered though it is a suboptimal choice because it is not very potent and HBV DNA may not be fully suppressed. The risk of ADV resistance rises if HBV DNA remains positive after 1 year of treatment. ETV monotherapy can also be used if one accepts the risk of M184 mutations for 3TC resistance. In the setting of prior 3TC exposure and probable M204 mutations, there is an increased risk for development of ETV resistance even if the higher 1 mg/day dose is used, particularly if HBV DNA cannot be fully suppressed by ETV within the first year of treatment.

If HBV currently does not need treatment, which is a rare event, there are many options for HIV therapy such that 3TC can be avoided, thereby avoiding selection of M204 mutations in HBV. Regimens using 3TC without TDF should be avoided. In most patients, both HBV and HIV need treatment. The current recommendation is to use 3TC or FTC in combination with TDF as a backbone for HIV therapy. This backbone is well tolerated in the majority of individuals. In those with intolerable GI side effects or renal disease, TDF use may not be possible. ETV 1 mg/day (without 3TC) may be used but it is a suboptimal salvage therapy. Those with underlying M204 mutations, especially if the HBV DNA is very high, have a high probability of treatment failure with subsequent ETV resistance. Treatment of HBV where the usual backbone of 3TC/FTC–TDF is not possible (e.g. presence of renal failure) must be individualized, balancing the relative risk of renal failure versus liver failure versus HIV control. Referral to an expert centre is suggested.

Drug-induced liver injury

Drug-induced liver injury (DILI) that leads to jaundice is dangerous, with a case fatality rate of 10–50% without liver transplant, as observed by Hy Zimmerman or "Hy's Law". This assumes that the jaundice is due to direct (conjugated) hyperbilirubinemia rather than the indirect (unconjugated) hyper-bilirubinemia and may be due either to drugs such as atazanavir, or hemolysis from use of ribavirin. In the setting of HIV infection where combinations of multiple drugs are routinely used, trying to determine which drug or drug combination is responsible can be challenging. A detailed drug history, including start times, stop times, and correlation with liver enzymes, is crucial. Early recognition so that the offending drug can be stopped is crucial for resolution of DILI.[7]

Mitochondrial toxicity through inhibition of DNA polymerase-γ is possible with all the NRTIs; the highest risks is with all the D drugs (ddC > ddI > d4T) but also reported with AZT and 3TC. This can manifest acutely and dramatically with liver failure associated with lactic acidosis, hepatic microvesicular steatosis, myopathy with very high creatine kinase, as well as pancreatitis. If the offending drug is stopped and the individual survives, it is not yet clear if long-term liver injury may result. Recently, the clinical finding of non-cirrhotic portal hypertension through the development of nodular regenerative hyperplasia has been reported in those with prior exposure to the D drugs. If the D drugs had been stopped many years before, the only management is supportive therapy for esophageal varices, ascites, and even hepatic encephalopathy.

Hypersensitivity reactions have been reported for the NRTI abacavir (ABC). ABC hypersensitivity is primarily a risk for those who are HLA-B*5701 positive and so this reaction is now rarely observed if HLA (human leukocyte antigen, the major histocompatibility complex in humans) testing is done prior to its use. All the NNRTIs can result in hypersensitivity reactions, particularly if initiating therapy in women with CD4 more than 250 cells/mm^3 or men with more than 400 cells/mm^3. Hypersensitivity reactions have also been reported with the NNRTI nevirapine, protease inhibitors darunavir, fosamprenavir, and the fusion inhibitor maraviroc.

Idiosyncratic drug reactions are, by definition, unpredictable but fortunately rare events. The parent drug compound is metabolized to intermediates that may be hepatotoxic. Many metabolic pathways are present for drug metabolism, and the major pathways in each individual are genetically determined. These intermediates are then further metabolized, once again in a genetically determined manner. If an individual relies on an uncommon pathway to metabolize a drug, toxic and hepatotoxic intermediates may accumulate. A number of adaptive mechanisms may then be induced to metabolize the reactive intermediate but, if unsuccessful, significant liver injury may result. Clinically, this usually manifests as new increase in liver enzymes after introduction of a new medication. The timing can be quite variable, from weeks to months, but usually less than 1 year. The key to diagnosis is to take a detailed history to correlate the timing of drug exposure to liver enzyme abnormality. If the liver enzymes subsequently normalize despite continued drug therapy, it is likely that the adaptive mechanisms were successfully induced. However, if the liver abnormalities persist and are followed by rising INR or bilirubin, both signs of severe liver dysfunction, all suspected offending agents must be stopped. There is no diagnostic test to confirm DILI but, in general, the reaction will recur if the drug is reintroduced (not recommended) as the subsequent reaction can be both rapid and very severe and so rechallenge is not recommended.

Cholangiopathy

AIDS cholangiopathy in untreated HIV is associated with poor median survival of less than 1 year.[8] The hallmark is elevation in alkaline phosphatase (ALP), usually without jaundice, usually in the setting of low CD4 less than 200 cells/μL. Investigations may show generalized thickening of the biliary tree, papillary stenosis, features of sclerosing cholangitis or strictures. The causes of these abnormalities are not always known but opportunistic infections of the biliary tree with cytomegalovirus, cryptosporidia, and microsporidia have been described. Biliary decompression and stenting may provide symptomatic improvement but has not been shown to improve survival. The survival of those with AIDS cholangiopathy has improved significantly with the introduction of effective HIV therapy to the point that biliary decompression is now rarely required.

Other liver diseases not related to HIV infection

Schistosomiasis is an infection with a parasitic worm of the genus *Schistosoma*. It is very common in Asia, Africa, and South America. The eggs of *S. mansoni* and *S. japonicum* can lead to obstruction of the microscopic portal veins, resulting in a syndrome of non-cirrhotic portal hypertension. In non-endemic areas, the imaging characteristics are frequently mistaken for cirrhosis. Although the infection is easy to treat, the long-term sequelae of portal hypertension remain. Fortunately, variceal bleeding tends to be less severe as the liver synthetic function tends to remain normal.

Iron overload from hereditary hemochromatosis is very common in those of Celtic ancestry. Serum ferritin is the usual test for assessing the total body iron load. However, ferritin is also an acute phase reactant that is frequently elevated in fatty liver. It can also be very high during a severe hepatitis flare with ALT greater than 500 IU/L. In hemochromatosis, iron saturation, calculated from serum iron and serum transferrin, is elevated through increases of both serum iron and serum transferrin in true iron overload states.

Autoimmune hepatitis (AIH) is a rare condition where the diagnosis is particularly difficult in those with HIV. There is no diagnostic test and the supportive tests can be affected by HIV infection. For example, IgG levels are increased in a polyclonal fashion both in AIH and untreated HIV. The autoantibodies, antinuclear antibody (ANA) and smooth muscle antibody (SMA), may be positive in both diseases. In the end, diagnosis requires an exclusion of all other liver diseases, especially drug reactions and viral hepatitis. A liver biopsy may be helpful.

Case study 18.1

A 52-year-old man with a past history of HIV, diagnosed in 1990, and hepatitis C diagnosed in 1992 (when HCV testing first became available) has been well until 2010, when he was treated for depression following the death of his mother. He has never had an opportunistic infection related to HIV; CD4 nadir was around 250 cells/μL. HIV is currently treated with 3TC–tenofovir–Kaletra (previously treated with ddI and d4T in the 1990s) and CD4 rebounded to the 400–500 cells/μL range. His hepatitis C has never been treated or investigated as serum ALT levels have been only moderately elevated at 53–72 IU/L. He now presents with ascites. In retrospect, his muscle mass has been noticeably decreasing around his face, chest, and arms over the last 6 months. Thrombocytopenia had been noted for the last 10 years and a rising INR and falling albumin had been noted for the last 3–4 years. He also has a history of significant alcohol use starting at age 20, increasing to 6–12 drinks a day when his HIV was diagnosed at age 30, with subsequent ongoing daily use (wine, one to two glasses) over the last 10 years.

Comment. This case history illustrates the very slow silent progression from initial liver injury to cirrhosis, and then hepatic decompensation that is often mistaken for a sudden onset of liver failure presenting as ascites. The fatigue and malaise that accompanies advanced cirrhosis may mimic depression. Hepatitis C is the major cause of cirrhosis in those with HIV. The prior exposure to ddI and d4T could have further injured the liver by either causing microvesicular steatosis (mitochondrial injury) or vascular injury, giving rise to portal hypertension through development of nodular regenerative hyperplasia. However, both "D drugs" had been stopped in the past and so nothing further can be done to optimize the patient now. The significance of alcohol history is often missed when current consumption is no longer obviously excessive. Excessive alcohol use in the early 1990s, when HIV infection was a fatal diagnosis, is not surprising. Identifying alcohol as a significant factor contributing to liver injury is important as alcohol cessation can lead to recovery of liver function and potential resolution of ascites. If liver function recovers 6–12 months after stopping alcohol, hepatitis C antiviral therapy can be considered but if treatment is not successful and he develops worsening liver failure, liver transplant should considered.

Case study 18.2

A 42-year-old man with a past history of HIV, diagnosed in 1997, has been treated with several different combination therapies since 1999, most recently Atripla (FTC–tenofovir–efavirenz). The CD4 nadir was around 200 cells/µL, rebounded to 600 cells/µL but has fallen to around 450–500 cells/µL over the last year. Furthermore, HIV viral load, which was initially undetectable, has been intermittently detectable and is now consistently positive at low levels, range from 100 to 1000 copies/mL. The serum creatinine had been slowly increasing over time and currently ranges between 90 and 110 µmol/L and the estimated glomerular filtration rate (eGFR) is down to 60 mL/min. Given the inadequate HIV suppression and worsening renal function, HIV therapy was switched to 3TC–abacavir–darunavir–ritonavir with good effect, that is HIV viral load became undetectable 3 months later. Routine blood tests 6 months after switching therapy demonstrated an "acute hepatitis" with ALT rising from 22 to 1630 IU/L though this man remained asymptomatic.

Comment. This case history illustrates an acute hepatitis after the introduction of a new medication(s). The usual assumption is that this is an idiosyncratic drug reaction leading to drug-induced liver injury (DILI). Although all of the current

(Continued)

medications have been reported to cause hepatitis, 3TC and low-dose ritonavir are unlikely to cause a hepatitis. Abacavir can cause a hepatitis as part of a hypersensitivity reaction, especially if this man is HLA-B*5701 positive. Darunvair has been reported to cause severe hepatitis. The role of therapeutic drug monitoring (TDM for drug levels) is unclear in this setting but may be suggestive if the drug levels are high. However, TDM is not available for most drugs and serum levels do not always reflect the intracellular drug concentrations. TDM is probably most informative if they are negative, that is the drug was not taken, so ruling out DILI. DILI remains a diagnosis of exclusion and is suggested if the hepatitis resolves when the offending drug is stopped. DILI is probable if hepatitis reappears when the offending drug is reintroduced, though this is rarely done because it may prompt a very severe, potentially fatal hepatitis.

The other major diagnosis to exclude is viral hepatitis. Everyone with HIV should have vaccination for hepatitis B and everyone with HIV with acute ALT elevations should be tested for new infections with hepatitis B and hepatitis C. Hepatitis B infection is common but frequently forgotten if liver enzymes have been normal in the past. Long-term exposure to 3TC without tenofovir invariably leads to HBV mutations (M204V/I) and drug resistance. If tenofovir is then stopped, usually because of concerns about renal function, HBV is essentially untreated even if 3TC is continued, allowing HBV viral load rebound, which leads to acute ALT elevation. Immune reconstitution inflammatory syndrome (IRIS) is a severe inflammatory state resulting from renewed immune attack against a previously acquired infection in the setting of AIDS where HIV suppression with effective therapy results in a rapid rise of CD4+ T cells from very low levels. Although IRIS is possible in those with concomitant HBV infection and "acute hepatitis", HBV viral load is usually seen to rise during the "acute hepatitis", more consistent with a diagnosis of ineffective HBV therapy, as opposed to falling, as would be expected in the setting of IRIS. New infection with viral hepatitis B or C is also possible. Behaviors that are associated with risk for viral transmission, such as unprotected sex, may change if the individual knows their HIV is controlled. When HIV control is suboptimal and then fully controlled with new agents, safer sexual practices may no longer be used. When the diagnosis of a new viral hepatitis infection is made, contact tracing should be done. It is possible that HBV infection in this setting may not be sensitive to 3TC monotherapy if the infection source was previously exposed to 3TC; in this situation, HIV therapy including tenofovir should be started, using appropriate dosing based on renal function (eGFR).

Multiple choice questions

1. A 48-year-old man with HBV–HIV coinfection has been taking FTC–tenofovir–darunavir/ritonavir for 1.5 years. Blood tests this month shows the following: HIV viral load is fully suppressed, CD4 285 cells/μL. HBsAg

remains positive, HBeAg positive, HBV DNA 2.53E3 IU/mL (2530 IU/mL). The most likely causes of ongoing HBV viremia are:

A. Tenofovir resistance in HBV
B. FTC resistance in HBV
C. FTC and tenofovir resistance in HBV
D. Inadequate potency of FTC–tenofovir
E. Imperfect adherence

2. A 43-year-old Somali woman presents with variceal bleeding. HIV has been controlled for many years and CD4 is 242 cells/μL, currently on Atripla (FTC–tenofovir–efavirenz). ALT 26 IU/L, AST 21 IU/L, ALP 103 IU/L, platelets 104×10^9/L, INR 0.98, albumin 42 g/L, bilirubin 12 μmol/L. HBsAg and anti-HBs are both negative but IgG anti-HBc is positive. Anti-HCV is negative. The most likely causes of liver disease are:

A. Hepatitis B
B. Schistosomiasis
C. Hepatitis C
D. Nodular regenerative hyperplasia
E. Hepatitis D

Answers

1. D. Inadequate potency of FTC–tenofovir. After a year of therapy, HBV DNA is not fully suppressed in 30–40% of those with HBV that is HBeAg positive. However, serial HBV DNA testing is required to be confident of this diagnosis—each subsequent HBV DNA reading should be lower. The next best answer is E. Imperfect adherence where adherence is adequate for HIV suppression but inadequate for HBV suppression. Tenofovir resistance has not yet been described. Those with FTC resistance should still be controllable if FTC is used in combination with tenofovir.

2. B and D. Schistosomiasis and nodular regenerative hyperplasia as the presentation is non-cirrhotic portal hypertension. She comes from an area where schistosomiasis is endemic. Nodular regenerative hyperplasia is also possible if she was treated with ddI and/or d4T in Africa. Serology shows prior exposure to hepatitis B that has resolved, cirrhosis from HBV is less likely given HBV resolution before age 50. Hepatitis C testing is negative and hepatitis D requires HBsAg to replicate.

References

1. FDA. Antiretroviral drugs used in the treatment of HIV infection. http://www.fda.gov/ForConsumers/byAudience/ForPatientAdvocates/HIVandAIDSActivities/ucm118915.htm. Accessed July 2011.
2. Palella FJ Jr, Baker RK, Moorman AC, et al. Mortality in the highly active antiretroviral therapy era: changing causes of death and disease in the HIV outpatient study. J Acquir Immune Defic Syndr 2006; 43: 27–34.

3. Soriano V, Puoti M, Sulkowski M, et al. Care of patients coinfected with HIV and hepatitis C: 2007 updated recommendations from the HCV-HIV International Panel. AIDS 2007; 21: 1073–89.

4. Tseng A, Toronto General Hospital Immunodeficiency Clinic. Drug information for healthcare professionals. http://www.hivclinic.ca/main/drugs_home.html. Accessed July 2011.

5. European AIDS Treatment Network (NEAT) Acute Hepatitis C Infection Consensus Panel. Acute hepatitis C in HIV-infected individuals: recommendations from the European AIDS Treatment Network (NEAT) consensus conference. AIDS 2011; 25: 399–409.

6. Marcellin P, Heathcote EJ, Buti M, et al. Tenofovir disoproxilfumarate versus adefovir dipivoxil for chronic hepatitis B. N Engl J Med 2008; 359: 2442–55.

7. Nunez M. Clinical syndromes and consequences of antiretroviral-related hepatotoxicity. Hepatology 2010; 52: 1143–55.

8. Ko W-F, Cello JP, Rogers SJ, Lecours A. Prognostic factors for survival of patients with AIDS cholangiopathy. Am J Gastroenterol 2003; 98: 2176–81.

Autoimmune hepatitis in adults and children

CHAPTER 19

Gideon M. Hirschfield

Division of Gastroenterology, Toronto Western Hospital, University Health Network, University of Toronto, Toronto, Ontario, Canada, and Centre for Liver Research, University of Birmingham, Birmingham, UK

Key points

- Autoimmune hepatitis (AIH) is a chronic and relapsing, immune-mediated liver injury.
- No single diagnostic test exists for AIH and in the absence of alternative liver disease, diagnosis rests on the presence of a constellation of laboratory and histological features.
- Successful treatment with steroids and azathioprine is generally very effective in the induction of disease remission and maintenance free of relapse.
- In children, overlap presentation with a biliary disease (just sclerosing cholangitis) occurs in approximately 50% of patients (but much less often in adults).
- Non-compliance with therapy is the commonest reason for treatment failure; management of this chronic disease must be sensitive to individual patient concerns and circumstances.

Introduction

Autoimmune hepatitis (AIH) describes a condition characterized by chronic and relapsing lymphoplasmacytic hepatitis, which is usually associated with positive autoimmune serology and elevated immunoglobulins.[1-4] More importantly, drug injury, viral hepatitis, Wilson disease, and metabolic liver disease need to be excluded to confirm diagnosis. This disease is protean in its presentation, ranging from fulminant liver failure through to chronic asymptomatic hepatitis. The generally excellent and durable response to steroids and azathioprine clinically distinguishes this disease. There is no such thing as a classic

Hepatology: Diagnosis and Clinical Management, First Edition. Edited by E. Jenny Heathcote.
© 2012 John Wiley & Sons, Ltd. Published 2012 by John Wiley & Sons, Ltd.

AIH patient. This disease is more prevalent in younger women but it is also clearly recognized in men, and in patients of all ages. Autoimmune serology is used to broadly classify patients into two groups, although these two groups are treated similarly: type 1 disease with positive antinuclear antibodies (ANA) or smooth muscle antibodies (SMA), and type 2 disease, a predominantly pediatric disease at presentation, with anti-liver–kidney–microsomal (LKM) antibodies. Type 2 AIH is distinctly uncommon in North America, most patients having type 1 disease.

Differential diagnosis

It is essential to consider other diagnoses before treating a patient for AIH, given the recognized deleterious side effects of immunosuppression. Exclusion of alternative etiologies for liver disease relies on a suitably detailed history from the patient that includes details of prescribed and unprescribed drug ingestion, as well a thorough liver screen. It is important to recognize that no single test can diagnose AIH, and one must appreciate the limitations of such tests.

Pediatric

Wilson disease. This is described in greater detail in Chapter 23. Particularly in a patient under the age of 21(but to some extent in all patients), Wilson disease must be carefully considered and excluded. Those with Wilson disease can have elevated IgG levels and positive autoimmune markers.

Minocycline hepatitis. Many drugs can give a hepatitic picture, and a few drugs can mimic all the features of AIH. In the pediatric age group, minocycline hepatitis must be considered as such patients may have a transaminitis, positive ANA or SMA, and elevated immunoglobulins (and patients respond to corticosteroids when removal of the offending drug is all that is needed).

α_1-antitrypsin deficiency. This entity is relatively straightforward to diagnose clinically—one can measure serum levels of α_1-antitrypsin and stain for α_1 inclusions on liver biopsy. Some patients with α_1-antitrypsin can present with a hepatitic picture, without a history of neonatal cholestasis.

Adults

Drug injury. As alluded to above, many prescribed drugs and herbal remedies can present with a hepatitis. Fortunately, the hepatitis is usually self limiting if the exposure to the offending agent is halted. The list of injurious agents is lengthy and increases each year. Usually, the injury is non-specific and does not have etiologic clues other than from the patient history. Nitrofurantoin is frequently used for the treatment of recurrent urinary tract infections and minocycline for acne; in a minority of patients, it has very characteristic acute and chronic hepatic side effects. In its classic form, nitrofurantoin hepatitis is entirely indistinguishable from AIH. Antitumor necrosis factor agents have also been reported to be associated with development of AIH.

Primary biliary cirrhosis. Whilst true overlap syndromes between different autoimmune liver diseases are distinctly rare, it is quite common for patients with primary biliary cirrhosis (PBC) to present with an elevated alkaline phosphatase that is accompanied by a transaminitis. Usually, the transaminases are less than five times the upper limit of normal. Liver biopsy in PBC can also frequently show an interface hepatitis. It is important to treat the predominant process, and usually ursodeoxycholic acid is sufficient. The serologic hallmark for PBC (AMA) may be detectable although rarely a true overlap with PBC is present.

Primary sclerosing cholangitis (PSC). At younger ages, PSC presentation can be more hepatitic, and in children (see Chapter 20), 50% of patients with AIH have a sclerosing cholangiopathy and vice versa. PSC should also be entertained as a differential diagnosis in patients who do not respond well to immunosuppression.

Non-alcoholic fatty liver disease (NAFLD). Low titer autoantibodies (ANA/SMA) alongside minor elevations in IgG are surprisingly common. Given the vast number of patients with NAFLD, it is therefore imperative to avoid over interpretation of such findings in patients with usually relatively minor elevations in transaminases. Additionally, accurate liver biopsy interpretation is important, given that steatohepatitis and Mallory bodies are not features of AIH.

Viral hepatitis. The exclusion of concomitant active viral liver disease is a prerequisite for making a diagnosis of AIH. An overlap between hepatitis C and AIH is not a common clinical reality, although making this distinction can be difficult. The frequent presence of autoantibodies (ANA, SMA) in hepatitis C is neither sufficient to diagnose AIH nor to be of any relevance in the management of the hepatitis C. Given the epidemiology of hepatitis B, there are inevitably patients at different stages of viral hepatitis that might also develop AIH. Such patients need to be evaluated on an individual basis, and have their hepatitis B treated first with oral nucleoside analogues if HBsAg positive before any corticosteroids are given.

Miscellaneous. AIH can present in a variety of ways from acute liver failure to anicteric asymptomatic transaminitis, and so metabolic and infiltrative disorders can sometimes be pertinent items on the differential diagnosis. Clinicians should avoid indiscriminate testing for autoantibodies if an appropriate diagnosis already exists; positive serology for ANA or SMA are far more common in the general population than is AIH.[5] Very rarely, severe untreated celiac disease can mimic autoimmune liver disease, so serologic testing and subsequent duodenal biopsy should be considered.

Making the diagnosis

Presentation

Clinically, the presentation of AIH spans the breadth of all liver disease— patients may present asymptomatically with only a biochemical transaminitis found incidentally, through to acute liver failure. At the time of histological diagnosis, AIH is usually a chronic inflammatory process, and one-third of patients are cirrhotic. When symptoms are present, they are usually non-specific, such as fatigue, arthralgias, and upper abdominal pain. If the patient is very cholestatic, they may be jaundiced but rarely complain of pruritus.

Pediatric perspective

Type 1 AIH accounts for two-thirds of the cases and usually presents during adolescence, while type 2 AIH presents at a younger age (<10 years) and also during infancy. In both types there is a female preponderance (75%). Children are more likely to have symptomatic disease, which triggers investigation. Systemic symptoms such as arthralgias are frequent; amenorrhea may be present. Acne may also flare. Type 2 AIH (LKM antibody positive) is more likely to be severe at presentation, with higher rates of cirrhosis. However, treatment for both types of AIH is the same.

Investigations

It should always be remembered that AIH is a diagnosis of exclusion. Clinical scoring systems (Table 19.1)[6] are helpful, but their intended purpose is often for research studies (i.e. uniformity in patient inclusion). Therefore, not all patients in all scenarios can necessarily be evaluated by these systems. Finally, no test in isolation can diagnose AIH. Seronegative disease is well described and behaves identically in terms of treatment response.

Table 19.1 Simplified autoimmune hepatitis scoring system[6]

Parameter	Classifier	Score
ANA or SMA	≥1:40	1
ANA or SMA	≥1:80	
or LKM	≥1:40	2
IgG	> ULN	1
	>1.10 × ULN	2
Liver histology	Compatible AIH	1
	Typical AIH	2
Absence of viral hepatitis	Yes	2

SCORE: ≥6 "probable" AIH; ≥7 "definite" AIH.
AIH, autoimmune hepatitis; ANA, antinuclear antibodies; LKM, anti-liver–kidney–microsomal antibodies; SMA, smooth muscle antibodies; ULN, upper limit of normal.

Diagnostic blood work. After the exclusion of common liver injuries such as hepatitis B and C, testing includes:

- Serum autoantibodies: type 1 AIH is characterized by the presence of ANA or SMA. Whilst ELISA-based assays for F-actin can reliably detect the antigen most associated with SMA, this is not the case for ELISA-based ANA assays, given the lack of ANA specificity in AIH. Therefore clinicians concerned about autoimmune liver disease should insist on immunofluorescence testing particularly for ANA.
- Type 2 disease, almost always a pediatric disease at presentation, is very uncommon in North America, and is characterized by LKM antibodies. Particularly in adults, clinicians should request immune serology in a sequential manner—ANA and SMA first, with additional testing for LKM antibodies only if the patient is ANA/SMA negative. In routine practice most clinicians do not have access to other specific AIH serology, for example anti-soluble liver antigen. Mitochondrial antibodies can be positive in AIH, especially when determined by immunofluorescence. Their presence does not necessarily mean the patient has an overlap syndrome with PBC, since true AMA-positive AIH is reported to behave identically to type I AIH.
- Immunoglobulins: most commonly, patients with AIH have elevated IgG values at presentation, usually at least twice the upper limit of normal. It is essential to measure IgG in all patients suspected of having AIH. If the presentation is very acute, IgG titers may be normal initially and thus should be repeated a few weeks later. Remember, non-specific elevations in IgG can be seen in any cause of cirrhosis as well as other systemic inflammatory conditions. It is important to measure IgG levels as relapse of disease can often be identified if the IgG begins to rise towards pretreatment levels. In children, IgG is usually raised at presentation, although 15% of children with type 1 AIH and 25% with type 2 AIH have normal levels, especially those with an acute presentation. IgA deficiency is common in type 2 AIH.
- α_1-Antitrypsin and ceruloplasmin levels should be measured in order to screen for rare patients with α_1-antitrypsin deficiency or Wilson disease. If the suspicion is high for Wilson disease (e.g. acute presentation of young patient with an unconjugated hyperbilirubinemia and a relatively low alkaline phosphatase) urine copper and ophthalmic evaluation for Kayser–Fleischer rings should be performed, as well as possibly measuring hepatic copper concentration.

Imaging. Baseline ultrasound imaging is usually sufficient in the workup of patients. Such imaging should always include Doppler interrogation of the portal and hepatic veins. Cross-sectional imaging is not usually needed unless there is doubt as to the diagnosis, or if malignancy is suspected. Given the high frequency of biliary disease in children with AIH, magnetic resonance cholangiopancreatography (MRCP) is indicated in all pediatric patients. The need for MRCP in all adult patients is debatable, for the frequency of overlap of AIH and biliary disease (namely PSC) is less than 10%. Thus, it can reasonably be reserved for those with clinical, laboratory, or histologic features of both AIH and biliary disease, or who fail to respond as expected to therapy. Cholestatic AIH is described predominantly in Africans.

Histology. There are no specific features on histology that are unique to AIH. The degree of histologic change is also affected by the severity of presentation and whether immunosuppressive treatment has been initiated prior to biopsy. However, there are recurrent patterns of inflammation, including an interface hepatitis, lymphoplasmacytic infiltration, and hepatocyte rosetting, and albeit rarely zone 3 necrosis which help focus attention towards AIH (Plates 19.1 and 19.2). Liver biopsy is generally recommended as part of the diagnostic work up in all patients, given the nature, duration, and potential side effects of treatment of AIH. Exceptions to this rule may include those with acute liver failure, ascites, and the very elderly, where treatment may be initiated on the basis of history and blood work alone. However, if histology is omitted in patients such as these, great attention needs to be given to treatment response; a failure to respond to treatment should raise the possibility of an incorrect diagnosis, and may heighten the need for liver biopsy. The pathologist must be given adequate clinical information in order to interpret the liver histology correctly. Also when discussing the findings with the pathologist, the clinician should probe for important differentials that must not be missed, such as viral inclusion bodies or malignant infiltration. When there is a marked hepatitis (i.e. significant hepatocyte necrosis and architectural collapse) fibrosis evaluation is difficult and should not be relied upon until treatment has resolved the active inflammation.

Endoscopy. Generally, endoscopy at presentation is not indicated. In patients with cirrhosis or decompensated disease, varices should be sought, as with any patient with advanced liver disease.

Bone density. It is sensible to establish the baseline bone density in adults either before starting therapy, or soon after. In combination with the patient's age, gender, past medical history, and treatment plan, prophylaxis against bone loss may be indicated, i.e. milk and vitamin D.

Associated autoimmune diseases. Routine screening for additional autoimmune disease is not normally pursued, although the presence of autoantibodies can be used as surrogate support for the diagnosis of autoimmune hepatitis. Thyroid disease, rheumatoid arthritis, ulcerative colitis, type 1 diabetes, and celiac disease are all associated with AIH.

Miscellaneous. Hepatitis B testing should always be part of the initial investigation, and particular attention should be paid to high-risk patients (e.g. Asians) to screen for current (HBsAg) and past (HBcAb) infection. Patients with risk factors for infectious disease exposure (e.g. travel, intravenous drug use) should be screened for *Strongyloides*, tuberculosis, and HIV before immunosuppression.

Pediatric perspective

The investigation for a pediatric patient is very similar to that of an adult. The most important difference is that Wilson disease must be aggressively excluded, and investigation must be timely and rapid as patients are often jaundiced and at risk of decompensated liver disease. MRCP is recommended for all patients as overlap with PSC is more common. Serologically false-positive associations are far less common, and for this reason autoantibody titers at a lower level (e.g. 1 in 20) carry diagnostic significance.

Management

In general, there are three phases to caring for a patient with AIH: (1) induction of remission (prednisone); (2) maintenance of remission (prednisone and azathioprine); and (3) prevention of relapse (azathioprine).

Because of the variability of patients, the paucity of current randomized data, and differences amongst experts, no one treatment algorithm is widely practiced. The AASLD guidance is a reasonable framework for non-hepatologists to use, with most people favoring joint therapy with prednisone and azathioprine (Table 19.2). On average, it takes 12–18 months (sometimes more) of

Table 19.2 Current AASLD treatment guidelines for AIH[1]

Weeks administered	Combination therapy			Prednisone therapy
	Prednisone (mg daily)	Azathioprine		Prednisone (mg daily)
		North America (mg daily)	Europe (mg/kg/day)	
1	30	50	1–2	60
1	20	50	1–2	40
2	15	50	1–2	30
Maintenance until end point, e.g. normal liver enzymes	10	50	1–2	20

Few people use prednisone as monotherapy; most adjust therapy based on treatment response rather than being protocol driven. The maintenance phase may last 12–18 months with respect to prednisone use (and longer for azathioprine), and the dose is usually around 5–10 mg/day. Pediatric practice typically uses prednisone initially at 2 mg/kg (maximum 40–60 mg/day). The so-called absolute criteria for treatment relate to the high mortality if no intervention occurs and include: serum AST or ALT > 10-fold ULN; serum AST or ALT > five fold ULN and IgG > two fold ULN; bridging necrosis or multiacinar necrosis on liver biopsy.

steroids, with azathioprine at 1–2 mg/kg per day, to induce complete disease remission with sustained normalization of liver enzymes and immunoglobulins. Steroid withdrawal at that point can usually be accomplished without a repeat biopsy, especially if all tests are normal. Most clinicians then maintain patients on monotherapy with azathioprine for 2–5 years, and in a non-cirrhotic patient, one chance off all treatment may be allowed, with monitoring. If the patient is cirrhotic, or if they have had an episode of relapse off treatment, long-term maintenance with azathioprine is generally indicated, which is usually life long. Relapses must first be managed with steroids again (Box 19.1).

For most patients, prednisone and azathioprine are the most appropriate medications. Alternatives may be needed for individual reasons or because of allergic reactions. Apart from intravenous steroids, which are rarely needed, budesonide is the only alternative steroid for which there are relatively good data to support its use. Certainly in patients *without* cirrhosis, who have mild–moderate disease, it is likely that budesonide is at least as effective as traditional prednisone and is generally associated with fewer side effects.[7] Alternatives to azathioprine (other than mercaptopurine) include mycophenolate mofetil, cyclophosphamide, and calcineurin inhibitors in particular. However, the number of patients needing such alternatives is small and so there are few randomized data to support or refute efficacy. Biologics have as yet not become established therapy but may become so in the future.

Overall guidelines for management of AIH

Given that AIH is relatively rare, few clinicians look after enough patients concurrently to become expert in all aspects of care. Collective wisdom provides some useful day to day tips and thoughts, and includes recognition of the following.

- Untreated severe disease is associated with significant mortality, particularly in children. It is a mistake to delay investigation of cryptogenic acute hepatitis in the belief that it is benign.
- AIH is a chronic and relapsing disease, with off treatment relapse in at least 90% of patients.
- Repeated relapses are associated with a poorer outcome, and a relapse in a cirrhotic patient can be fatal.
- "Short, sharp" treatment is not a useful paradigm in AIH: slow is generally good and steroids are generally needed for 12–18 months at least from presentation.
- Histologic resolution of liver injury lags behind biochemical resolution by about 3–6 months and relapse can still occur if histology on treatment is normal.
- The presence of bridging collapse on histology identifies a high-risk group who should be treated.
- Bile duct injury can be seen without true overlap with another biliary disease being present and a cholestatic presentation of disease is reported in Africans and African Americans.

Box 19.1 Management algorithm for acute severe autoimmune hepatitis*

- Initiate prednisone at dose of 20–40 mg orally per day; screen, counsel, and monitor patient for side effects.
- Monitor CBC, LFT, IgG approximately every 2 weeks (more often if INR elevated).
- Look to initially see a transaminase drop; bilirubin and IgG fall more slowly; follow trends not individual tests.
- Expect to see a drop in transaminases rapidly and a significant drop (more than 50%) by 2–4 weeks.
- By 1 month the patient is usually still on 20 mg prednisone and assuming they are responding add azathioprine; delay azathioprine if jaundice significantly >100 μmol/L.
- Generally start at 50 mg azathioprine orally per day and build up to at least 1 mg/kg within 1 month; consider aiming for 2 mg/kg depending on individual patient.
- Monitor for hematologic side effects of azathioprine; in particular, weekly full blood count for 4 weeks, monthly for 3 months, and 3 monthly for life.
- Based on the degree of biochemical response and the individual patient factors (e.g. age, comorbidities, risk of side effects, azathioprine tolerance), keep prednisone at 10–20 mg daily for first 3 months.
- Taper the steroids down to about 5–7.5 mg daily if doing well by approximately 12 months.
- Aim to get the patient to normal tests by approximately 6 months (ALT, IgG, and bilirubin) on prednisone and azathioprine, but don't be surprised if it takes 12–18 months.
- If the patient has persistently normal tests including IgG by about 18 months, consider stopping steroids *but* maintaining azathioprine. Liver biopsy at this point can help but if the enzymes and immunoglobulins have been persistently normal for 3–6 months it is unusual to be contributory; relapse can occur even after a normal biopsy is seen.
- Monitor liver biochemistry for relapse off steroids initially monthly (for 3 months) then 3 monthly (maintain on azathioprine and regularly check CBC).
- In a non-cirrhotic patient consider azathioprine for 2–5 years total before offering a single chance at cessation of all drugs.
- In a cirrhotic patient, or an individual who would be at high risk from further steroids, expect to prescribe azathioprine, with long-term monitoring for life.

*For patients with probable or definite AIH by international consensus. This algorithm is intended to be applied in a patient-specific manner, and it is recommended that a hepatologist manage such patients long term, and also advise if second-line therapies are indicated by treatment intolerance or failure.

- In the original studies, one-third of patients demonstrated progressive liver fibrosis over time, despite treatment.
- The persistence of normal enzymes and normal immunoglobulins is usually associated with good resolution of liver injury and normalization of enzymes should be the goal of treatment.
- The failure to see a significant improvement in liver biochemistry within the first 4 weeks of therapy should lead to a careful re-appraisal of the diagnosis.
- The original, pivotal, placebo-controlled studies by Cook et al. used a dose of only 15 mg of prednisolone and showed a survival benefit; high-dose prednisolone therapy is fraught with side effects.
- Steroids are used to treat the active inflammation and azathioprine is employed to prevent relapse; therefore, it is quite reasonable and often logical to delay introducing azathioprine by about 1 month after treatment is initiated.
- The original studies of azathioprine generally used a target dose of 2 mg/kg at the outset, with tapering back towards 1 mg/kg over time.
- The putative benefits of budesonide over prednisone are lost in cirrhotic patients and one-third of patients at presentation have cirrhosis.
- Patients differ (age, ethnicity, comorbidities, disease severity) and treatment must be tailored to the individual and their response to immunosuppression, whilst weighing up the individual risks and benefits and costs of treatment.
- Some data support a benign course for mild disease or that which is asymptomatic; treatment is therefore not necessarily needed for everyone but those not treated still need follow up (Fig. 19.1).
- Inactive cirrhosis due to AIH does not usually need treatment. In this setting, confident diagnosis of AIH is difficult because burnt-out non-alcoholic steatohepatitis (NASH) is far more common than AIH, and patients may have positive immune serology of no significance and elevated IgG levels are common in all causes of cirrhosis.
- Immunosuppression carries real risks and side effects. Patient education and involvement in the management of this chronic disease is paramount to success (Table 19.3).
- The most common reason for apparent treatment failure or disease relapse is lack of adherence to treatment.
- Overlap with sclerosing cholangitis is much more common in children than adults, but should be considered in adults who do not respond optimally to therapy.
- Before intensifying treatment beyond dual therapy with prednisone and azathioprine, careful thought must be given to whether the risks are greater than the benefits and whether transplant is a better option.
- The risk of sepsis from steroids in acute liver failure is genuine and in that setting management should be in conjunction with a transplant program.
- Subacute liver failure can fully reverse with steroids if due to AIH but patients need close monitoring.

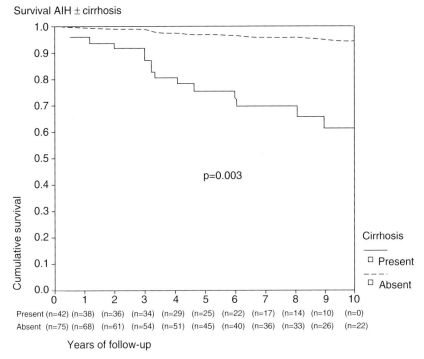

Fig. 19.1 Survival of autoimmune hepatitis patients with or without cirrhosis. Reproduced from Feld et al. Hepatology 2005; 42: 53 with permission from VG Wort.

Table 19.3 Monitoring required during IST for autoimmune hepatitis

Baseline	CBC, blood and urine glucose, chest X ray (? old tuberculosis)
	Stool culture ova and parasites (*Strongyloides*)
	Systemic blood pressure
	Bone mineral density
	Eye exam
	EGD if cirrhotic
	Check HBsAg status, pneumococcal vaccination
	HIV
During therapy	WBC and platelets
	ALT/AST
	IgG
	Repeat baseline measurements annually
	? Liver biopsy at end of treatment
	If cirrhotic: ultrasound surveillance for HCC
	EGD surveillance for varices

ALT, alanine aminotransferase; AST, aspartate aminotransferase; EGD, esophagogastroduodenoscopy; HCC, hepatocellular carcinoma.

> **Box 19.2 Preventative measures while on steroid with or without azathioprine**
>
> - Advice about how to avoid weight gain
> - Calcium + vitamin D supplements ± bisphosphonates?
> - Check stools: ova + parasites (and advice regarding travel)
> - Monitor complete blood count (on azathioprine)
> - Annual checks: blood pressure, urine sugar, cataract, bone mineral density
> - If cirrhotic: avoid sedation (cautious anesthesia), infection, non-steroidal anti-inflammatory drugs
> - Discuss pregnancy issues
>   Wear medic alert bracelet

- Pregnancy-induced flares of AIH are most common postpartum, although they are rarely seen during the pregnancy.
- Treatment is best continued during and after pregnancy without modification; it is traditionally taught that breast feeding is contraindicated for those on azathioprine but this is not supported by practical experience.
- In children, non-compliance during puberty can be challenging and avoiding changes to treatment over this time is sensible.
- In children, there is no benefit in terms of side-effect profile to alternate-day dosing of steroids but there is a greater likelihood of non-compliance and a high relapse rate, requiring increased steroid doses, with attendant more severe side effects and growth impairment.

Non-disease-specific management (Box 19.2)

Cirrhosis surveillance. Patients with cirrhosis are at risk for hepatocellular carcinoma, and generally all cirrhotic patients should be considered for ultrasound surveillance every 6 months. Hepatocellular carcinoma in AIH is reported, albeit rarely.

Endoscopic surveillance. Most patients who develop varices with autoimmune liver disease are cirrhotic and portal hypertension commonly persists after active inflammatory disease has been well treated. Spleen size and platelet count ($<150 \times 10^9$/L) are reasonable indicators for elective gastroscopy.

Vaccination. Patients with chronic liver disease should be vaccinated against hepatitis A and B. Patients with cirrhosis should receive the annual influenza vaccination in particular, as well as periodic pneumococcal vaccination. Patients on azathioprine cannot receive live vaccines.

Presurgery advice. Caution in those with cirrhosis and portal hypertension is recommended. Avoidance of perioperative hypotension and postoperative fluid overload can minimize risks of postoperative decompensation.

Pregnancy. Becoming pregnant is not contraindicated but added caution is recommended if patients have portal hypertension. All cirrhotic patients should be checked for varices during the second trimester. Generally fetal outcomes are good, and are relate to the mother's own health. Patients should generally not stop their immunosuppression for conception or pregnancy, with the exception of mycophenolate mofetil, which has been associated with an increased risk of spontaneous abortion in the first trimester and congenital malformations. Flares are most commonly seen postpartum and monitoring the mother in the first 3 months postpartum is important, although inconvenient. Intensification of immunosuppression, usually by increased steroids, is usually sufficient if a flare occurs.

Need for and timing of transplant referral

Transplantation is quite uncommon nowadays for patients with ΛIH. The common scenarios where it is still relevant is in patients with a fulminant presentation, in whom steroid response is unlikely to work and treatment potentially undesirable as sepsis may be precipitated, in those with burnt-out end-stage disease with portal hypertensive complications, and in those with a biliary overlap from sclerosing cholangitis, for whom liver injury will persist and progress despite adequate immunosuppression. The model for end-stage liver disease (MELD) score, and its equivalents, are generally effective tools for predicting the need for transplant, although those patients with a subacute presentation can fully improve with steroids. This subgroup of patients should be managed in close liaison with a transplant program.

Pediatric perspective

Treatment of pediatric AIH is generally very similar to that for adults, but is more sensitive to issues regarding compliance, growth, and side effects. Treatment is initiated with prednisone at 2 mg/kg per day (maximum 40–60 mg/day). This dose is gradually decreased over a few months, guided by the decline of transaminase levels, to a maintenance dose of 2.5–5 mg/day. Some clinicians aim for an 80% decrease of the transaminase levels by the first 2 months of treatment, and not their complete normalization, which may take many months. Azathioprine is added variably in some centers, if the transaminase levels stop decreasing on steroid treatment alone, or in the presence of steroid side effects, at a starting dose of 0.5 mg/kg per day. In the absence of signs of toxicity, the dose is increased up to a maximum of 2.0–2.5 mg/kg per day. Other centers use azathioprine at a dose of 0.5–2 mg/kg per day, in all cases after a few weeks of steroid treatment when the serum aminotransferase levels begin to decrease. In those with a biliary overlap, it remains commonplace to give ursodeoxycholic acid although evidence for efficacy is absent.

Case study 19.1

A 35-year-old woman presents to her local gastroenterologist with a recent onset of jaundice, not associated with pain or any new medication use. She complains of fatigue and arthralgias. On examination, apart from her jaundice, she has mild ascites and spider telangiectasia. She was not encephalopathic. Her bilirubin was 300 μmol/L, ALT 950 IU/L, INR 1.5, and platelets 150 × 10^9/L. IgG was significantly elevated at 35 g/L, and ANA was strongly positive at 1:360. SMA was positive at 1:80. Viral screens were negative and ceruloplasmin normal. Imaging showed a small liver with ascites but nil focal. Transjugular liver biopsy revealed a chronic hepatitis, with significant hepatocyte loss and bridging collapse. There was an interface hepatitis with a predominant lymphoplasmacytic infiltrate. No viral inclusion bodies were seen and the infiltrate was polyclonal. Fibrosis could not be evaluated.

What is the diagnosis?

This woman meets standard criteria for severe type 1 AIH, given the absence of viral liver disease (e.g. hepatitis A, B, and C negative), no known drug triggers, and the presence of a hepatitic illness with positive immune serology, raised globulins, and a consistent liver biopsy. Untreated she would have a likely mortality of approaching 100% within 1 year. Due to her severe presentation, the initial management should be in hospital under the guidance of an experienced gastroenterologist/hepatologist. Prednisone should be initiated promptly and is predicted to be highly effective at reversing the inflammation and allowing resumption of liver function. Azathioprine would likely not be introduced until her bilirubin was less than 100 μmol/L given its hepatotoxicity. If she fails to improve or her clinical status were to deteriorate, transplant should be considered, and a transplant program should be consulted at the time of her admission and be informed of her progress periodically from the outset.

Multiple choice questions

1. A 58-year-old woman presents with jaundice and abdominal discomfort. You are the internist evaluating her in the rapid access ambulatory clinic. In evaluating her history, which of the following factors are likely relevant?
   A. Use of acetaminophen for a simple headache (two tablets) 3 days ago
   B. Family history of rheumatoid arthritis in her mother
   C. Occupation as a secretary in a travel agency
   D. Recent course of nitrofurantoin for an uncomplicated urinary tract infection
   E. A history of increasing pruritus over the prior 2 weeks

2. You are the family doctor of a young woman with established, well-treated AIH. She sees you because she wants to discuss family planning and future

plans for pregnancy. In guiding her through the issues, which factors are most relevant to your discussion?

A. The choice of oral contraceptive is limited to progesterone-only containing preparations as estrogens are always contraindicated in liver disease.

B. Her present medication with azathioprine as maintenance therapy poses a serious concern to future pregnancy.

C. Clarifying whether there is underlying cirrhosis is essential.

D. The risk of disease transmission is high and she should see a genetics councilor.

E. Disease relapse during pregnancy is likely and therefore a cause for concern.

Answers

1. B and D. AIH is a disease without a specific diagnostic test. In evaluating patients for autoimmune liver disease an appropriately detailed history is essential. This should focus on identifying risk factors for alternative diagnoses (drugs, toxins, viral infection) and for any autoimmune predisposition. Acetaminophen is only toxic if taken in overdose, or with sustained high doses. A family history of autoimmunity is relevant to note and should be considered carefully. Occupation can be a relevant factor in the history for exposure to viral hepatitis, e.g. health-care workers, sanitation workers, school teachers. Some drugs are prone to give a syndrome indistinguishable from AIH. Nitrofurantoin is one such drug. Symptoms of liver disease such as abdominal discomfort, fatigue, and itch are usually not specific to one etiology.

2. C. Patients with AIH are frequently concerned about family planning and pregnancy. Whilst there may be some theoretical concerns about associations between cholestasis and estrogen-containing contraception, broadly speaking, in the presence of preserved liver function there are no absolute restrictions on choice of contraceptive pill. For patients with symptomatic biliary disorders there does remain the possibility that an estrogen-containing product can exacerbate cholestasis and appropriate monitoring in this setting is needed. Azathioprine is an immunosuppressant and does have side effects. However, in most settings the benefit of maintaining disease remission is greater than the risks posed. In terms of specific pregnancy concerns, there is good observational data for safe use at conception and during pregnancy. Cirrhosis is a risk factor for adverse outcomes in pregnancy and thus it is important to know if a women planning pregnancy is cirrhotic, as this would define the pregnancy as high risk, and lead to specific monitoring (e.g. risk of varices). One-third of patients with AIH are cirrhotic at presentation. Therefore evaluation for cirrhosis by bloods (platelet count), imaging, non-invasive markers (FibroScan, FibroTest), and possibly even liver biopsy need to be considered. Whilst AIH is certainly a disease with a genetic influence, it is not a heritable trait in the traditional sense, and with

the exception of truly rare syndromes of familial autoimmunity, no genetic screening is either appropriate (or available). Like many autoimmune diseases, the disease course during pregnancy is often characterized by remission. Postpartum biochemical monitoring for flares of activity is more important, as certainly for AIH, significant biochemical flares in disease (even in the absence of any symptom) can be seen, requiring increased therapy.

References

1. Manns MP, Czaja AJ, Gorham JD, et al. Diagnosis and management of autoimmune hepatitis. Hepatology 2010; 51: 2193–213.
2. Mieli-Vergani G, Heller S, Jara P, et al. Autoimmune hepatitis. J Pediatr Gastroenterol Nutr 2009; 49: 158–64.
3. Czaja AJ, Manns MP. Advances in the diagnosis, pathogenesis, and management of autoimmune hepatitis. Gastroenterology 2010; 139: 58–72, e4.
4. Decock S, McGee P, Hirschfield GM. Autoimmune liver disease for the non-specialist. BMJ 2009; 339: 3305.
5. Zeman MV, Hirschfield GM. Autoantibodies and liver disease: uses and abuses. Can J Gastroenterol 2010; 24: 225–31.
6. Hennes EM, Zeniya M, Czaja AJ, et al. Simplified criteria for the diagnosis of autoimmune hepatitis. Hepatology 2008; 48: 169–76.
7. Manns MP, Woynarowski M, Kreisel W, et al. Budesonide induces remission more effectively than prednisone in a controlled trial of patients with autoimmune hepatitis. Gastroenterology 2010; 139: 1198–206.

Chronic cholestatic liver disease and its management in adults and children

CHAPTER 20

Gideon M. Hirschfield[1] and Binita M. Kamath[2]

[1] Division of Gastroenterology, Toronto Western Hospital, University Health Network, University of Toronto, Toronto, Ontario, Canada, and Centre for Liver Research, University of Birmingham, Birmingham, UK
[2] University of Toronto, and Division of Gastroenterology, Hepatology and Nutrition, The Hospital for Sick Children, Toronto, Ontario, Canada

Key points

- Nowadays, most adult patients with cholestatic liver disease are first diagnosed when asymptomatic; this is not the case for children.
- In adults, testing for antimitochondrial antibodies (AMA) can rapidly diagnose primary biliary cirrhosis without the need for further investigation, except in the appropriate context.
- Cholangiography by MRI is indicated if AMA negative or in those with pre-existing risk factors for primary sclerosing cholangitis, such as inflammatory bowel disease.
- Early surgery in infants with biliary atresia is important in order to derive greatest benefit from biliary surgery; this underscores the need to *rapidly* investigate jaundice in babies.

Introduction

Cholestasis arises whenever impairment of hepatobiliary excretion occurs and normal biliary constituents appear in the circulation. If marked, jaundice and pruritus are notable, but, when milder, abnormal liver biochemistry and non-specific symptoms such as fatigue may be the only evidence. Generalized pruritus can occur at any stage of cholestatic liver disease. In addition to the systemic presence of biliary constituents, tissue cholestasis is seen at the level of hepatocytes, with retained bile acids proving toxic to the liver.[1,2]

Hepatology: Diagnosis and Clinical Management, First Edition. Edited by E. Jenny Heathcote.
© 2012 John Wiley & Sons, Ltd. Published 2012 by John Wiley & Sons, Ltd.

The etiologies of cholestasis can be found at either the level of the hepatocyte, the small bile duct, or the large bile duct, and can be considered to be either acute and self-limiting or chronic, with irreversible duct loss and/or progressive biliary fibrosis. Mechanisms of injury include toxins, genetic defects, inflammation, immune mediated or obstruction, although some conditions are characterized by more than one process.

The characteristic biochemical features of chronic cholestasis are an elevated alkaline phosphatase (ALP), or, more reliably in children, by elevation in γ-glutamyl transpeptidase (GGT). Transaminases may be elevated, but generally cholestasis is characterized by a ratio of ALP:ALT (alanine transaminase) of greater than 3. In very acute cholestasis, such as that sometimes seen in pregnancy, elevated transaminases are predominant. Jaundice in cholestatic liver diseases may be due to direct biliary obstruction, hepatocyte injury and subsequent failure to excrete bilirubin, or end-stage liver disease.

Differential diagnosis

Chronic cholestatic syndromes are prevalent but have a lower annual incidence than acute processes such as drug toxicity, gallstone disease, or severe hepatitis with consequent cholestasis. Traditionally, "chronic" is applied when the pathology appears to persist for greater than 6 months. In childhood, however, cholestatic syndromes represent the most common class of liver disease. Pediatric illnesses within this umbrella include biliary atresia (BA), Alagille syndrome (ALGS), and the inherited biliary transporter disorders (previously collectively labeled as the progressive familial intrahepatic cholestatic (PFIC) syndromes). In adults, chronic cholestatic liver disease is largely restricted to two inflammatory syndromes. Primary biliary cirrhosis (PBC) a classic autoimmune disease, and primary sclerosing cholangitis (PSC), an autoinflammatory disease, commonly associated with inflammatory bowel disease. Other etiologies can give rise to secondary biliary disease, which include chronic biliary obstruction and secondary cholangiopathies consequent to ischemia, infection, residual drug toxicity, inherited biliary abnormalities, or inflammation.

Pediatric

In childhood the distinction between acute and chronic disease is less valuable, compared to a consideration of the age at presentation (see Chapter 3).

Biliary atresia. BA is the most common cause of end-stage liver disease and liver transplantation in children. It is a progressive sclerosing inflammatory process of extrahepatic *and* intrahepatic bile ducts causing complete biliary obstruction in the first 3 months of life. It has an incidence of 1 in 10 000 live births. The etiology is unknown but postulated to be an immune-mediated perinatal insult in 80% of cases and syndromic in 20%, in which case it is associated with other congenital anomalies such as situs inversus, cardiac defects, malrotation, and polysplenia. BA is uniformly fatal unless a Kasai portoenterostomy is rapidly performed, in which a Roux-en-y jejunostomy is formed to establish bile drainage from the hilar plate. This surgery has the best outcomes if performed within the first 60 days of life. Nevertheless, even in children who do establish biliary flow, there is progressive hepatic fibrosis. Approximately 50% of all children with BA undergo liver transplantation by the age of 2 years and more than 90% of young adults with BA who have their native liver have hepatic fibrosis.[3]

Alagille syndrome. ALGS is the most common inherited cause of conjugated hyperbilirubinemia in the neonatal period. It is a multisystem, autosomal dominant disorder characterized by cholestatic liver disease and bile duct paucity on liver biopsy, congenital cardiac defects, typically peripheral pulmonary stenosis, renal anomalies, vascular abnormalities, characteristic facies (broad forehead, deep-set eyes, and a pointed chin), posterior embryotoxon of the eye on slip-lamp examination, and skeletal anomalies, commonly butterfly vertebrae. In the majority of patients (>93%) a mutation in *JAGGED1* can be identified whilst a smaller number of ALGS individuals have mutations in *NOTCH2*. Mutations are inherited in 40% and *de novo* in the remainder.[4]

Progressive familial intrahepatic cholestasis syndromes. This group of three biliary transport disorders that were previously categorized as PFIC1, PFIC2, and PFIC3, are now better described by their molecular terminology.
- PFIC1/FIC1 deficiency: this is an autosomal recessive condition that presents with cholestasis in early childhood. It is caused by mutations in *ATPB81*, encoding an aminophospholipid flippase which is widely expressed throughout the body. As a consequence, in addition to severe pruritus, it is manifest by failure to thrive, diarrhea, sensorineural hearing loss, and pancreatic dysfunction.
- PFIC2/BSEP deficiency: the presentation is similar to FIC1 deficiency though it is caused by mutations in another canalicular transporter gene, *ABCB11*. However, the bile salt export pump is only expressed in the liver and therefore there are no extrahepatic manifestations. It is characterized by cholestasis, gallstones, and a higher incidence of hepatocellular carcinoma, which is otherwise very unusual in childhood.
- PFIC3/MDR3 deficiency: this condition is also inherited as an autosomal recessive trait and is a defect of biliary phospholipid secretion. Although it may present in early life with cholestasis, it has a broader range of presentations, including recurrent choledocholithiasis in older children and adults, and some cases of intrahepatic cholestasis of pregnancy.
- Benign recurrent cholestasis: this causes episodic cholestasis (rarely progressive) and is associated with *ATP8B1* and *ABCB11* mutations.

Miscellaneous. Immune-mediated processes such as PSC also present in older children, with some similarity to adults. Of note, in children with autoimmune hepatitis, upwards of 50% of them will have a cholangiopathy; this is often described as an "overlap" syndrome, termed autoimmune sclerosing cholangitis. Metabolic liver diseases such as α_1-antitrypsin deficiency and cystic fibrosis-related liver disease may present with cholestasis in early childhood, although these are not classically considered cholestatic diseases.

Adults

Primary biliary cirrhosis. As the commonest adult chronic cholestatic liver disease, PBC is an archetypal autoimmune biliary disease, in which the overwhelming majority of patients are women in middle age who have circulating antimitochondrial antibodies (AMA). One in 1000 Caucasian women over the age of 40 are estimated to have the disease. Histologically, disease is evident as a granulomatous lymphocytic cholangitis, in which small bile duct loss progresses alongside an interface hepatitis. Biliary cirrhosis is the end result. Clinically, presentation is usually asymptomatic and is identified by blood work alone, but symptoms of pruritus in particular may be evident.[5]

Sclerosing cholangitis. PSC is a progressive inflammatory disease of the large bile ducts, which is more common in men. It is frequently associated with inflammatory bowel disease. Its prevalence is probably about half that of PBC. It is a disease that can affect children as well as adults, although typically patients present with symptoms in their 40s. With incidental screening, the age at diagnosis is ostensibly falling. The disease is usually diagnosed by imaging criteria (cholangiography by MRI or endoscopically); liver biopsy changes can be patchy and is therefore not usually needed. Histologically, a fibro-obliterative process may be seen surrounding larger bile ducts, with so-called "onion skin" fibrosis. Disease is predominantly driven by this obstruction to biliary drainage, although, as with PBC, a component of liver injury is from an interface hepatitis. Patients are commonly asymptomatic upon diagnosis, which is a result of screening biochemistry in "at-risk" populations. As disease progresses to secondary biliary cirrhosis, cholangitis, portal hypertension, and liver failure are common.[6]

Secondary sclerosing cholangitis is the term used when a recognized etiology for large duct cholangiopathy can be identified, and occurs because there appears to be a common pathway to biliary injury such that a variety of insults cause sclerosing cholangitis.[7] Many secondary causes are recognized including, but not limited to, autoimmune pancreatitis, biliary ischemia (arterial or secondary to chronic portal vein thrombosis), an infected choledochal cyst, and recurrent intrahepatic choledocholithiasis or infective cholangitis, particularly in patients with various immunodeficiencies. Before the label *primary* is applied to patients, clinicians should assiduously consider secondary etiologies, in particular IgG4-associated autoimmune pancreatitis, a disease that is multisystem and exquisitely sensitive to steroids, unlike PSC (Fig. 20.1).

Idiopathic ductopenia. Histologically, the only positive finding is of small bile duct loss. The cholestatic disease course is usually but not always progressive.

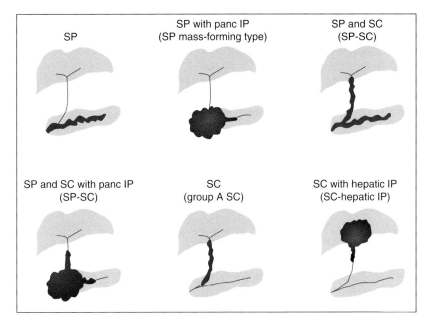

Fig. 20.1 A spectrum of IgG4-associated sclerosing cholangitis. IP, idiopathic pancreatitis; SC, sclerosing cholangitis; SP, sclerosing pancreatitis. From: Björnsson E, Chari ST, Smyrk TC, Lindor K. Immunoglobulin G4 associated cholangitis: description of an emerging clinical entity based on review of the literature. Reproduced from Björnsson et al. Hepatology 2007; 45: 1547–54 with permission from VG Wort.

Drug exposure must be carefully excluded as should paraneoplastic syndromes, especially those of lymphoma. Overall, this rare syndrome is likely a collection of diseases including genetic triggers and unidentified toxin exposure.

Adult presentations of inherited disease. Benign recurrent intrahepatic cholestasis is usually a variant of PFIC2 (low GGT cholestasis). Patients may experience recurrent episodes of symptomatically intense, histologically bland cholestasis, which is sometimes triggered by infection or medication. MDR3 (PFIC3) mutations can also have a varied presentation in adulthood, including cryptogenic biliary cirrhosis, recurrent intrahepatic choledocholithiasis, and cholestasis of pregnancy. Pediatric patients with ALGS and biliary atresia successfully managed by Kasai portoenterostomy may transition to adult care. Those with ductal plate malformations such as Caroli disease, in addition to having portal hypertension, can have cholestatic disease as well as renal disease; either polycystic or medullary sponge kidneys may be present.

Miscellaneous. These include chronic graft versus host disease following bone marrow transplant, any severe hepatitis including autoimmune hepatitis, resolving hepatitis A, hepatitis E, or EBV infection, hepatic infiltration including sarcoidosis, amyloidosis, tuberculosis, any granulomatous liver injury, and malignancies such as lymphoma and adenocarcinoma; severe recurrent hepatitis B or C post-liver transplant and post-transplant chronic rejection can also give rise to chronic cholestasis.

Making the diagnosis

Presentation
Adult perspective
In adult practice, presentation can be asymptomatic or symptomatic. Asymptomatic presentations are increasingly common. In adults, the usual observation is a disproportionate elevation in ALP. GGT is usually also elevated; although GGT is a very sensitive biochemical marker of liver injury, the majority of patients with an elevated GGT do not have a cholestatic liver disease. Additionally, fatty liver can present with an isolated elevation in ALP. The utility of GGT is of course the exact opposite in children, where ALP is not very helpful because it is also produced in bone. Other asymptomatic presentations occur when patients with associated autoimmune diseases are specifically screened by their clinicians for either PBC or PSC (e.g. in those with Sjögren syndrome, scleroderma, and inflammatory bowel disease). When symptomatic, patients with cholestatic liver disease may present with jaundice (but this is increasingly uncommon as dark urine and pale stools are usually recognized before scleral icterus), pruritus (a broad differential, but this is a specific symptom of cholestasis), or fatigue (a very non-specific symptom). Patients with PBC commonly complain of eye, mouth, or vaginal dryness. More often than not this reflects a non-specific sicca complex syndrome, as opposed to primary Sjögren syndrome. Cholangitis (which is clinically manifested as right upper quadrant pain and fever) is a medical emergency regardless of etiology and prompt treatment with antibiotics trumps investigation initially. It is *not* a feature of small bile duct disease, and indeed it should be noted that *de novo* cholangitis in PSC is uncommon, usually only occurring after there has been an intervention such as endoscopic retrograde cholangiopancreatography (ERCP). This may not be the case in some secondary forms of cholangitis, for example portal biliopathy (Fig. 20.2). Additionally, an elevated white cell count whilst common is not universal; patients with severe cholangitis can have a normal white blood cell count. A dull ache over the liver is not infrequently noted by women with PBC, and perhaps this is just a reflection of the hepatomegaly of cholestasis.

Pediatric perspective
Cholestatic liver disease in children is invariably symptomatic. Infants will typically present with jaundice and conjugated hyperbilirubinemia. The GGT is an important discriminator between different groups of diseases. Infants with BA and ALGS present with high-GGT cholestasis. They can be further

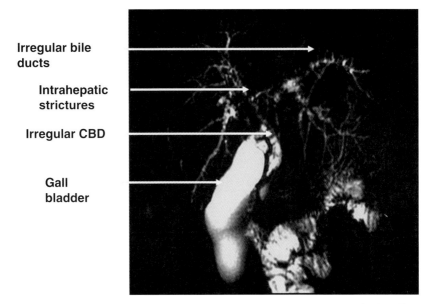

Irregular bile
ducts

  Intrahepatic
  strictures

Irregular CBD

  Gall
  bladder

Fig. 20.2 Portal biliopathy at magnetic resonance cholangiopancreatography (MRC). Definitive therapy is retroperitoneal splenorenal anastomosis. CBD, common bile duct.

differentiated by the presence of other characteristic congenital anomalies in ALGS. However, since variable expression is a hallmark of ALGS, extrahepatic involvement may be subtle and other investigations are required (see below). Children with BA progress to end-stage liver disease within a few months of life without surgical intervention. Children with ALGS and cholestatic liver disease usually develop intense pruritus and xanthomas (Plate 20.1) in the first few years of life. The liver disease of ALGS does not have onset outside early childhood, though it may progress or improve with time. Infants with FIC1 and BSEP deficiency present with low-GGT cholestasis and usually present outside the neonatal period but in the first 2 years of life with intense pruritus. They do not have xanthomas.

Investigations
Investigation is aimed at diagnosis, estimating disease severity, and looking for associated complications (Box 20.1). In addition to a pertinent and comprehensive history from the patient (which must include family history of autoimmunity/biliary disease and a careful drug history), thorough clinical examination remains important, even if nowadays no abnormal physical findings are likely to be evident. Findings may not be specific but patients may be jaundiced, and/or have hepatomegaly and splenomegaly, as well as other signs of chronic liver disease/portal hypertension, such as spider telangiectasia, ascites, and muscle wasting. Occasionally, overt skin damage from chronic

---

Box 20.1 Cholestasis: investigation and treatment algorithm for adult patients with cholestasis

1 Perform baseline standard liver screen (including viral markers, immunoglobulins) and exclude drug injury by history; note features to suggest prior cholangitis and pregnancy-related symptoms in addition to present symptoms such as pruritus.
2 Arrange an ultrasound of the liver with Doppler studies, to identify overt biliary obstruction, focal lesions or infiltration:
   (a) proceed to ERCP only if jaundiced with dilated biliary tree; ideally perform cross-sectional studies before any biliary intervention.
3 Request antimitochondrial and antinuclear antibodies:
   (a) if PBC is diagnosed, commence treatment with UDCA at 15 mg/kg.
4 If AMA negative, and no specific ANA reactivity, proceed to MRCP:
   (a) if large duct cholangiopathy on imaging, ensure secondary etiologies such as IgG4-associated autoimmune pancreatitis/sclerosing cholangitis are excluded;
   (b) if PSC is diagnosed, ensure pancolonoscopy with biopsies is performed, and consider use of UDCA at 15–20 mg/kg.
5 If MRCP shows no large duct disease, proceed to liver biopsy to identify AMA-negative PBC, small duct PSC, granulomatous disease, infiltration and vanishing bile duct syndrome/idiopathic ductopenia:
   (a) consider genetic studies as appropriate for PFIC syndromes, and treat with UDCA at 15 mg/kg;
   (b) consider empiric UDCA at 15 mg/kg for persistent idiopathic cholestatic syndromes.
6 *Arrange ongoing gastroenterology or hepatology follow-up* as appropriate, to include disease surveillance and monitoring for associated complications (including bone and colonic disease).

---

itching can be evident, as well as skin xanthelasma and xanthomas. Undue lymphadenopathy should prompt one to consider lymphoma.

Usually, the first clue that there is cholestasis in adults is an elevation in ALP. This should then be confirmed as biliary in origin by measurement of GGT. ALP isoenzymes are now rarely requested. If cholestasis is confirmed, investigation should then focus on further blood tests and imaging (ultrasound, MRI). Liver biopsy is rarely needed to make a diagnosis but does still have a role to play in selected circumstances.

Diagnostic blood work. As usual, after first excluding common liver diseases, as well as ruling out an unconjugated hyperbilirubinemia, testing should include:
- **Antimitochondrial antibodies:** more than 95% of patients who have PBC are AMA positive. The positive predictive value of finding PBC by histology if there is cholestasis and a positive AMA and the ALT or AST is less than

five times the upper limit of normal is over 90%. If AMA testing is by immunofluorescence, then it is advisable to confirm any positive finding with a specific ELISA assay. If AMA testing is used in settings other than cholestasis, it must be recognized that specificity is lost, as other conditions such as autoimmune hepatitis, drug injury, or acute liver failure can cause a positive AMA.

- **Antinuclear antibodies** (by immunofluorescence): most patients who have so-called "AMA-negative PBC" are ANA positive with distinct immunofluorescent patterns, namely multiple nuclear dot and membrane rim pattern. Automated ANA assays are unlikely to detect these highly specific ANA reactivities, and laboratories should be asked to perform immunofluorescence if specific ELISA-based assays for gp210 and sp100 are not available. In contrast, patients with PSC may have ANA reactivity that is non-specific. This can include perinuclear antineutrophilic cytoplasmic antibody (p-ANCA), which is not disease specific and is not of any value as a routine investigation.
- **Immunoglobulins:** an elevated IgM is a sensitive but not specific feature of PBC. Elevations in IgG are possible in all patients with cirrhosis, and also in those with autoimmune liver disease. Marked elevations of IgG (>two times ULN) should lead the clinician to consider whether there could be an autoimmune hepatitis overlap component, to their PBC/PSC, although reaching the diagnosis of a so-called overlap syndrome should be carefully considered, as outside of pediatric practice, it is quite rare. In patients presenting with sclerosing cholangitis, it is recommended that IgG4 subclasses are measured to ensure the treatment-responsive and systemic disease, IgG4-associated autoimmune pancreatitis, is identified.

Imaging. All patients should have a baseline ultrasound, particularly focusing on the gallbladder and biliary tree. In PBC the biliary imaging is expected to be normal. In PSC, gallstones, biliary wall thickening (particularly common bile duct), and biliary dilation are important features to ascertain. Choledochal cysts are usually easily visible on ultrasound; they are a risk factor for cholangiocarcinoma and thus require resection. Gross cirrhosis with splenomegaly may be evident, but at initial presentation this is uncommon in adults. Hepatomegaly is a feature of cholestatic liver disease but is not specific. Another common finding in chronic liver disease, particularly when immune mediated, is lymphadenopathy, which is often periportal. This is almost always innocent, and pursuit of lymphoma should only be carried out if there are striking radiological or clinical concerns. In those with persistent cholestasis, but negative serologic screening for PBC and a normal biliary tree on ultrasound, magnetic resonance cholangiopancreatography (MRCP) should be performed. There is little, if any, role for purely diagnostic ERCP, although the individual center's experience in reporting MRCP should be taken into account. ERCP is more sensitive to early biliary changes in sclerosing cholangitis, but it is accompanied by too many risks to support its use diagnostically in the era of MR imaging.

MRI also has the advantage of being a cross-sectional imaging modality, and therefore provides greater information about parenchymal liver injury and pancreatic changes, in particular. If a patient is jaundiced and has a dilated biliary tree or gallstones, therapeutic ERCP should be considered.

Histology. Particularly for biliary disease, liver biopsy samples are prone to sampling variation and are rarely used for diagnostic purposes for either PBC or PSC. If a patient is AMA negative and has a normal MRCP, then biopsy may be appropriate with the intent to identify AMA-negative PBC or small-duct PSC (a variant of PSC with normal cholangiography and a different natural history). Estimates of disease severity can be made from histology, but the clinician must be aware that errors of plus or minus one stage of fibrosis are commonly encountered (Plate 20.2). If patients wish to have a concept of disease severity then consideration of FibroScan, although not validated in cholestasis, may be appropriate (transient elastography).

Endoscopy. Evaluation for varices is usually reserved for those with cirrhosis; the majority of patients with cholestatic liver disease who have varices are cirrhotic, but not all (as some may have presinusoidal portal hypertension). Although guidelines suggest screening all cirrhotic patients by endoscopy, the greatest yield in those with cholestatic liver disease is either for those with thrombocytopenia (e.g. $<200 \times 10^9$/L), splenomegaly, or who have elevated risk scores such as the Mayo PBC score.

Bone density. Osteoporosis is a frequent concern in normal postmenopausal women, as well as in those with inflammatory bowel disease. Cholestatic liver disease is likely associated with a low bone turnover state, and certainly in advanced disease osteoporosis and sometimes osteomalacia can be found. Appropriate screening at diagnosis and follow-up is usually advised. Bone density measurements should be interpreted in the context of the patient's sex, age, history of fragility fractures, family history, as well as use of steroids in particular.

Associated autoimmune diseases. Particularly in PBC, associated autoimmune diseases may be relatively common (>10%).Therefore, where easy screening and intervention exist, they should be sought. This applies particularly to celiac and thyroid disease.

Pediatric perspective
Unlike in adults, the GGT is a useful pediatric diagnostic discriminator and a liver biopsy is a key step in establishing the diagnosis (Box 20.2). The liver biopsy in BA reveals bile duct proliferation, suggestive of large duct obstruction, whereas it is characteristically shows bile duct paucity in ALGS. Ultimately, the gold standard for diagnosing BA is an intraoperative cholangiogram, which demonstrates the atretic extrahepatic biliary tract. In any infant with high-GGT cholestasis, an echocardiogram, slit-lamp examination, and spinal

---

Box 20.2 Investigation and treatment for pediatric patients with cholestasis

1 Take a careful history of jaundice as well as associated systemic symptoms, from parents, and carefully examine the baby/child (to include evaluation for syndromic features).
2 Perform a baseline liver screen to include direct and indirect bilirubin, GGT, immunoglobulins, autoantibodies, α_1-antitrypsin levels, metabolic and sepsis screens as appropriate.
3 Arrange a baseline ultrasound to exclude choledochal cyst, in particular.
4 Consider liver biopsy and MRCP as appropriate to individual findings.
5 Ensure early referral for surgery (by 6–8 weeks of age) if biliary atresia likely.
6 Optimize nutrition to include fat-soluble vitamin supplementation (vitamins A, D, E, and K).
7 *Refer for expert ongoing management* to include consideration of genetic testing/ family screening, prescription of UDCA and/or antibiotics, symptom management, and surgical therapies.

X-ray for butterfly vertebrae are also needed. Mutational analysis of *JAGGED1* is also commercially available. The liver biopsy in FIC1 and BSEP deficiencies can be bland (i.e. no inflammatory component) on light microscopy but electron microscopy is more revealing, demonstrating coarse, abnormal bile. These disorders can be indistinguishable except for clinical course and mutational analysis.[8]

Management

Management focuses on disease-specific interventions, symptom control, routine management of the patient with chronic liver disease, and timing of transplant referral. The natural history of PBC is progression to cirrhosis and liver failure. With appropriate therapy, ursodeoxycholic acid (UDCA), this is increasingly uncommon. The natural history of PSC is progression to liver transplantation in about 50% of patients after about 10–15 years of symptomatic disease; to date, no intervention has changed this.

Medical management
Disease-specific management
PBC. The only licensed treatment for PBC is the choleretic and hydrophilic bile acid, ursodeoxycholic acid. At treatment doses of 13–15 mg/kg per day the consensus is that UDCA slows the progression of disease and reduces the chances of developing liver failure. Clinical trials have not shown it to be effective in treating symptoms such as itch. The greatest efficacy is in those demonstrating a biochemical response to treatment. This is variably defined, but it

includes either normalization of ALP at 1 year, a 40% decline of ALP from baseline at 1 year, or a bilirubin less than normal *and* AST less than two times ULN *and* ALP less than three times ULN at 1 year. UDCA has a good safety profile at this dose. Thinning of the hair, some weight gain, and bloating are reported. Medication can be taken either all together prior to bedtime, or if desired split over the day. If patients are concurrently using cholestyramine, care must be taken to adequately space medications. There are no proven second-line therapies if UDCA is ineffective. Many agents have been suggested but lack a robust evidence base to justify their use routinely. Patients without an appropriate biochemical response should be considered for clinical trials.

PSC. There are no proven medical therapies for PSC. The only drug to have been repeatedly evaluated is UDCA. There is, however, no consensus on the efficacy of UDCA in this setting. High-dose therapy (28–30 mg/kg per day) has been discredited by a randomized study that suggests increased adverse events in those treated with UDCA, possibly because of increased lithocholic acid levels, without any clinical benefit even in those with a biochemical response. Treatment at 20 mg/kg per day is nevertheless felt by some to be appropriate and certainly it is quite likely that PSC as a disease is heterogeneous, and therefore subgroups may benefit from interventions in different ways. However, the pathology of this disease (Plate 20.3) likely suggests that response to any medical therapy will be minimal. A therapeutic role for routine ERCP is controversial, and the center's experience is relevant, but certainly those with tight dominant proximal strictures warrant consideration for intervention.

Management of associated symptoms/disease
Pruritus. Itch can be a devastating symptom and the severity of itch need not correlate with the severity of the biliary injury. If an identifiable obstructive component is contributing to cholestasis (i.e. in PSC, this is *not* of course relevant to the pruritus of PBC), relief of this via ERCP maybe important. Dominant strictures (in which malignancy must be excluded) are best treated with just balloon dilation if possible, as stenting may precipitate biliary sepsis. Medical therapy will usually ameliorate the symptoms of itch. A stepwise approach is recommended with response to treatment driving the need for additional therapy: cholestyramine (bile acid resin, 4 g twice daily, before and after breakfast); rifampin (150–300 mg b.i.d., with appropriate hematologic, renal, and hepatic screening blood tests at 6 weeks, and then periodically); sertraline (serotonin reuptake inhibitor, 50–100 mg daily); and naltrexone (opiate antagonist, 50 mg orally). UV light therapy, plasmapheresis, MARS (albumin dialysis), and liver transplant can be occasionally needed.

Cholangitis. The constellation of fever, jaundice, and right upper quadrant pain should raise the suspicion of cholangitis. Cholangitis is a relative medical emergency that necessitates prompt broad-spectrum antibiotics (e.g. ciprofloxacin or third-generation cephalosporin). Biliary drainage may be appropriate—patients with PSC who develop sudden-onset jaundice that does not rapidly settle when antibiotics are given (rather than a progressive jaundice of liver failure) generally should have ERCP to exclude stones, sludge, and malignancy. Providing patients with antibiotics such as ciprofloxacin or moxifloxacin to keep at home, or when traveling, is a sensible strategy.

Fatigue. Many patients with liver disease, cholestatic diseases included, complain of tiredness. Whilst certainly a prevalent symptom, it is not specific to one disease and has a multifactorial etiology. Exclusion of treatable causes of fatigue is important and these include thyroid disease, anemia, depression, drug side effects (beta-blockers, sedatives), and adrenal failure. Specific interventions are limited. Some suggest modafinil, a stimulant, but this should be used only if the clinician has appropriate experience. Exercise seems a simple, risk-free intervention, and is reported by patients to be helpful.

Inflammatory bowel disease in PSC. There is a high prevalence of inflammatory bowel disease (IBD) in those with PSC (not with secondary etiologies), that approaches 75% in some studies. All patients diagnosed with PSC should undergo a screening colonoscopy including biopsies, if they are not already known to have IBD. The colitis of PSC can be distinctive, in that it is often milder (including microscopic only at times), right sided, exhibits rectal sparing, and backwash ileitis. The concern principally is the high rate of colorectal cancer—approaching 25% in patients with PSC and IBD in some series over the lifetime of a patient. For this reason, in addition to optimal management of the IBD (e.g. 5-ASA products, azathioprine), approximately yearly surveillance colonoscopy is recommended. Some data suggest that UDCA has a preventative role in reducing colon cancer rates, and this is given as a reason for its use in PSC. For patients needing colectomy, issues of timing may be challenging, since surgery before the complications of cirrhosis and portal hypertension arise is safer. Ectopic varices can develop at the sites of stomas and prove hard to treat, therefore pouch surgery is attractive if possible. There are also some data to suggest that recurrent PSC post liver transplant is less likely if colectomy occurs pre- or peritransplant.

Gallbladder disease and PSC. Malignancy in PSC is a real concern, and this includes gallbladder cancer. Annual imaging of the biliary tree by ultrasound is sensible and elective cholecystectomy is appropriate if the patient is symptomatic with gallstones, or has focal lesions such as polyps. Generally, in any patient with cirrhosis, the presence of symptomatic gallstones should prompt consideration of early elective cholecystectomy, prior to any complications.

Cholangiocarcinoma and PSC. The risk of cholangiocarcinoma over their lifetime for a patient with PSC is less than 10%. Most patients with cholangiocarcinoma do not have PSC. No effective screening exists and treatments remain challenging. Serum markers such as CA19.9 and radiologic/endoscopic investigation are sufficiently imperfect that no consensus exists over their routine use. Over one-third of patients who have PSC and cholangiocarcinoma present with the cholangiocarcinoma. It is therefore uncommon to develop cholangiocarcinoma in established PSC, and patients should be reassured by this. Secondary sclerosing cholangitis, particularly if associated with recurrent stones from parasitic infection, also has a heightened cholangiocarcinoma risk.

Bone disease. Routine supplementation with calcium (best as milk) and vitamin D is advisable, as is encouragement of weight-bearing exercise. Treatment with bisphosphonates (or other agents) may be indicated if the individual fracture risk suggests benefit.

Fat malabsorption. This is very rare nowadays since the advent of transplantation, but night blindness secondary to vitamin A deficiency is reported if patients have prolonged jaundice.

Non-disease-specific management
Cirrhosis surveillance. Patients with cirrhosis are at risk for hepatocellular carcinoma, and generally all cirrhotic patients should be offered ultrasound surveillance every 6 months.

Endoscopic surveillance. Most patients who develop varices with cholestatic liver disease are cirrhotic, although a minority may not be. Spleen size and platelet count are reasonable indicators for elective gastroscopy, as discussed above.

Vaccination. Patients with any cause of chronic liver disease should be vaccinated against hepatitis A and B. Patients with cirrhosis should receive annual influenza vaccination, in particular.

Presurgery advice. Caution in those with cirrhosis and portal hypertension is recommended. Avoidance of perioperative hypotension and postoperative fluid overload can minimize risks of postoperative decompensation.

Pregnancy. This is not contraindicated but added caution is recommended if patients have portal hypertension. Generally, fetal outcomes are good and relate to the mother's own health. UDCA treatment is considered safe during pregnancy, although some choose to stop taking UDCA during the first trimester. Itch can be the greatest challenge. Cholestyramine, rifampin, sertraline, and in treatment-resistant cases plasmapheresis have all been used in pregnancy. Endoscopy in the second trimester is usually recommended if patients are known to be cirrhotic. Ultrasound examination is also sensible.

Timing of transplant referral
In the absence of hepatocellular carcinoma (or very early cholangiocarcinoma) the Model for End-stage Liver Disease (MELD) score is a reasonable means of

determining the need for transplant, with a cutoff of 15 usually triggering evaluation. As a rule of thumb, if a patient with cholestatic liver disease persistently has a bilirubin over 100 µmol/L they have disease likely to need transplant. Occasionally symptoms such as pruritus or intractable cholangitis may necessitate transplant.

Pediatric perspective
The pruritus of cholestasis in children is managed similarly from a medical standpoint to adults. However, special attention must be paid to nutritional aspects of cholestasis in childhood. Infants are switched to medium-chain triglyceride formulas and almost all cholestatic children require fat-soluble vitamin supplementation, especially vitamin D. A vitamin preparation containing vitamins A, D, E, and K is commonly used. Many children will require nutritional supplementation via a nasogastric tube or gastrostomy.

Surgical management
From the adult perspective, apart from transplantation, surgical intervention is not commonly of value. Occasional patients with localized biliary stones may benefit from surgical resection and individual patients with extrahepatic biliary obstruction may need tailored biliary diversion surgery.

Pediatric perspective
Surgical management of pediatric cholestatic liver diseases includes two unique procedures. The Kasai portoenterostomy is described above and is life-saving in BA. Children with severe cholestasis and intense pruritus (ALGS, PFIC) may benefit from an external biliary diversion in which a loop of jejunum is fashioned into a conduit between the gallbladder and the skin, interrupting enterohepatic circulation. Liver transplantation is widely performed for all cholestatic diseases, largely with excellent outcomes.

Case study 20.1

A 39-year-old woman referred to a gastroenterologist with itch and abnormal liver biochemistry, that started during her third pregnancy, 6 months prior to the consultation. Other than hypothyroidism she was well and on no medications other than thyroxine. Her itch began in the last trimester of her last pregnancy, and persisted post-partum. Topical therapies only had been tried and she had scarring on both her legs from excoriations. Apart from this clinical examination was unremarkable.

Bloods: ALP 450 IU/L (normal <150), AST 150 IU/L (normal <40), ALT 175 IU/L (normal <40), Bilirubin 17 µmol/L (normal <24), IgG 18 g/L (normal <14), IgM 4 g/L (normal <2), Hb 14 g/L (normal >13), platelet 225 × 10^9 (normal >150); AMA, seen by immunofluorescence; ANA, multiple nuclear dot pattern; antismooth muscle negative; Hepatitis B immune, Hepatitis C negative. Ultrasound, coarse liver, normal spleen size.

(Continued)

What is the diagnosis?
AMA-positive primary biliary cirrhosis; no further investigation is required in routine care to determine therapy. Defining the AMA as AMA-M2 is not necessary because she has a specific ANA pattern of PBC. Liver biopsy is not necessary as the positive predictive value of having PBC on biopsy with this presentation is well over 90%. The elevated transaminases and IgG do not mean this woman has overlap autoimmune hepatitis—it is quite common for patients with PBC to have interface activity. If after appropriate therapy her transaminases were still very abnormal (particularly if >5 × ULN) then further investigation may be appropriate, assuming no drug injury is present (e.g. statins, non-steroidal anti-inflammatory drugs, antibiotics). Management is with ursodeoxycholic acid (see above), and symptom control, as described earlier, is very important.

Case study 20.2

A 3-week-old baby is seen by his pediatrician for unremitting jaundice. Born normally without concern, the mother reported jaundice from day 2 that did not resolve. She also noticed increasingly dark urine and pale stools. The baby fed well but was small for his age and on examination had hepatomegaly. Cardiac examination was normal, and no syndromic features were evident. Blood tests revealed a direct bilirubin of 120 μmol/L, GGT of 650 IU/L (normal <25), ALT of 80 IU/L (normal <30), ALP of 750 IU/L (normal <420). Albumin, prothrombin time, and glucose were normal. Metabolic screening, including α_1-antitrypsin levels, was negative. Imaging by ultrasound was unremarkable, with no choledochal cyst and no overt biliary changes. The patient was referred to a tertiary center urgently and liver biopsy showed features of bile duct obstruction (ductular proliferation, portal tract edema, bile plugging). Nutritional support was optimized, including fat-soluble vitamins, and pediatric surgery consulted.

What is the diagnosis?
This baby presents with unremitting conjugated hyperbilirubinemia, with an elevated GGT and features of bile duct obstruction on biopsy. The diagnosis is therefore most likely biliary atresia. At laparotomy, on table cholangiography, confirmed an atretic extrahepatic biliary tree and a successful portoenterostomy, with resolution of jaundice postoperatively, was performed at 6 weeks of age.

Investigation of persistent jaundice in this setting is essential and should be *rapid* and thorough. The success of portoenterostomy is dependent on the age at which surgery takes place. Ideally, the diagnosis should be arrived at by the time the baby is 5–7 weeks of age, and the Kasai portoenterostomy performed by 6–8 weeks. By the age of 14 weeks it is probably ineffective. In expert centers, 80% of children with optimally timed surgery, and supportive medical care (including nutrition and ursodeoxycholic acid), can survive without transplant for 8–10 years, sometimes even longer (i.e. to adulthood).

Multiple choice questions

1. You are asked to review a 50-year-old man with primary sclerosing cholangitis who is attending his local emergency room with increasing jaundice, itch, and abdominal pain, alongside development of a new fever in the last 24 hours. In your evaluation which two factors are important to consider?
   A. Bacterial cholangitis requiring prompt treatment with antibiotics.
   B. A full blood count is important because if the white cell count is normal that excludes cholangitis and facilitates discharge.
   C. Primary sclerosing cholangitis is commonly associated with cholangiocarcinoma in the majority and this is the most likely etiology here.
   D. Endoscopic intervention should be considered in the presence of new jaundice in patients with primary sclerosing cholangitis.
   E. Antihistamines are the first-line treatment for cholestatic pruritus.

2. Which of the following is *not* true about biliary atresia?
   A. Biliary atresia is the leading indication for pediatric liver transplantation.
   B. Biliary atresia is associated with congenital anomalies such as situs inversus and malrotation in approximately 20% of cases.
   C. Biliary atresia usually presents with high-GGT cholestasis.
   D. Biliary atresia is associated with characteristic facial features.
   E. A liver biopsy in biliary atresia typically reveals bile duct proliferation.

Answers

1. A and D. Primary sclerosing cholangitis is usually a slowly progressive, large bile duct disease that culminates in secondary biliary cirrhosis, which may be complicated by liver failure and portal hypertension. Biliary tract infection is common. Bacterial cholangitis is potentially life threatening and very prompt treatment is essential. Initial management includes fluid resuscitation, blood cultures, and antibiotics. Diagnosis is made on the basis of the history as well as laboratory and imaging studies. A high white cell count need not be present, especially in the setting of chronic biliary disease with cirrhosis. Whilst cholangiocarcinoma is definitely seen at increased rates in patients with primary sclerosing cholangitis, the lifetime risk is still relatively low (<15%), so most patients will not develop this dreaded complication. Endoscopic treatment of biliary disorders remains important to consider, so long as the risks and benefits of therapeutic intervention are apprised carefully. In the presence of new jaundice in a patient with primary sclerosing cholangitis, concern over dominant strictures, biliary stones, and sludge are real, and therefore consultation with an interventional endoscopist may be appropriate. Cholestatic pruritus does not usually respond adequately to antihistamines. Therapies such as cholestyramine and rifampin need to be considered as first-line interventions.
2. D

References

1. Decock S, McGee P, Hirschfield GM. Autoimmune liver disease for the non-specialist. BMJ 2009; 339: b3305.
2. Hirschfield GM, Heathcote EJ, Gershwin ME. Pathogenesis of cholestatic liver disease and therapeutic approaches. Gastroenterology 2010; 139: 1481–96.
3. Hartley J, Harnden A, Kelly D. Biliary atresia BMJ 2010; 340: c2383.
4. Kamath BM, Loomes KM, Piccoli DA. Medical management of Alagille syndrome. J Pediatr Gastroenterol Nutr 2010; 50: 580–6.
5. Lindor KD, Gershwin ME, Poupon R, et al. Primary biliary cirrhosis. Hepatology 2009; 50: 291–308.
6. Chapman R, Fevery J, Kalloo A, et al. Diagnosis and management of primary sclerosing cholangitis. Hepatology 2010; 51: 660–78.
7. Abdalian R, Heathcote EJ. Sclerosing cholangitis: a focus on secondary causes. Hepatology 2006; 44: 1063–74.
8. van der Woerd WL, van Mil SW, Stapelbroek JM, et al. Familial cholestasis: progressive familial intrahepatic cholestasis, benign recurrent intrahepatic cholestasis and intrahepatic cholestasis of pregnancy. Best Pract Res Clin Gastroenterol 2010; 24: 541–53.

Vascular diseases of the liver

CHAPTER 21

Jordan J. Feld

Division of Gastroenterology, Toronto Western Hospital, University Health Network, University of Toronto, Toronto, Ontario, Canada

---

Key points

- Portal vein thrombosis is common in patients with cirrhosis.
- The main complication of portal vein thrombosis is variceal bleeding.
- Acute portal vein thrombosis without cirrhosis should be treated with anticoagulation.
- Anticoagulation in the setting of cirrhosis for portal vein thrombosis remains controversial but is likely safe.
- Budd–Chiari syndrome is almost always associated with an underlying predisposing condition (JAK2 tyrosine kinase mutations are the most common).
- Acute Budd–Chiari syndrome is a medical emergency.
- Transjugular intrahepatic portosystemic shunt (TIPS) is first-line therapy for acute Budd–Chiari syndrome.
- Sinusoidal obstruction syndrome (formerly called veno-occlusive disease) is usually a complication of stem-cell transplantation.
- Treatment options for sinusoidal obstruction syndrome are limited but prophylactic ursodeoxycholic acid appears beneficial.

Vascular anatomy

The liver is unique in that its primary blood supply is venous blood entering the liver through the portal vein. The hepatic artery supplies 30% of the blood volume but provides 90% of the oxygenated blood to the liver. The veins of the entire gastrointestinal tract drain into the portal vein, which then branches into the left and right portal vein as it enters the liver. The portal vein branches into smaller and smaller units until portal venules, which supply individual portal tracts, finally flow into the hepatic sinusoids.

Hepatology: Diagnosis and Clinical Management, First Edition. Edited by E. Jenny Heathcote.
© 2012 John Wiley & Sons, Ltd. Published 2012 by John Wiley & Sons, Ltd.

The sinusoids are lined by sinusoidal epithelial cells but are not true blood vessels as the sinusoids are fenestrated, allowing nutrients and waste to diffuse between the blood stream and the hepatocytes. The sinusoids drain into hepatic venules, which drain into larger and larger hepatic veins, which drain into the right, middle, and left hepatic veins.

The hepatic veins drain into the inferior vena cava (IVC). The caudate lobe of the liver has its own venous outflow, which empties directly into the IVC. As a result, in the setting of hepatic vein outflow obstruction (e.g. Budd–Chiari syndrome), the caudate lobe enlarges as blood from the other lobes of the liver is rerouted to the caudate to allow it to drain into the IVC and thereby return to the heart.

Portal vein thrombosis—with cirrhosis

Cirrhosis is present in 25–28% of cases of portal vein thrombosis (PVT). PVT is common in patients with cirrhosis, particularly as the disease progresses. Sluggish flow through the liver and possibly an imbalance between prothrombotic and antithrombotic factors in the liver increase the risk of PVT in patients with cirrhosis.

Although typically patients with cirrhosis are thought to be at increased risk of bleeding, it is important to note that although the liver makes clotting factors, it also makes antithrombotic factors such as protein C and protein S. Even when the PT/INR is elevated (this is the only parameter that is easily measurable), patients may actually be hypercoagulable.

Thrombophilic tendencies are identified in 40 to 70% of patients with cirrhosis and PVT. These include the Factor V Leiden mutation as well as mutations in the methylene–tetrahydrofolate and prothrombin genes.

Prevalence data estimate 10–25% of patients with cirrhosis have PVT.[1] Old studies suggest an incidence of less than 1% per year in patients with compensated cirrhosis, but PVT occurs much more frequently with more advanced liver disease. In patients on the liver transplant waiting list, PVT develops in 7 to 16% annually. The risk of PVT is highest with hepatocellular carcinoma (HCC), with rates as high as 35%. In contrast, PVT occurs in 16% of alcohol or viral-related cirrhosis, 8% in primary biliary cirrhosis, and 3.5% in primary sclerosing cholangitis.[2]

Presentation
Acute
Acute PVT is very variable, ranging from an asymptomatic incidental finding on imaging to precipitation of acute life-threatening hepatic decompensation. Symptoms may include GI bleeding from varices or portal hypertensive gastropathy (approximately 40%) and abdominal pain (approximately 18%) with possible extension to the mesenteric veins with intestinal infarction (a potentially fatal complication). Ascites is relatively uncommon unless patients

already have advanced cirrhosis. Ascites may develop with fluid resuscitation after a GI bleed.

It may be difficult to differentiate whether symptoms are from PVT or progression of underlying advanced cirrhosis.

Chronic

Typically, chronic PVT is found incidentally on radiologic investigation done for another purpose (e.g. HCC surveillance); however, it may also lead to a symptomatic presentation, usually with acute variceal hemorrhage. Esophageal varices are present in 85–90% of patients with PVT and 30–40% also have gastric varices. Variceal hemorrhage occurs at least once in 50–70% of patients over time and in 30% of patients on more than one occasion. Varices may also develop in atypical locations. Isolated splenic vein thrombosis usually leads to the development of just gastric varices. Splenomegaly is common with PVT and may be massive.

Diagnosis

The diagnosis is usually made with ultrasonography with Doppler evaluation. Contrast-enhanced ultrasonography (if available) is more sensitive but unnecessary in most cases.

Computed tomography (CT) or magnetic resonance imaging (MRI) allow better evaluation of the extent of the PVT and also may be used to evaluate for the presence of HCC in the liver and/or portal vein. Spontaneous shunts may develop between the splenic vein and left renal vein to decompress the portal system, which also are better visualized with CT or MRI.

Prognosis

The natural history of PVT in cirrhosis is not well documented. In a study of 37 patients with non-malignant PVT in the setting of cirrhosis, 5-year survival was only 45%.[3]

Recanalization of both acute and chronic PVT may occur. If recanalization occurs with acute PVT, there may be no evidence of its past occurrence and recurrence appears to be relatively infrequent. In the presence of cirrhosis, recanalization of the portal vein is uncommon. Cavernous transformation, in which collateral vessels develop to maintain blood flow in a hepatopedal direction, is typical of non-cirrhotic PVT. In contrast, with cirrhosis, PVT may persist or alternatively a spontaneous shunt may develop between the portal vein and the left renal vein, which decompresses the portal system but may lead to severe encephalopathy, out of keeping with the degree of liver dysfunction, due to marked portosystemic shunting.

PVT may progress from the large vessels to the small intrahepatic veins. Even if recanalization of the large vessels subsequently occurs, the intrahepatic microthrombi may lead to worsening of cirrhosis due to so-called "parenchymal extinction".

A trial of prophylactic low-molecular weight heparin (LMWH) (doses similar to deep vein thrombosis prophylaxis) in patients with advanced cirrhosis to prevent PVT showed that not only did patients have a lower incidence of PVT but also a lower rate of hepatic decompensation, reinforcing the concept that microthrombi in the liver may worsen cirrhosis.[4] Whether patients awaiting liver transplant should receive daily prophylactic heparin is currently unknown.

Management

Optimal management of PVT in the setting of cirrhosis is unknown. No randomized controlled trials have been performed. Anticoagulation is the most common treatment employed, with the primary goal of preventing extension of the clot rather than necessarily achieving recanalization (Fig. 21.1). In acute PVT without cirrhosis, early introduction of anticoagulation is advised, with 80% recanalization and a reduced risk of future thrombotic events or progression of clot to the mesenteric system. In patients with cirrhosis, the main concern is that if variceal hemorrhage were to occur, bleeding may be much more severe with anticoagulation. However, anticoagulation is unlikely to directly precipitate variceal hemorrhage. In a small study of 29 patients on the liver transplant waiting list, anticoagulation led to PVT recanalization in 8 of 19 compared to 0 of 10 who were left untreated. Transplant outcome was also improved, likely because the presence of PVT significantly complicates liver transplant surgery.[5] Anticoagulation with LMWH may be preferred to warfarin. Warfarin affects the INR and therefore makes the MELD score unreliable. Although a modification of MELD is made for patients on anticoagulation, LMWH may have other advantages such as less need for monitoring because

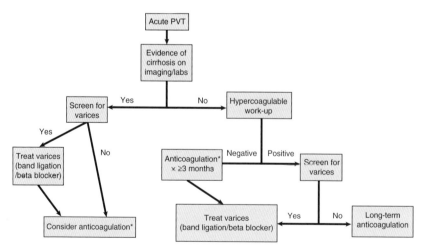

Fig. 21.1 Management of acute portal vein thrombosis (PVT). *Optimal anticoagulant is unclear—consider warfarin, low-molecular weight heparin, or new oral anticoagulant agents.

of weight-based dosing. New oral anticoagulants may offer similar advantages; however, their effects cannot be easily reversed with fresh frozen plasma and therefore should be used with caution in patients with cirrhosis.

If anticoagulation is used, variceal screening should be performed. The optimal therapy for varices in the setting of PVT with anticoagulation is unknown (beta-blockers vs. band ligation). Some advocate band ligation prior to starting anticoagulation, particularly if the varices have high-risk features (e.g. red spots). The risk of such an approach is bleeding from postbanding ulceration. Other therapeutic options for PVT include thrombectomy (minimal data) and transjugular intrahepatic portosystemic shunt (TIPS). Thrombectomy is followed by intraportal thrombolysis. TIPS is feasible if the intrahepatic PV branches are patent. TIPS placement is followed by anticoagulation and should serve as a bridge to liver transplantation.

Portal vein thrombosis—without cirrhosis

Approximately 75% of patients with PVT do not have underlying cirrhosis. The most common causes of non-cirrhotic PVT are abdominal surgery, abdominal sepsis (usually in childhood), pancreatitis, and hypercoagulability. Myeloproliferative disorders are the most common thrombophilic states seen with PVT. PVT may also occur due to childhood infections such as omphalitis. Neoplastic causes of PVT with tumor thrombus, particularly from renal cell carcinoma, should be excluded with imaging.

Presentation
Like in cirrhosis, PVT ranges from asymptomatic to life-threatening if intestinal infarction occurs from clot extension. Development of varices is common, with a high risk of bleeding. Variceal hemorrhage is much better tolerated in patients with non-cirrhotic PVT because of preserved liver synthetic function. In addition to atypical varices, patients often develop splenomegaly, which may be massive. Cavernous transformation, in which collateral vessels develop to maintain blood flow in a hepatopedal direction, often develops, particularly when PVT occurs in childhood. Cavernous transformation is usually easily seen on abdominal imaging. Even with recanalization or cavernous transformation, the spleen may remain enlarged. If so, patients, particularly children and adolescents, should be advised to avoid contact sports or be fitted with a splenic guard to prevent splenic rupture.

Prognosis
The major problem with non-cirrhotic PVT is variceal bleeding. Long-term survival is excellent with a 5-year mortality rate of 5 to 10%. Complications and fatalities are more commonly due to the underlying illness precipitating the PVT than to complications of the PVT itself.

In acute non-cirrhotic PVT, anticoagulation is recommended. Therapy should be continued for at least 3 months, but if a hypercoagulable risk factor is identified, longer-term (potentially indefinite) anticoagulation is necessary. Recanalization is reported to occur in from 40% to as high as 80% of patients when treatment is started at diagnosis.[6]

Anticoagulation is likely less useful in chronic PVT. The largest study showed a higher risk of bleeding (12.5 per 100 patient years) than thrombosis (5.5 per 100 patient years) in patients anticoagulated for chronic non-cirrhotic PVT.[7] Guidelines recommend anticoagulation for those with non-cirrhotic PVT and an identifiable thrombophilic predisposition that cannot be corrected. Screening for varices with institution of appropriate therapy (beta-blockers or band ligation) is recommended prior to starting anticoagulants. Band ligation is usually preferable as there are no data on beta-blocker therapy in PVT and, as the pathophysiology is different from that for varices secondary to portal hypertension due to cirrhosis, the efficacy may differ.

Portal biliopathy

Patients with chronic PVT (usually without cirrhosis) may develop bile duct abnormalities visible on cholangiogram that typically present with cholestatic jaundice. Biliary findings on imaging include: biliary stenosis, upstream dilatation, wavy appearance to the biliary tree, and angulation of the common bile duct. Gallbladder and choledocal varices are common in patients with biliopathy, however bleeding is very uncommon.

Portal biliopathy is thought to occur in the setting of long-standing PVT, but the precise mechanisms responsible are not well understood. Ursodeoxycholic acid is used empirically to treat portal biliopathy. Endoscopic retrograde cholangiopancreatography (ERCP) with stenting may be useful if significant strictures develop. Rarely mesocaval or other surgical shunts are performed to increase portosystemic shunting to reduce portal inflow and thus portal pressure.

Budd–Chiari syndrome

Budd–Chiari syndrome (BCS) usually refers to a thrombosis of the hepatic veins or suprahepatic inferior vena cava (see also Chapter 24). The largest series of BCS included 237 patients from four centers in three countries. It was found that BCS was more common in woman (67%), especially during or shortly after pregnancy, and the median age of presentation was 35 years old (range 13–76). Obstruction was in the hepatic veins in 62%, the IVC in 7%, and both in 31%, and 14% had associated PVT.[8]

Presentation
Patients may present with acute, subacute, or chronic BCS.
- Acute (20%): usually very symptomatic, classically with new-onset ascites, severe right upper quadrant pain, and tender hepatomegaly that may progress to fulminant hepatic failure. Mixed elevation of alanine

aminotransferase (ALT) and alkaline phosphatase (ALP), with subsequent development of jaundice, is common.

- Subacute (40%): symptoms for less than 6 months with no evidence of cirrhosis.
- Chronic (40%): signs and symptoms for more than 6 months with evidence of portal hypertension and cirrhosis at diagnosis.

Subacute and chronic BCS are often only mildly symptomatic or entirely asymptomatic. Some patients recall a period of abdominal pain with or without distension in the past. The chronic congestion associated with hepatic outflow obstruction leads to cirrhosis. In chronic BCS, the caudate lobe hypertrophies because of shunting of blood from the rest of the liver to the caudate lobe to allow drainage through its unique direct connection to the IVC. With time, the hypertrophied caudate lobe may compress the IVC, worsening the venous return and increasing portal hypertension.

Complications of cirrhosis may develop and notably up to 28% of patients have been reported to develop the "hepatopulmonary syndrome" with intrathoracic right to left shunts. The explanation for the association between BCS and hepatopulmonary syndrome is unknown.

Etiology

An underlying disorder is identified in more than 80% of patients (Box 21.1). Up to half may have more than one thrombophilic abnormality. The most common conditions associated with BCS are the myeloproliferative disorders, with polycythemia vera occurring most frequently.[9]

In the chronic form of BCS, if portal hypertension is already present, features of an underlying myeloproliferative disorder may be masked by hypersplenism. Mutations in the JAK2 tyrosine kinase are common in all myeloproliferative disorders and particularly polycythemia vera. Patients with BCS may have JAK2 mutations alone without other features of a myeloproliferative disorder. JAK2 should be assessed in all patients presenting with BCS. Solid tumor malignancy accounts for about 10% of BCS, with HCC being the most common

---

Box 21.1 Underlying conditions in Budd–Chiari syndrome

Myeloproliferative disorder with or without JAK2 mutation

Isolated JAK2 mutation

Solid tumor malignancy

High estrogen state: pregnancy, birth control pill, hormone replacement therapy (see Chapter 24)

Hypercoagulable state (Factor V Leiden, antiphospholipid, protein C and S, paroxysmal nocturnal hyperbilirubinemia)

Liver lesion (abscess, hydatid cyst)

Inferior vena cava web

Other diseases (vasculitis, inflammatory bowel disease)

tumor identified. High estrogen states, particularly pregnancy and use of oral contraceptives, are associated with BCS. BCS has been reported in the setting of most hypercoagulable states (Factor V Leiden (most common), antiphospholipid syndrome, protein C and S deficiency, paroxysmal nocturnal hemoglobinuria, etc.). Less commonly, infections and space-occupying lesions in the liver may alter the hepatic and subsequently vascular architecture sufficiently to lead to clot formation. Examples include hepatic abscess and hydatid disease. Membranous IVC webs are found occasionally in North America but are much more frequent in India and Africa. Patients may present with severe varicosities in the legs before the development of ascites or other symptoms. The webs are presumed to be congenital anomalies and respond well to radiological interventions. Other rare causes of BCS have been described, including vasculitis and inflammatory bowel disease, and up to 20% remain idiopathic.

Diagnosis
The diagnosis can usually be confirmed with ultrasonography and Doppler examination, however CT with contrast may show more specific findings of BCS. A patchy appearance to the liver may reflect increased central relative to peripheral contrast. Rapid clearance of contrast from the caudate lobe is suggestive of BCS. Venography is the gold standard for diagnosis and is helpful for assessing patency of hepatic veins, a factor that may influence the durability of response to radiological therapy. A liver biopsy may be useful for diagnosis if imaging is unclear. The major features are centrilobular congestion, necrosis, and hemorrhage, with or without cirrhosis.

Prognosis
In the largest series to date (n = 237, as above), patients were divided into categories (Class I to III) based on a score calculated at initial presentation.[8] The score included: ascites (0 or 1), encephalopathy (0 or 1), INR above 2.3 (0 or 1), and bilirubin as a continuous variable. The hazard score was calculated as:

$$1.27 \times encephalopathy + 1.04 \times ascites + 0.72 \times prothrombin\ time + 0.004 \times bilirubin\ (\mu mol/mL)$$

Class I = 0–1.1
Class II = 1.1–1.5
Class III = >1.5
Five-year survival rates ranged from 89% in Class I to 74% in Class II and 42% in Class III.

Management
Medical treatment
Anticoagulation is useful but often inadequate as a lone therapy except in patients with mild disease (Class I) (Box 21.2). In the setting of pregnancy, heparin must be used as warfarin is contraindicated. Diuretic therapy and salt

---

Box 21.2 Management of acute Budd–Chiari syndrome

Medical therapy
   Anticoagulation
   Thrombolysis (limited data)
   Symptomatic (diuretics)
Radiological therapy
   TIPS
   Angioplasty
Surgical therapy
   Shunt surgery
   Liver transplantation

---

restriction are used to control ascites; however, paracentesis may be necessary. Thrombolytic agents may be used. Data are limited to case reports and small case series. Thrombolytic therapy should only be considered in acute or possibly mild subacute BCS. The likelihood of success in chronic BCS is too low to justify the risks associated with the therapy (bleeding).

Radiological treatment

Angioplasty may be used, particularly for webs in the IVC; however, reocclusion is common. Insertion of an expandable stent may be possible; however, data are limited and stents may complicate subsequent liver transplantation. TIPS may be performed with fairly high success rates and good long-term survival (88% 1-year survival and 78% 5-year survival) and is now considered to be the first-line therapy.[10] Occlusion of TIPS and rarely extension of clot to the portal vein may be problematic. TIPS may be technically difficult in late-term pregnancy. Long-term anticoagulation should be given unless a reversible cause of BCS is identified (e.g. high estrogen state).

Surgical treatment

Surgical shunts to decompress the portal system may be successful but are often technically very challenging. Portocaval, mesocaval, and even splenorenal shunts are possibilities. Difficulty finding surgeons with experience with these procedures may also limit their utility. Compression of the IVC by the enlarged caudate lobe may complicate the surgery. Recurrent thrombosis is not uncommon, particularly if synthetic grafts are used to bypass a compressed IVC. In patients with shunt surgery performed prior to development of cirrhosis, long-term survival is very good (up to 90% at 5 years). Liver transplantation is an alternative option, although the clot may significantly complicate the surgery itself. Notably, patients who developed BCS due to protein C, protein S, or antithrombin III deficiency will be cured of their hypercoagulable state as the new liver will make adequate amounts of these proteins.

Therapeutic options, particularly transplant, may be limited in patients with an underlying myeloproliferative disorder as the cause for BCS.

Sinusoidal obstruction syndrome/ veno-occlusive disease

Sinusoidal obstruction syndrome (SOS) was previously referred to as veno-occlusive disease (VOD). The name was changed to reflect the underlying pathology. SOS is thought to be an injury to the sinusoidal epithelium, which typically occurs in the setting of potent chemotherapy used for hematopoietic stem cell transplantation. The process begins in the centrilobular region of the liver acinus (zone 3) and is characterized by deposition of fibrinogen in sinusoids, which ultimately leads to congestion and eventually occlusion of venules with resulting hepatic necrosis. A procoagulant state may develop in severe instances as well.

Etiology

SOS occurs almost exclusively in the setting of hematopoietic stem cell transplantation but has also been described with other chemotherapeutic regimens, alkaloid toxins (bush tea), high-dose radiation therapy, and liver transplantation. A number of risk factors predisposing to SOS have been identified, including:[11]

- Pre-existing liver disease: HCV may increase risk, cirrhosis markedly increases risk. Hemochromatosis increases risk (8.6-fold for C282Y homozygotes).
- Radiation dosage: doses of 13–15.75 Gy and single rather than fractionated dosing schedules increase the risk of SOS.
- Alkaloid agents: many have been associated with SOS but busulfan and cyclophosphamide carry the highest risk in a dose-dependent manner.
- Reduced lung diffusing capacity: may reflect existing endothelial dysfunction, thus increasing the risk of SOS.
- Female sex: SOS is more common in women than men and the use of progesterone prior to transplant may increase the risk further.

Prevalence and prognosis

The incidence of SOS varies considerably, at least partially based on the definitions used. Mild SOS may occur in up to 50% of stem cell transplants but fortunately severe disease is less common. With mild SOS, survival rates are more than 90% at 100 days post transplant compared to 77% in moderate SOS; in severe SOS (up to 25% of cases) survival is rare.[12]

Presentation

Symptoms and signs usually develop within 3 weeks of the stem cell infusion. Abdominal pain (epigastric or right upper quadrant) with abrupt weight gain and hepatomegaly are often the first signs (3 to 6 days post transplant). Edema develops in about half of patients and ascites in 20%. Jaundice develops later, usually after day 6, but earlier jaundice portends a worse prognosis. Severe disease often includes other organ systems with renal failure, confusion, heart failure, and systemic bleeding. The cause for these features is not well understood but is thought to relate to the liver disease directly.

Diagnosis

In the correct clinical context, that is within 3 weeks of stem cell transplantation, diagnosis of SOS is strongly suggested by:
- hyperbilirubinemia more than 34 mmol/L;
- hepatomegaly with right upper quadrant pain;
- rapid weight gain (>2% baseline weight).

Other diagnostic considerations should be considered such as graft-versus-host disease, acute viral infections, and sepsis. Mild reductions in antithrombin III and protein C (but not S) are associated with SOS. Other markers of coagulation status, such as plasminogen activator inhibitor 1, may also be useful diagnostic tools but more data are needed. Liver biopsy is usually unnecessary to diagnose SOS. Notably, the risk of bleeding is significantly higher in this setting (18% in one trial) and thus liver biopsy confirmation should be considered cautiously. If a liver biopsy is performed, the transjugular approach may reduce the consequences of hemorrhage, provided the catheter is able to pass the obstruction.

Management

For mild and even moderate SOS, most patients do well with no specific therapy. For severe disease, tissue plasminogen activator (tPA) with heparin and defibrotide have been used but the prognosis is very poor.

Tissue plasminogen activator

The association with a procoagulative state provided the rationale to try thrombolytic and anticoagulant therapy. Response rates of 30–40% with tPA and heparin have been reported but frequent bleeding has limited the utility of this approach. The risk of severe bleeding in patients with multiorgan failure is high.

Defibrotide

Defibrotide is a polydeoxyribonucleotide with antithrombotic and fibrinolytic properties by activating endogenous tPA. Small studies have suggested a beneficial effect to defibrotide, with up to 40% of patients with severe SOS and multiorgan failure recovering with this therapy.[13] Other therapies that have been tried in small studies include antithrombin (in patients with antithrombin deficiency), prostaglandin E1, and antioxidants.

Primary prevention

Ursodeoxycholic acid (600 to 900 mg daily) has been shown in a randomized placebo-controlled trial to reduce the rate of SOS in patients undergoing hematopoietic stem cell transplant. There was a non-significant trend towards improved survival, leading many centers to use this agent routinely prior to transplant.[14] Unfractionated heparin infusion has been used prior to transplant with somewhat conflicting results. The largest randomized controlled trial showed a lower rate of SOS but other studies have not consistently found any benefit from this agent. LMWH is currently being evaluated for prevention of SOS. Defibrotide has also been evaluated as prophylactic therapy and small uncontrolled trials have shown complete prevention of SOS in treated patients. Randomized controlled trials have not yet been performed.

Arteriovenous malformations

Large arteriovenous malformations (AVMs) may develop between the hepatic artery and hepatic vein. In extreme cases, AVMs may cause a hemodynamically significant left to right shunt that may cause a steal syndrome, precipitating angina or other forms of ischemia. Large AVMs are more common in patients with hereditary hemorrhagic telangiectasia (HHT) or Osler–Weber–Rendu syndrome. Patients with HHT may develop high-output cardiac failure with portal hypertension. Biliary lesions may occur in patients with HHT as well, likely due to small AVMs affecting the biliary tree.[15] Although there was initial enthusiasm for arterial embolization with coils for large AVMs, because of a high rate of complications this should only be considered if liver transplantation is available as a salvage therapy.

Case study 21.1

A 32-year-old woman presents to the emergency room with abdominal swelling and right upper quadrant pain 3 weeks after a normal vaginal delivery following an uncomplicated pregnancy. Her past medical history is unremarkable, she takes no regular medications, and the baby is healthy. Examination reveals scleral icterus, moderate ascites, and tender hepatomegaly. Laboratory investigations are notable for an ALT of 834 IU/L, AST of 945 IU/L, ALP of 245 IU/L, bilirubin of 72 mg/dL, INR of 2.6, and albumin of 34 g/L. Ultrasound examination revealed an enlarged liver with moderate ascites.

Comment

The case described is a classic example of acute Budd–Chiari syndrome related to the hypercoagulable state associated with pregnancy. The increased risk of thrombosis is greatest in the postpartum period. Based on the severity score described in the chapter, this woman has relatively poor prognosis with a score 1.77 (5 year survival 47%). However, although she should be screened for coagulation defects, particularly JAK2, this presentation is likely related to her recent pregnancy and therefore provided she survives the initial episode, she is at lower risk of recurrence. Ultrasound with Doppler or CT with contrast should be used to confirm the diagnosis and she should be aggressively treated with TIPS insertion and anticoagulation. Whether she should consider another pregnancy is controversial but it would be reasonable to consider LMWH prophylaxis if she were to conceive.

Case study 21.2

A 45-year-old woman born in rural India is found to have large esophageal varices at the time of an endoscopy for dyspeptic symptoms. Aside from her upper GI complaints, she is asymptomatic with no history of upper GI bleeding or known liver disease. Lab tests reveal an isolated elevation of ALP (453 IU/L) and γ-glutamyl transferase (GGT 325 IU/L) with normal transaminases, bilirubin, INR, and albumin. She has no significant past medical or family history and takes no regular medications or herbal preparations. Imaging reveals a large portal vein with cavernous transformation, marked splenomegaly, and a coarse liver with no biliary dilatation.

Comment

This woman has a chronic portal vein thrombosis. Although the thrombosis likely resulted from neonatal sepsis or omphalitis, a condition reported with much greater frequency in the Indian subcontinent than elsewhere, she should still have a hypercoagulable work-up. Provided she does not have an identifiable thrombophilic condition, anticoagulation is likely of little value and is associated with an increased risk of bleeding. She has had cavernous transformation and fortunately has not bled despite the presence of large esophageal varices. Varices should be managed with primary band ligation rather than beta-blocker therapy. The elevation of her ALP and GGT likely reflects portal biliopathy, which may develop in the setting of longstanding portal vein thrombosis and is usually evident on MR cholangiography. Ursodeoxycholic acid may improve ALP and GGT, although it is unknown if treatment changes the natural history of this condition.

Multiple choice questions

1. Common complications of portal vein thrombosis include all of the following *except*:
   A. Splenomegaly
   B. Bile duct abnormalities
   C. Massive ascites
   D. Thrombocytopenia
   E. Variceal hemorrhage

2. The most common abnormality associated with Budd–Chiari syndrome is:
   A. Protein C deficiency
   B. Antithrombin III deficiency
   C. Factor V Leiden
   D. JAK2 mutation
   E. Antiphospholipid syndrome

Answers

1. C
2. D

References

1. Okuda K, Ohnishi K, Kimura K, et al. Incidence of portal vein thrombosis in liver cirrhosis. An angiographic study in 708 patients. Gastroenterology 1985; 89: 279–86.
2. Amitrano L, Guardascione MA, Brancaccio V, et al. Risk factors and clinical presentation of portal vein thrombosis in patients with liver cirrhosis. J Hepatol 2004; 40: 736–41.
3. Englesbe MJ, Kubus J, Muhammad W, et al. Portal vein thrombosis and survival in patients with cirrhosis. Liver Transpl 2010; 16: 83–90.
4. Villa EZR, Marietta M, Bernabucci V, et al. Enoxaparin prevents portal vein thrombosis (PVT) and decompensation in advanced cirrhotic patients: final report of a prospective randomized controlled study. Hepatology 2011; 54 (Suppl. S1).
5. Amitrano L, Guardascione MA, Menchise A, et al. Safety and efficacy of anticoagulation therapy with low molecular weight heparin for portal vein thrombosis in patients with liver cirrhosis. J Clin Gastroenterol 2010; 44: 448–51.
6. Plessier A, Darwish-Murad S, Hernandez-Guerra M, et al. Acute portal vein thrombosis unrelated to cirrhosis: a prospective multicenter follow-up study. Hepatology 2010; 51: 210–8.
7. Condat B, Pessione F, Hillaire S, et al. Current outcome of portal vein thrombosis in adults: risk and benefit of anticoagulant therapy. Gastroenterology 2001; 120: 490–7.
8. Darwish Murad S, Valla DC, de Groen PC, et al. Determinants of survival and the effect of portosystemic shunting in patients with Budd–Chiari syndrome. Hepatology 2004; 39: 500–8.
9. Darwish Murad S, Plessier A, Hernandez-Guerra M, et al. Etiology, management, and outcome of the Budd–Chiari syndrome. Ann Intern Med 2009; 151: 167–75.
10. Eapen CE, Velissaris D, Heydtmann M, et al. Favourable medium term outcome following hepatic vein recanalisation and/or transjugular intrahepatic portosystemic shunt for Budd Chiari syndrome. Gut 2006; 55: 878–84.
11. Maradei SC, Maiolino A, de Azevedo AM, et al. Serum ferritin as risk factor for sinusoidal obstruction syndrome of the liver in patients undergoing hematopoietic stem cell transplantation. Blood 2009; 114: 1270–5.
12. McDonald GB, Hinds MS, Fisher LD, et al. Veno-occlusive disease of the liver and multiorgan failure after bone marrow transplantation: a cohort study of 355 patients. Ann Intern Med 1993; 118: 255–67.
13. Richardson PG, Murakami C, Jin Z, et al. Multi-institutional use of defibrotide in 88 patients after stem cell transplantation with severe veno-occlusive disease and multisystem organ failure: response without significant toxicity in a high-risk population and factors predictive of outcome. Blood 2002; 100: 4337–43.
14. Essell JH, Schroeder MT, Harman GS, et al. Ursodiol prophylaxis against hepatic complications of allogeneic bone marrow transplantation. A randomized, double-blind, placebo-controlled trial. Ann Intern Med 1998; 128: 975–81.
15. Garcia-Tsao G, Korzenik JR, Young L, et al. Liver disease in patients with hereditary hemorrhagic telangiectasia. N Engl J Med 2000; 343: 931–6.

Approach to metabolic and storage diseases

CHAPTER 22

Hemant A. Shah[1] and Eve A. Roberts[2]

[1] Division of Gastroenterology, Toronto Western Hospital, University Health Network, University of Toronto, Toronto, Ontario, Canada
[2] Departments of Paediatrics, Medicine, and Pharmacology, University of Toronto, and Division of Gastroenterology, Hepatology and Nutrition, The Hospital for Sick Children, Toronto, Ontario, Canada

Key points

- Metabolic liver diseases have a wide clinical spectrum of presentation and are often asymptomatic in adults. A high index of suspicion must be maintained in order to achieve a diagnosis.
- In children and adults, metabolic disease is often insidious, progressing silently to cirrhosis and subsequent liver failure.
- There have been many therapeutic advances for the metabolic liver diseases but good outcome depends upon early detection.
- In the pediatric population, enzymatic deficiencies of the essential metabolic pathways cause severe liver disease with or without neurologic disease.
- Diagnosis in the pediatric population usually requires direct enzyme analysis or genetic testing.
- Liver transplantation corrects only the hepatic phenotype abnormality in metabolic diseases due to enzymatic deficiency, but often this is sufficient for generally improved health.

The liver has numerous metabolic functions. Metabolic liver disease includes a wide variety of clinical disorders and pathophysiology (Table 22.1). Most are due to inherited enzymatic abnormalities, which result in storage disorders, errors of metabolism, and transport defects. These diseases can manifest as acute and life-threatening illnesses in the neonatal period or as chronic liver illness in adolescence or adulthood. In the pediatric population, up to 20% of liver transplants are performed for complications resulting from a metabolic

Hepatology: Diagnosis and Clinical Management, First Edition. Edited by E. Jenny Heathcote.
© 2012 John Wiley & Sons, Ltd. Published 2012 by John Wiley & Sons, Ltd.

Table 22.1 Selected metabolic diseases with mainly adult or child/adolescent presentation

Disease	Age of presentation	Distinguishing clinical features	Distinguishing laboratory features	Diagnostic testing
Hereditary hemochromatosis type 1	Adulthood	Arthritis, hypogonadism (infertility), heart failure, diabetes	High iron saturation, high ferritin	Mutation analysis, liver biopsy
α_1-antitrypsin deficiency	Infancy to adulthood	Panacinar emphysema	Abnormal pulmonary function tests, low serum AAT levels	Liver biopsy, phenotype analysis, mutation analysis
Amyloidosis	Adulthood	Variable dependent upon organ involvement	Variable	Tissue biopsy with identification of abnormal fibrils
Gaucher disease type 1	Childhood to adulthood	Splenomegaly, skeletal disease	Erlenmeyer flask deformity of distal femur	Enzyme analysis, mutation analysis, Gaucher cells in bone marrow
Gaucher disease type 3	Childhood	Supranuclear gaze palsy, myoclonus	Audiometric testing to identify brainstem disease	Enzyme analysis, mutation analysis
Glycogen storage diseases 1, 3, 4, 6, 9	Mainly childhood	Hepatomegaly, hypoglycemia; hepatic adenomas in GSD1	Splenomegaly with GSD3	Enzyme analysis
Cystic fibrosis	Childhood to adulthood	Pulmonary infections, poor growth, malabsorption	Sweat chloride, nasal potential difference (PD)	Mutation analysis
MDR3 deficiency	Childhood to adulthood	Childhood: chronic biliary disorder Adulthood: bile duct stones, pruritus of pregnancy	Abnormal cholangiogram	Mutation analysis
Citrullinemia type 2	Adulthood	Fatty liver	None	Enzyme analysis
Urea cycle defects	Varies	Neonatal respiratory alkalosis	Very high serum ammonia levels	Quantitative plasma amino acid analysis, enzyme activity in fibroblasts

liver disease whereas in the adult population it is approximately 5%. Metabolic liver diseases are great mimics. For example, citrullinemia type 2 (discussed here) and Wilson disease (Chapter 23) can both resemble non-alcoholic fatty liver disease (NAFLD; Chapter 17). To diagnose metabolic disease, a structured approach is required, which includes consideration of the age at presentation, symptoms, laboratory abnormalities, and specific diagnostic testing.

Hereditary hemochromatosis

Hemochromatosis is a clinical syndrome of iron overload, which may be due to genetic abnormalities or to exogenous iron overload by transfusion or food contamination. Hereditary hemochromatosis (HH) comprises several inherited disorders of iron homeostasis, all of which lead to increased intestinal iron absorption and tissue iron deposition. Classic (type 1) HH is the well-known form of iron overload due to *HFE1* ("high Fe") gene defects. It affects 0.5% of Caucasians and currently is most often detected during the work-up for arthritis or infertility or other disease (such as heart failure or diabetes) with biochemical markers of increased iron stores. It should be considered in all Caucasians with unexplained abnormal liver tests (Fig. 22.1). Several other

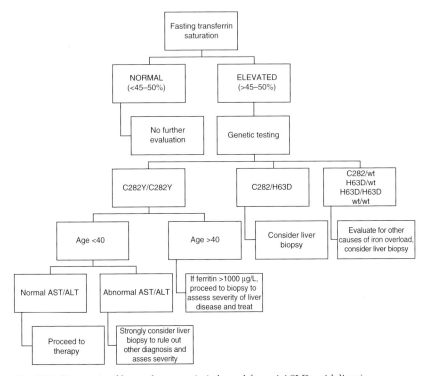

Fig. 22.1 Diagnosis of hemochromatosis (adapted from AASLD guidelines).

genetic disorders of iron metabolism that cause HH have been identified but are much less common (Table 22.2).

Type 1 HH is the most prevalent inherited metabolic disease in Caucasians. The only important mutations of the *HFE1* gene are C282Y and H63D. Both C282Y/C282Y homozygotes and C282Y/H63D compound heterozygotes can manifest disease, although penetrance is markedly higher in homozygotes than compound heterozygotes. C282Y homozygotes account for 90% of type 1 HH. Phenotypic expression of disease depends upon non-genetic factors such as amount of iron consumption and/or blood loss; for example, women develop clinical consequences of iron overload four to eight times less frequently than men and 10–20 years later due to menstruation.

HFE1 gene defects lead to increased intestinal iron absorption. Usually, only 10% of daily iron intake (1–2 mg) is absorbed in the small bowel. However, individuals with C282Y homozygosity may absorb up to 40% of their daily iron intake (4–8 mg). The mechanism by which this occurs is through the circulating peptide hormone, hepcidin. In normal patients, hepcidin is produced in the liver and increases in response to increased levels of circulating iron, signaling to intestinal cells to decrease iron absorption. However, in patients with classic hereditary hemochromatosis, hepcidin production in the liver is impaired and leads to uncontrolled intestinal iron absorption. Organ damage occurs when iron stores approach 10 g and thus it may take many years before clinical end-organ damage is detected. Patients with clinical end-stages of disease typically have 20–30 g of iron stores.

Iron overload in the liver induces lipid peroxidation, and membrane-dependent functions of mitochondria, microsomes, and lysosomes become abnormal. There is a clear relationship between the degree of lipid peroxidation and hepatic fibrosis. As liver disease progresses, cirrhosis can develop. Late non-hepatic manifestations include hyperpigmented "bronzing" of skin, heart failure, hypogonadism, and diabetes.

Transferrin saturation is a more accurate indicator of iron overload than serum ferritin. High transferrin saturation usually precedes increases in ferritin. Transferrin saturation should be measured in the fasting state. A fasting transferrin saturation above 50% in women and above 60% in men will detect over 90% of patients with homozygous HH1. Ferritin is an acute phase reactant as well as an indicator of increased iron stores; low values can be found with iron deficiency and thus it used to monitor therapeutic response to therapy. In patients with elevated transferrin saturation, genetic testing for *HFE* gene mutations should be performed. Liver biopsy can be a useful adjunct to serum diagnostic testing because hepatic iron concentration can be measured and values higher than 71 μmol/g are highly suggestive of HH. For patients less than 40 years old, who are homozygous for C282Y and have no clinical features to suspect advanced fibrosis, biopsy is usually not indicated (Fig. 22.1).

Screening. The rationale for screening for hemochromatosis is that treatment of asymptomatic disease prior to significant iron overload will prevent

Table 22.2 Classification of hemochromatosis

Type	Inheritance pattern	Genetic defect	Clinical characteristics
Hereditary hemochromatosis			
HH1	AR	HFE protein	Classic hereditary hemochromatosis, low penetrance and late presentation
HH2	AR	Hemojuvelin (2A) and hepcidin (2B)	Juvenile hemochromatosis, 100% penetrance, rapid iron loading, early onset of hypogonadism and cardiac disease
HH3	AR	Transferrin receptor 2	Rare condition, described in a few families, clinical manifestations similar to classical hereditary hemochromatosis
HH4	AD	Ferroportin-1	Highly variable disorder, manifestations can include minimal hepatic iron deposition or disease similar to classical hereditary hemochromatosis
HH5	AD	H-ferritin	Described in a single Japanese family
HH6	AD	L-ferritin	High levels of ferritin associated with bilateral congenital cataracts, no hepatic iron deposition
Secondary hemochromatosis			
Chronic anemias: Beta-thalassemia, sickle cell disease, myelodysplastic syndrome, other hereditary hemolytic anemias			
Multiple red blood cell transfusions			
Long-term oral intake of high amounts of iron (including therapeutic misadventure with Fe supplementation)			
Iron overload in Bantu Africans (dietary)			
Aceruloplasminemia			
Unclassified types of hemochromatosis (including perinatal hemochromatosis—alloimmune liver disease)			

AD, autosomal dominant; AR, autosomal recessive; HH, hereditary hemochromatosis.

> **Box 22.1 Recommendations for treatment of hereditary hemochromatosis (HH1)**
>
> - Begin with one phlebotomy (500 mL) once or twice per week
> - Check hematocrit prior to each phlebotomy; hematocrit should not fall by more than 20% of prior level
> - Check serum ferritin every 10 to 20 phlebotomies
> - Reduce frequency of phlebotomies with ferritin 100 μg/L
> - Continue ferritin every 1 to 6 months to keep ferritin at approximately 50 μg/L
>   NB. The phlebotomized blood may be transfused to others as long as it is appropriately screened as per usual protocols.

end-organ damage. Thus, screening (with iron saturation and/or *HFE1* gene testing) is recommended for first-degree relatives of affected individuals. Population screening is not recommended.

Treatment. Treatment for HH is mainly medical. The most uncomplicated and cost-effective treatment for hemochromatosis in non-anemic patients with iron overload is therapeutic phlebotomy (Box 22.1). Each 500 mL of blood removed contains 200 to 250 mg of iron. Most patients (even those with established cirrhosis) with HH1 or any genetic hemochromatosis will benefit from therapeutic phlebotomy unless their life expectancy is short for other reasons. Phlebotomy itself can be performed at a blood bank or medical facility, and the blood that is removed can be safely transfused to other individuals (provided that it passes other screening tests). While the optimal schedule is patient-dependent, in general iron should be depleted as rapidly as possible. Most male patients will tolerate 1 to 2 units of blood removed per week, while others may tolerate less. The goal of therapy is to deplete total body iron stores, which is achieved when the ferritin level drops to between 50 and 100 μg/L or the patient develops iron deficiency anemia. It is not uncommon to need 70 to 100 phlebotomies to deplete iron stores adequately before a maintenance phlebotomy schedule is put in place.

Patients with hemochromatosis are often concerned about consuming excess iron in their diet. However, given that most ingested iron is not absorbed, avoiding iron-containing foods is unnecessary. The one caveat to this principle is that excess alcohol consumption should be avoided as it is significantly associated with increased iron absorption and progression of liver disease.

Iron chelation therapy is available but usually not needed for genetic hemochromatosis. It is most commonly used for secondary hemochromatosis in patients who receive chronic transfusion therapy for anemia. Iron chelation therapy can be cumbersome when it requires continuous subcutaneous or intravenous infusion. Deferoxamine is a widely used infusional agent. Side effects include visual loss and ototoxicity. However, oral agents are now available, which are effective in most conditions. Deferasirox is a commonly used oral agent.

Hemochromatosis is an uncommon indication for liver transplantation. It is only considered for patients with end-stage hepatic disease and preserved cardiac function. Hepatocellular carcinoma may develop in cirrhotic HH1.

α_1-Antitrypsin deficiency

α_1-Antitrypsin (AAT) deficiency leads to an increased risk of both lung and liver disease. AAT is a protease inhibitor that binds to the serine proteases in serum and tissues and promotes their degradation. The most important of the serine proteases is elastase. Loss of serum AAT activity leads to uninhibited neutrophil elastase activity and is the primary mechanism for the development of emphysema. Lung disease is characterized by the development of panacinar emphysema and its presence is independent of liver manifestations. Liver disease presents as an inactive cirrhosis and is caused by structural misfolding and polymerization of mutant AAT in the liver, leading to its retention in the endoplasmic reticulum of hepatocytes. It is not known exactly how AAT retention leads to liver injury.

The pattern of inheritance is codominant. Variants of the AAT allele produce gene products that can be distinguished by electrophoresis. Protease inhibitor MM (PI MM) is the normal allelic representation. The PI Z variant produces a mutant protein and homozygosity of the allele (PI ZZ) is the most common form of AAT deficiency leading to liver disease. More than 70 naturally occurring allelic variants have been described, but only some lead to chronic liver failure and cirrhosis in adults. More than 90% of all AAT is produced in the liver, and each allele contributes to the total amount of AAT produced. Thus individuals with the PI MZ phenotype have approximately half as much AAT as normal, and those with PI SZ have less than half and may develop clinical liver disease. AAT is an acute phase reactant. Serum levels of AAT may be artificially elevated by hepatic inflammation, and therefore phenotyping is the reliable diagnostic method. Genetic testing is an option; the mutation responsible for the Z protein is lysine replacing glutamic acid at position 342.

Diagnosis of AAT deficiency should be made with phenotypic analysis of the enzyme. While AAT levels can be measured, it should be noted that AAT is an acute phase reactant and thus levels can rise in pregnancy, with stress, or injury, even in PI ZZ patients. A liver biopsy is not universally recommended but should confirm the diagnosis if performed. Histologically, in infants, the biopsy can show bile duct loss, intracellular cholestasis, and mild inflammatory changes, but few of the characteristic periodic acid–Schiff (PAS)-positive globules. In adults, PAS-positive, diastase-resistant globules are usually seen. The inclusions are most prominent in periportal hepatocytes. Cirrhosis may be present.

The prevalence of PI Z is highest in populations derived from northern European ancestry, though many racial subgroups may be affected. About 10% of newborns with PI ZZ present with conjugated hyperbilirubinemia, and up to 50% have elevated serum aminotransferase levels by age 3 years (though most are asymptomatic). In adults lung disease generally precedes the development of liver disease. Even though liver disease is generally mild during infancy, patients with AAT deficiency have an eightfold higher risk of developing cirrhosis during adulthood. Additionally, homozygous AAT deficiency increases the risk of hepatocellular carcinoma. The diagnosis of AAT deficiency should be considered in any patient presenting with signs of cirrhosis. The presence of PAS-positive globules in hepatocytes on liver biopsy is almost always due to AAT deficiency, and this staining should be performed routinely on all liver biopsies.

Medical treatment is limited to lung disease. Most medical therapies for AAT deficiency are targeted at restoring AAT levels in the lung. No effective medical therapy is currently available to prevent progressive liver damage, although drugs that promote proper protein folding are being investigated. Gene therapy to restore the normal function of AAT to deficient human cells requires more study. Liver transplantation is reserved for patients with end-stage hepatic disease. It may be performed in conjunction with lung transplantation. Transplantation of a liver from a PI MM individual restores the normal hepatic phenotype as donor livers will produce and secrete AAT.

Amyloidosis

Amyloidosis presents in a myriad of ways. By infiltration into organs it can cause renal failure, heart failure, gastrointestinal bleeding, motor and sensory neuropathy, muscular pseudohypertrophy, bleeding diathesis, tracheobronchial fistulization, and pleural effusions. In the liver, it typically presents as massive hepatomegaly, with or without splenomegaly, or as mild chronic hepatitis. Amyloidosis refers to the extracellular deposition of fibrils composed of low molecular weight subunits of a variety of circulating proteins.

Several types of amyloid are hereditary and result from missense mutations of precursor proteins. Virtually all of the hereditary forms of amyloid are codominantly inherited heterozygous disorders, where both wild type and mutant molecules are identified in the amyloid deposits. There are several types of amyloidosis. AL (primary) amyloidosis is due to deposition of protein derived from immunoglobulin light chain fragments. This condition is a plasma cell dyscrasia in which a monoclonal immunoglobulin is detectable in serum. It can occur alone but is often associated with multiple myeloma, Waldenström macroglobulinemia or non-Hodgkin lymphoma. AA (secondary) amyloidosis occurs as a complication of a chronic inflammatory disease such as rheumatoid arthritis, spondyloarthropathy, inflammatory bowel disease, chronic infections, or periodic fever syndromes. Dialysis-related amyloidosis is a result of deposition of β_2-microglobulin fibrils found in long-term hemodialysis patients. Other types of amyloidosis include familial amyloid polyneuropathy, age-related amyloidosis, and organ-specific amyloidosis.

Diagnosis of amyloidosis requires tissue biopsy in the suspected involved organ. If hepatomegaly is present, the liver has a thick, rubbery feel to it. The sensitivity of a liver biopsy in systemic amyloid disease when hepatomegaly is present is approximately 90%. Of note, liver is not the preferred site for tissue sampling because these patients have slightly higher than normal postbiopsy bleeding rates (though liver biopsies are not contraindicated). Biopsies of abdominal fat or rectal tissue have high sensitivity. The amyloid deposits appear as amorphous hyaline material deposited around hepatocytes on light microscopy; with Congo red staining they have green birefringence under polarized light. In some cases, immunohistochemical staining can help differentiate the various types of amyloid.

Treatment of amyloidosis varies with the type of fibrils. AL amyloid is treated by management of the plasma cell dyscrasia. AA amyloid is treated by management of the underlying condition leading to fibril formation (i.e. optimized control of rheumatoid arthritis). For the hereditary amyloidoses where mutant protein is produced by the liver, early liver transplantation can prevent further fibril deposition and lead to long-term regression of deposits.

In particular, liver transplantation has shown promise for familial amyloid polyneuropathy when performed based upon the severity of the sensorimotor neuropathy.

Gaucher disease

Gaucher disease (GD) is an error of metabolism that results from a deficiency of the lysosomal enzyme glucocerebrosidase, leading to deposition of glucosylceramide and other glycolipids in lipid-laden macrophages of the reticuloendothelial system. In the liver, pathologic accumulation of these lipid-laden macrophages leads to an inflammatory and hyperplastic cellular response. GD, an autosomal recessive disorder, is the most common lysosomal storage disease and is most prevalent in the Ashkenazi Jewish population. For affected individuals, testing of all first-degree relatives with enzymatic functional assays and gene sequencing is recommended.

GD involves the visceral organs, bone marrow, and bone in all affected persons. Presenting features are variable and can present at any age. There are three subtypes of GD. Hepatomegaly is a feature in all three subtypes, and approximately 60% of patients at presentation have a liver volume of two to three times normal.

Type 1 GD is characterized by variability in age of onset; while it can present in infancy, some patients have no symptoms until adulthood. In addition to hepatomegaly, splenomegaly is the most common presenting sign with a median spleen size of 15 times normal. While hepatic fibrosis occurs, cirrhosis and liver failure are uncommon (but do occur). Patients with type 1 GD also develop skeletal disease (bone pain, avascular necrosis, joint collapse, osteolytic lesions, pathologic fractures), growth and developmental problems, interstitial lung disease, peripheral polyneuropathy, and are at increased risk of hematologic malignancies. Ninety percent of all GD patients have type 1 disease.

Type 2 GD is characterized by early onset of disease, typically within the first year of life. The first sign of disease is usually central nervous system disease (such as oculomotor dysfunction). Visceral involvement is extensive and severe.

Type 3 GD typical presents in childhood as a neurologic disease and visceral organ involvement, and varies by subtype. Type 3b has severe visceral involvement (hepatomegaly, bone disease) whereas type 3c has little visceral disease.

Diagnosis. Diagnosis of GD is suspected after identification of "Gaucher cells" in the blood; Gaucher cells are macrophages filled with lipid material. Other laboratory findings include anemia, thrombocytopenia, mild liver enzyme elevations, and increased levels of angiotensin converting enzyme. Radiologic findings of an "Erlenmeyer flask" deformity of the distal femur, fractures, and lytic lesions may also be seen. Diagnosis is confirmed by the finding of reduced glucocerebrosidase activity, usually in peripheral leukocytes, in a patient with clinical features consistent with GD. Mutation analysis can be performed and may have a role in predicting clinical course.

Treatment. The goal of medical treatment of GD is to improve symptoms and quality of life while preventing irreversible damage. GD is one of very few conditions that can be treated with enzyme replacement therapy (ERT). ERT with recombinant glucocerebrosidases is the preferred treatment of patients with type 1 and type 3 GD. It is not used for type 2 GD. ERT is very expensive (approximate cost of $US400000 per year for a 70-kg person) and guidelines have been developed for its use. In general, it is used for type 1 GD patients presenting as children with symptoms, or in any patient with severe disease (i.e. platelets $<60000 \times 10^9/L$, liver greater than 2.5 times normal size, spleen greater than 15 times normal size, or radiologic evidence of skeletal disease). ERT is also recommended for patients with type 3 GD who present before the onset of any neurologic symptoms. ERT has varying degrees of effectiveness in each individual. A second-line medical therapy is substrate reduction therapy. Miglustat, an inhibitor of glucosylceramide synthetase, reduces glycoplipid accumulation by decreasing the synthesis of glucocerebroside. Finally, hematopoietic stem cell transplantation can be performed and is curative for this condition.

With respect to surgical treatment, splenectomy used to be a mainstay of therapy prior to ERT. Now, it is reserved primarily for life-threatening thrombocytopenia.

Glycogen storage disease

Glycogen is the stored form of glucose, and inborn errors of glycogen metabolism result from virtually all of the proteins involved in its synthesis, degradation, and regulation. There are over 10 types of this disease, with five involving the liver: types 1, 3, 4, 6, and 9 (Table 22.3).

Type 1 glycogen storage disease

Type 1 glycogen storage disease (GSD1) is the most common inborn error of glycogen metabolism. It results from a deficiency of a two-component enzyme system involved in the transport of glucose-6-posphate into endoplasmic reticulum and subsequent cleavage by glucose-6-phosphatase. Most patients with GSD1 present in infancy with growth failure, a protruding abdomen, hypotonia, and delayed psychomotor development. Physical examination reveals

Table 22.3 Glycogen storage diseases affecting the liver

Disease	Age of presentation	Distinguishing clinical features	Distinguishing test features	Diagnostic test
Type 1	Infancy	Protruding abdomen, epistaxis 1b: leukopenia	High lactic acid levels	DNA testing, liver biopsy and enzyme assay
Type 3	Early childhood	Hepatomegaly Splenomegaly Hypotonia	Abnormal electromyography	Fibroblast or liver enzyme assay; DNA testing
Type 4	Intrauterine, neonatal, and childhood	Intrauterine death; cardiomyopathy	Creatine kinase elevation	Fibroblast, muscle, or liver biopsy; DNA testing
Type 6	Early childhood	Improvement with age	Postprandial lactic acidemia; increased biotinidase activity	Enzyme activity, DNA testing
Type 9	Early childhood	Hypoglycemia	Elevated lipids	Enzyme activity, DNA testing

hepatomegaly, which results from increased glycogen storage in the liver. Metabolic derangements include high lactic acid levels, metabolic acidosis, low phosphorus levels, and hyperuricemia. In addition to hepatomegaly, patients demonstrate mild elevations in aminotransferases. The most accurate diagnostic measure is direct analysis of glucose-6-phosphatase enzyme activity performed on fresh liver tissue; however, histochemical staining for glucose-6-phosphatase can be highly informative. Patients with GSD1 are prone to hepatic adenomas. The risk of such adenomas undergoing malignant transformation is poorly defined but certainly not negligible.

Nutritional supplementation has become the mainstay of therapy for GSD1. For infants, formula that does not contain fructose or galactose should be used. Frequent daytime feedings with high-carbohydrate meals and continuous night-time enteral feedings (with uncooked corn starch) are required at a rate of approximately 8 mg/kg body weight per min. As solids are introduced, high-carbohydrate foods should be emphasized, but most children continue to need regular cornstarch supplementation throughout the day. Target preprandial blood glucose is higher than 4.3 mmol/L. Prevention of metabolic derangements can allow for normal psychological development.

GSD1 patients who develop multiple hepatic adenomas require evaluation for liver transplantation whereas a single adenoma may be suitable for resection. Tightening metabolic control sometimes slows the rate of growth of an adenoma. Renal insufficiency and problems relating to lipid metabolism persist after liver transplantation and may complicate management. Improved linear growth may occur.

There are two variant forms of GSD1.Glycogen storage disease 1b (GSD1b), due to a defect in the glucose-6-phosphatse transporter enzyme, displays neutropenia. In addition to management of features of GSD1, prophylaxis with antibiotics is recommended for GSD1b patients who have neutropenia and recurrent bacterial infections. Granulocyte-macrophage colony stimulation factor has also been used with success in these patients to reduce morbidities associated with severe bacterial infections.

Type 3 glycogen storage disease

Type 3 glycogen storage disease (GSD3) results from a deficiency of glycogen debranching enzyme, which impairs the cleavage and transfer of dextrin from glucose molecules, subsequently restricting glucose release by phosphorylase. Since gluconeogenesis is not impacted by GSD3, the clinical course is milder than that of GSD1; however, hepatic fibrosis and splenomegaly can occur. Serum lactic acid and uric acid levels are normal. Aminotransferases may be mildly elevated. Hepatic adenomas can develop in up to 25% of these patients. Muscle weakness is often a prominent feature of this condition, which worsens with activity. The diagnosis can be confirmed by direct enzyme analysis of muscle or liver tissue of peripheral leukocytes.

Medical treatment is dietary. A high-protein and low-carbohydrate diet has been recommended to normalize metabolic activity. This diet can allow adequate gluconeogenesis and reduces the need for glycogen storage. In cases of patients with refractory hypoglycemia, night time continuous feeding of corn starch may be needed.

Type 4 glycogen storage disease

Type 4 glycogen storage disease (GSD4) is a deficiency of the branching enzyme. It results in glycogen and amylopectin accumulation in hepatocytes. It is quite rare. Clinical presentation varies; a severe congenital form results in fetal hydrops, neonatal hypotonia, and fetal death, while a childhood subtype manifests as cardiomyopathy and abnormal neuromuscular development. The diagnosis of GSD4 can be made by direct enzyme analysis of liver tissue or fibroblasts. There is no known effective treatment and most patients die within the first 3 years. High-protein and low-carbohydrate diets have been used and are associated with improved growth but do not prevent liver involvement. Liver transplantation appears to be the best strategy. It has been used successfully to prolong life.

Types 6 and 9 glycogen storage disease

These two types are glycogen storage disease are somewhat related. Type 6 glycogen storage disease (GSD6) is a deficiency of the liver isoform of phosphorylase. Patients typically present early in life with hepatomegaly and growth retardation. The disease improves with age and hepatomegaly resolves. Type 9 glycogen storage disease (GSD9) is a deficiency of phosphorylase kinase. Clinical manifestations are similar to that of GSD6 with hypoglycemia as a more prominent feature. Cirrhosis may occur, predominantly with GSD9.

Cystic fibrosis

Thanks to the increased effectiveness of respiratory and nutritional treatment in childhood cystic fibrosis (CF), more children are surviving to adulthood. Chronic liver disease has become the second most common cause of death in CF. The mutant protein in CF, encoded by the cystic fibrosis transmembrane conductance regulator (*CFTR*) gene, is expressed in the biliary and gallbladder epithelium. *CFTR* is not expressed in hepatocytes and other liver cells. *CFTR* gene mutations affect the c-AMP inducible chloride channels in bile duct epithelium.

While the epidemiology of liver disease in CF is not well characterized, postmortem series have demonstrated hepatobiliary pathology in up to 72% of patients. Amongst living patients, approximately 30% will have liver enzyme abnormalities, and 1–2% will develop cirrhosis. The most severe liver disease tends to occur in the pediatric population, and hence most liver transplantation for CF is in the pediatric group.

Despite all patients with CF having abnormalities in bile flow (bile tends to be thick and viscous leading to obstruction), only some develop disease. Hence, other genes may also play a role. A spectrum of hepatobiliary lesions are seen in CF. Presentation in infancy is usually as cholestatic jaundice and transient hepatomegaly. Presentation at any age can also include asymptomatic elevations in liver enzymes, hepatosplenomegaly, GI bleeding, or abdominal pain. Diagnosis can usually be made clinically or with appropriate imaging tests (ultrasound, CT, MRI/magnetic resonance cholangiopancreatography (MRCP)) and liver biopsy is rarely needed. Consequences of CF-associated liver disease include hepatic steatosis, focal biliary cirrhosis, diffuse cirrhosis, cholelithiasis and cholecystitis, secondary sclerosing cholangitis, and bile duct stenosis. Once cirrhosis develops, the usual complications can occur.

Management of CF-associated liver disease includes nutritional correction of deficiencies of fat soluble vitamins (A, D, E, K), essential fatty acids, carnitine, and choline. Ursodeoxycholic acid (UDCA) has been used as a specific therapy to delay the progression of liver disease and is administered at a dose of 20 mg/ kg per day. There is no consensus on which patients will benefit the most from UDCA, and whether it should be used for early disease. However, early administration may delay the onset of liver disease.

Patients with end-stage liver disease should be evaluated for liver transplantation. The overall outcomes of well-selected CF patients post liver transplant appear to be similar to other patients.

Multidrug resistance protein 3 deficiency

Although most of the recognized genetic defects of bile formation are very rare, multidrug resistance protein 3 (MDR3) deficiency (also known as progressive familial intrahepatic cholestasis type 3, PFIC3) is fairly common and has a wide range of clinical presentations, including subtle liver disease in adults. MDR3 is a P-glycoprotein thought to replenish phosphatidylcholine in the outer lipid membrane of the bile canaliculus. In the absence of MDR3 (homozygous disease), bile acids damage the canalicular membrane resulting in destruction of small bile ducts. This condition is associated with marked elevations in γ-glutamyl transpeptidase (GGT) and can lead to biliary cirrhosis. Heterozygous mutations in the *ABCB4* gene coding for MDR3 can result in higher risk for cholesterol stones, sludge, and low-phospholipid associated cholestasis.

Patients with homozygous *ABCB4* mutations usually present in childhood with cholestasis, jaundice, and failure to thrive. However, delayed presentation in adolescence or adults has been reported. Patients presenting with cholelithiasis prior to age 40, sludge or microlithiasis, and recurrent stones after cholecystectomy should be suspected to have heterozygous *ABCB4* mutations. Many patients report a history of intrahepatic cholestasis of pregnancy, or cholelithiasis in a first-degree relative. Overall, one of every three adult patients presenting with cholestasis of unknown origin has an *ABCB4* mutation.

Treatment of these patients should include nutritional correction of the fat-soluble vitamins. For patients with recurrent stones, UDCA may help prevent formation and can be used at a dose of 15 mg/kg per day. Pruritus can be severe and often unresponsive to conventional therapies such as UDCA, cholestyramine, antihistamines, and rifampin. In refractory cases, surgical interruption of the enterohepatic circulation may be necessary. Liver transplantation is reserved for patients with end-stage liver disease or refractory pruritus.

Hereditary citrullinemia type 2

Unlike citrullinemia type 1 (a urea cycle disorder discussed below), type 2 citrullinemia occurs in both adults and children. Type 2 citrullinemia has a prevalence of 1 in 100 000 to 1 in 230 000 individuals. In infants, it may cause a neonatal intrahepatic cholestasis caused by citrin deficiency (NICCD). In adults, it can resemble non-alcoholic fatty liver disease clinically, though the primary organ targeted is the nervous system (symptoms include confusion, lethargy, hallucinations, delusions, tremors, and coma). Treatment of choice is liver transplantation for advanced disease.

Urea cycle defects

The urea cycle consists of five enzymes that process ammonia derived from amino acid metabolism to urea. Genetic defects have been reported in all of these enzymes. The syndromes caused by these defects are not associated with severe liver disease, but they can mimic other metabolic liver diseases. All of the urea cycle disorders present as acute, life-threatening events in infancy and early childhood, though adult presentations have also been reported. A common early sign in newborns is central hyperventilation leading to respiratory alkalosis. Clinical manifestations vary significantly (adults may present only with neurologic symptoms), but all affected have very high serum venous and arterial ammonia levels (may exceed 2000 mmol/L, normal <50 mmol/L). Tests performed should include serum ammonia, arterial blood gases (expect a respiratory alkalosis), urine organic acids, serum amino acids, and urinary orotic acid. Direct enzyme analysis in liver tissue, fibroblasts, and red blood cells can be performed and is useful in patients presenting in adulthood.

Treatment of urea cycle defects is mainly medical. The immediate goal of therapy in patients presenting with newly diagnosed urea cycle defects is to restore ammonia levels in blood to normal. Oral lactulose can be used but may not be effective given the high levels of serum ammonia. Usually hemodialysis or hemofiltration is required. Alternative metabolic pathways for waste nitrogen disposal can be utilized by intravenous administration of sodium benzoate (caution in cirrhotic patients in whom a paradoxical rise in serum ammonia can be seen) and sodium phenylacetate. Once a patient stabilizes, long-term therapy with protein restriction can be initiated and individually tailored. Essential amino acid supplementation is necessary. Liver transplantation is recommended for patients who deteriorate despite therapy. Transplanted patients have normalization of their enzyme activity and ammonia levels and can tolerate a normal diet. Some patients with severe enzyme deficiencies may benefit from early transplantation, even though the liver is structurally normal.

Muscular dystrophies

Duchenne muscular dystrophy and other genetic disorders classified as muscular dystrophy do not affect the liver. Some patients, mainly young children, present clinically with extremely subtle muscular involvement but prominently abnormal serum aminotransferases, usually AST greater than ALT. When it is established that the liver is normal, finding an extremely elevated serum creatine phosphokinase (CPK) can point to the correct diagnosis. Consultation with a neurologist or specialist in muscle disease is the next step in clinical management.

Metabolic liver disorders presenting as conjugated hyperbilirubinemia in early infancy

At least one-quarter of all infants who develop conjugated hyperbilirubinemia in the first 3 months of life have a metabolic liver disease. A few hepatic metabolic disorders, like the urea cycle defects, may present without conjugated hyperbilirubinemia. Any infant presenting with neuromuscular disease, developmental delay, failure to thrive, hepatomegaly, or elevated serum aminotransferases should be evaluated for acidosis, hypoglycemia, bleeding diathesis, and hyperammonemia. Parental consanguinity, recurrent miscarriages, or early infant deaths of previous siblings suggest inherited liver disease. A family pedigree displaying unexplained liver disease, neurologic disease, or muscle disease should also raise suspicion for inherited metabolic problem.

Not all hepatic metabolic diseases present with conjugated hyperbilirubinemia in the neonatal period. There is an extensive differential diagnosis of nonmetabolic disorders that also can present with conjugated hyperbilirubinemia at this time, such as biliary atresia, certain congenital infections, and Alagille syndrome. Therefore methodical and extensive clinical evaluation is important. Early, accurate diagnosis is always important for best clinical outcome.

Selected diseases of note are described in Table 22.4.

With disorders that can present in infancy or later, affected infants often have some distinctive features. In AAT deficiency approximately one-quarter of infants have very severe cholestasis. They may have acholic stools and, exceptionally, infants are found to have both AAT deficiency and biliary atresia. Infants whose jaundice is severe and slow to resolve generally have a poor overall prognosis and need early liver transplantation. Likewise, some infants with citrulinemia type 2 (citrin deficiency) have very severe neonatal hepatitis and have some metabolic features suggestive of galactosemia. Differentiation from galactosemia is important because treatment of the two disorders differs. Infants with CF may present with severe neonatal hepatitis with ductopenia or extrahepatic bile duct damage approximating biliary atresia or severe fatty liver. Those with meconium ileus are more likely to have liver involvement. Of the glycogen storage disorders, type 4 is the only one that presents with neonatal conjugated hyperbilirubinemia.

Galactosemia

Galactose is a sugar found in human and bovine milk primarily as the disaccharide lactose. Altered metabolism of galactose caused by deficient enzyme activity results in elevations in blood levels of galactose, called galactosemia. Galactosemia can result from three different enzyme deficiencies: galatose-1-phosphate uridyl transferase (GALT), galactokinase (GALK), and uridine diphosphate galactose-4-epimerase (GALE). Each enzyme deficiency has a different phenotype.

Classic galactosemia is caused by severe deficiency of GALT. It is the most common and severe. Affected individuals usually present in the first few days of life with jaundice, vomiting, hepatomegaly, failure to thrive, poor feeding, and lethargy. Examination can reveal hypotonia and lenticular cataracts. Laboratory abnormalities will include increased plasma galactose, increased blood and urine galactitol levels, liver dysfunction, metabolic acidosis, and hemolytic anemia. Gold standard for diagnosis is demonstration of absence of GALT activity in red blood cells.

Table 22.4 Selected metabolic liver diseases presenting in infancy with conjugated hyperbilirubinemia

Name	Clinical presentation	Gene mutated or enzyme deficient	Investigations	Treatment
AAT deficiency	Conjugated hyperbilirubinemia, up to 50% have elevated serum AST by age 3 years	*AAT* gene	Serum AAT concentration; PI type; liver biopsy may not show PASD globules in early infancy	None; breast feeding may be advantageous
Cystic fibrosis	Cholestatic jaundice, transient hepatomegaly	*CFTR* gene	Sweat chloride, immunoreactive trypsin	UDCA
Galactosemia	Jaundice, vomiting, hepatomegaly, failure to thrive, poor feeding, lethargy	Galactose-1-phosphate uridyltransferase gene	Galactose-1-6-phosphate uridyltransferase	Lactose-free formula
Hereditary tyrosinemia type 1	Neonatal liver failure, neonatal hepatitis	Fumaryl acetoacetate hydrolase gene (*FAH*)	Urine succinylacetone; serum tyrosine, methionine; α - fetoprotein	NTBC, formula low in tyrosine and phenylalanine
Hereditary fructosemia	Recurrent hypoglycemia and vomiting following weaning	Aldolase B (fructose biphosphate aldolase)	Liver biopsy: electron microscopy, enzyme activities	Fructose-free diet; medications free of fructose/sucrose
Citrullinemia type 2 (NICCD)	Neonatal intrahepatic cholestasis	*SLC25A13* which encodes a mitochondrial aspartate glutamate carrier (citrin)	Serum amino acids; genetic testing	Lactose-free low-protein high-carbohydrate formula

(Continued)

Table 22.4 (*Continued*)

Name	Clinical presentation	Gene mutated or enzyme deficient	Investigations	Treatment
Glycogen storage disease type 4	Fetal hydrops, neonatal hypotonia, fetal death OR Childhood cardiomyopathy and abnormal neuromuscular development	Brancher enzyme deficiency (α-1,4-glycan 6-glycosyltransferase)	Liver biopsy; genetic testing	Liver transplantation
Niemann–Pick type A	Infantile feeding difficulty, recurrent vomiting, hepatosplenomegaly	Lysosomal sphingomyelinase deficiency	Jaundice unusual; bone marrow aspirate, sphingomyelinase	
Niemann–Pick type C	Neonatal prolonged jaundice, hepatosplenomegaly, developmental delay, neurological symptoms	NPC1 (involved in cholesterol esterification)	Storage cells in bone marrow aspirate; liver, rectal biopsy; genetic testing (fibroblasts)	
Wolman disease	Feeding difficulties, diarrhea, hepatosplenomegaly, failure to thrive	Lysosomal acid lipase deficiency	Jaundice unusual; abdominal X-ray of adrenal glands	(Supportive)
Bile canalicular transport disorders	Pruritus, cholestasis, failure to thrive, diarrhea	Type 1: FIC1 Type 2: BSEP (ABCB11) Type 3: MDR3 (ABCB4)	GGT normal GGT usually normal GGT elevated Total serum bile acids (elevated); genetic testing	UDCA, rifampin
Zellweger syndrome	Hypotonia, poor feeding, seizures, liver dysfunction, liver cysts	PEX1 and PEX6	Dysmorphic facies; severe hypotonia; very-long-chain fatty acid studies; C_{27} bile acids	(Supportive)

AAT, α_1-antitrypsin; CFTR, cystic fibrosis transmembrane conductance regulator; GGT, γ-glutamyl transpeptidase; NICCD, neonatal intrahepatic cholestasis caused by citrin deficiency; NTBC, 2-nitro-4-trifluoro-methylbenzoyl-1,3-cyclohexanedione; UDCA, ursodeoxycholic acid.

GALK and GALE deficiency are far less common. GALK deficiency presents with lenticular cataracts and rarely as pseudotumor cerebri. Deficiency of GALE is restricted to erythrocytes and so systemic disease is not seen.

Management of galactosemia includes minimal intake of dietary galactose (by excluding milk and dairy products from the diet), use of soy-based infant formula, and calcium supplementation. If identified early (by a newborn screening program) and adequate dietary therapy is instituted immediately, most patients will have a normal childhood. However, there still remains an increased risk of neuropsychological and ovarian problems in teenage years.

Hereditary tyrosinemia type 1

Hereditary tyrosinemia type 1 (HT1) is an autosomal recessive condition caused by an enzymatic defect in fumarylacetate hydrolase, which leads to accumulation of the intermediates fumarylacetoacetate and maleylacetoacetate, which are then converted to toxic metabolites within the liver. Patients usually present with neonatal liver failure or chronic liver disease. Some infants, however, present with neonatal hepatitis and a few present with unexplained chronic liver disease with hepatic synthetic dysfunction later in the first 6 months of life. Typical biochemical features include abnormal standard tests of liver function, elevated levels of tyrosine and methionine, and serum α-fetoprotein is greatly elevated in the 40000–70000 IU/L range. The most informative test is the presence of succinylacetone in the urine. Those with the chronic form of HT1 have milder features and usually present after age 1 year old. These children may have hepatomegaly, rickets, nephromegaly, and systemic hypertension. Acute neuropathy resembling a porphyric crisis may occur. Hepatocellular carcinoma may develop in any child with HT1. In addition to the amino acid profile and urinary succinylacetone, definitive diagnosis of this condition is confirmed by genetic testing or measuring fumarlyacetate hydrolase levels in lymphocytes, erythrocytes, or liver tissue.

Treatment of tyrosinemia has been revolutionized by the introduction of NTBC (2-nitro-4-trifluoro-methylbenzoyl-1,3-cyclohexanedione) in the 1990s. NTBC, a herbicide, is a potent inhibitor of one of the initial steps in the degradation of tyrosine. The downstream toxic intermediates therefore do not accumulate. Nutritional therapy is still required with NTBC treatment. It consists of removing tyrosine and phenylalanine from the diet. This dietary restriction minimizes adverse effects of NTBC treatment, prevents or reverses renal damage, and improves metabolic bone disease.

Liver transplantation corrects the phenotype of this disease and restores normal fumarylacetate hydrolase activity. Previously, liver transplantation was one of the mainstays of management but this need has greatly declined with the use of NTBC.

In places where HT1 is highly prevalent, newborn screening programs have proved highly effective. Infants are diagnosed very early in life and started on NTBC. Early treatment with NTBC has been very successful at improving the hepatic clinical course of patients with tyrosinemia. With delayed treatment, however, the risk of hepatocellular carcinoma persists.

Hereditary fructose intolerance (fructosemia)

Fructosemia is an autosomal recessive disorder due to the deficiency of fructose-1-phosphate aldolase, isozyme b. Deficiency of this enzyme leads to the accumulation of fructose-1-phosphate and subsequent inhibition of hepatic phosphorylase and gluconeogenesis. As a result, patients present with recurrent hypoglycemia and vomiting following weaning, which is when fructose or sucrose is typically added to an infant's diet. Some infants who are formula fed may present earlier due to the sucrose content of some brands. As disease progresses, additional manifestations include jaundice, hepatomegaly, lactic acidosis, fructosuria, aminoaciduria, and failure to thrive.

Diagnosis has historically required a liver biopsy and measurement of enzyme levels. However, biopsy can now generally be avoided due to the availability of genetic testing of the aldolase B gene on chromosome 9q. Therapy involves elimination of fructose from the diet, which can be difficult since it involves eliminating sucrose. Pharmacists can advise as to medications free of sucrose. Adherence to this diet will tend to reverse and prevent additional manifestations of disease.

Neonatal liver failure

Some metabolic disease cause severe liver disease which presents as neonatal liver failure (Table 22.5). The clinical picture may resemble adult acute liver failure or end-stage chronic liver failure, the latter apparently due to liver

Table 22.5 Metabolic disorders that can present as neonatal liver failure resembling acute liver failure ("acute pattern") or chronic liver failure ("chronic pattern")

Acute pattern (Jaundice, extremely elevated serum aminotransferases, fixed coagulopathy)	Chronic pattern (Jaundice, near-normal serum aminotransferases, low serum albumin, fixed coagulopathy)
Hereditary tyrosinemia, type 1	Hereditary tyrosinemia, type 1
Galactosemia	Galactosemia Hereditary fructosemia
Mitochondrial disorders	Mitochondrial disorders Inborn error of bile acid synthesis: Δ^4-3-oxosteroid-5β-reductase Perinatal hemochromatosis

disease beginning antenatally in the fetus. Early recognition and intervention are critically important for such infants. Management should include elemental formula to remove potentially toxic sugars from the diet; exclusion of tyrosine and phenylalanine may also be instituted pre-emptively. Nutritional therapy can be revised once the relevant diagnoses have been ruled out. Since both bacterial and viral infection can cause a similar picture, diagnosis and management of infection are important. Perinatal hemochromatosis, which is usually due to an alloimmune process, can be investigated by serum ferritin, MRI of liver and abdominal organs, and bone marrow inspection to exclude hemophagocytosis. Perinatal hemochromatosis usually, but not invariably, affects the second and subsequent children in a family.

Case study 22.1

A 54-year-old Caucasian man complains of fatigue and is found to have abnormal liver biochemistry. He gives no history for any potential causes of liver disease. He denies any edema, jaundice, or pruritus. Other than type 2 diabetes, he is well. His HbA1C is within target just on oral metformin 500 mg once daily. He is a 20-pack year smoker. Otherwise, his health history is unremarkable apart from mild arthritis. There is no family history of liver disease but his father had type 2 diabetes. Physical exam reveals an obese man (BMI 32.2) with no other contributory findings.

Laboratory tests show: Hb 168 g/L (normal 140–170), WBC 4.4×10^9/L (normal 4–9), platelets 164×10^9/L (normal 150–400), AST 78 IU/L (normal <40), ALT 68 IU/L (normal <40), bilirubin 16 μmol/L (normal <24), INR 1.04 (normal 0.90–1.20), fasting transferrin saturation 0.65, ferritin 1982 μg/L (normal <200); *HFE* gene testing: C282Y/C282Y.

Imaging: abdominal ultrasound shows fatty liver with coarse echotexture with suggestion of nodularity.

Comment:

At first glance, it appears that this patient may have iron overload and coexistent fatty liver disease (likely NAFLD). However, he is a homozygous for the major mutation of the *HFE* gene. It is often difficult, without invasive testing, to determine whether fatty liver disease influences the natural history of another chronic liver disease. In this case a liver biopsy will be helpful as it can determine the degree of iron overload in the liver (liver iron quantification) as well as whether there are features of non-alcoholic steatohepatitis (NASH). If he does have iron overload, then phlebotomy to rapidly lower ferritin to below 100 μg/L is necessary followed by 3–6 monthly phlebotomies as maintenance therapy. In any case, lifestyle modification must be encouraged for his fatty liver seen on ultrasound.

Case study 22.2

A young mother brings her toddler to see you. She is obviously upset, although nothing appears wrong with her son. You know both of them well: you managed her through this first pregnancy; labor and delivery went well; the baby had great Apgars. You last saw the child when he was 18 months old when you suggested that it might be timely to stop breast feeding. You note that they missed the 2 year old well-baby visit, which should have happened a couple of months ago. When you ask why the mother has brought the child into clinic today you get an excited torrent of information: "He is the world's worst picky eater! My sister says that he has a big tummy and looks just like the kids with kwashiorkor she has seen in Peru. She says I am a hopelessly bad mother!" You are aware that this older sister is unmarried, a career missionary; it is a close-knit family and in fact this mom is married to her cousin. When you ask what the child refuses to eat, she says: "You mean, what will he eat? Bagels and potato chips and milk! I should never have weaned him." You mention that they missed the last appointment and she says that they were vacationing in South America. You ask how that went—nice mangos and papayas in South America. The mother says that her child proved that you could live by bread alone, would not touch all that beautiful fruit, finally broke down and drank goat's milk, and partway through the trip got gastroenteritis with vomiting. On physical examination, the child is not jaundiced but has a slightly firm liver edge felt 4 cm below the right costal margin. His weight remains on his previous percentile. "What about candy?" you ask, and the mother says that the child refuses candy but mentions that no one in her family is big on candy. "Apple juice?" you ask, thinking of the gallons consumed by most of the children in your family practice. "Oh no," she replies, "he pushes it away. Should I make him drink it? After all it does have vitamin C in it. Maybe he has scurvy."

Liver tests show elevated serum aminotransferases, serum albumin at the low end of the normal range, and normal coagulation. You check for celiac disease although you pretty certain it is not the diagnosis, given the history (tests come back negative). You arrange for a liver biopsy to be performed and suggest that in the meantime the little boy should eat whatever he wants and however much of it he wants. Two weeks later the mother and little boy return for the results of the liver biopsy, which had been uncomplicated. The biopsy shows findings on electron microscopy consistent with the diagnosis of hereditary fructose intolerance; there is also moderate fibrosis and a little fatty infiltration. You explain that her son has a certain "wisdom of his body" and knows what foods make him sick and therefore he steers clear of them. You explain that the liver can make some fructose from other sugars and thus it is impossible to avoid all liver damage, but you reassure her that on a diet containing no fructose *and no sucrose* he will do nicely. A consultation with a dietician, prescription for multivitamins, and a list of sucrose-free mediations complete the immediate management plan.

Multiple choice questions

1. Which of the following may point toward a metabolic liver disease in an infant?
   A. Family history of early death in children
   B. Parental consanguinity
   C. Neurodevelopmental delay
   D. Failure to thrive
   E. All of the above

2. A liver biopsy from a patient with abnormal liver tests and a family history of early-onset emphysema reveals PAS-positive, diastase-resistant globules in hepatocytes. Which phenotype will not explain this result?
   A. PI ZZ
   B. PI MZ
   C. PI M$_{Malton}$Z
   D. PI MM
   E. PI SZ

Answers

1. E
2. D

Further reading

Bals R. Alpha-1-antitrypsin deficiency. Best Pract Res Clin Gastroenterol 2010; 24: 629–33.

Moini M, Mistry P, Schilsky ML. Liver transplantation for inherited metabolic disorders of the liver. Curr Opin Organ Transplant 2010; 15: 269–76.

Pietrangelo A. Hepcidin in human iron disorders: therapeutic implications. J Hepatol 2011; 54: 173–81.

Pietrangelo A. Hereditary hemochromatosis: pathogenesis, diagnosis, and treatment. Gastroenterology 2010; 139: 393–408, 408, e1–2.

Roy A, Finegold MJ. Hepatic neoplasia and metabolic diseases in children. Clin Liver Dis 2010; 14: 731–46.

Wilson disease: when should you think of Wilson disease?

CHAPTER 23

Eve A. Roberts[1] and Gideon M. Hirschfield[2]

[1]Departments of Paediatrics, Medicine and Pharmacology, University of Toronto, and Division of Gastroenterology, Hepatology and Nutrition, The Hospital for Sick Children, Toronto, Ontario, Canada
[2]Division of Gastroenterology, Toronto Western Hospital, University Health Network, University of Toronto, Toronto, Ontario, Canada, and Centre for Liver Research, University of Birmingham, Birmingham, UK

Key points

- Wilson disease (WD) is a rare, but treatable, autosomal recessive disorder of hepatic copper disposition.
- Onset of clinical disease can occur at any age, though mainly between 3 and 55 years old. Age alone is not a reason for discounting the diagnosis of WD.
- WD can present as hepatic disease, neurological movement disorders, or psychiatric disease.
- In a patient with liver disease or typical neurologic features, the combination of subnormal serum ceruloplasmin (preferably <140 mg/dL) and elevated basal 24-h urinary copper excretion (>0.6 μmol/24 h or >40 μg/24 h) is highly suggestive of WD.
- Genetic diagnosis is definitive but requires skilled interpretation.
- Treatment is lifelong. Early diagnosis and treatment provide the best outlook. Discontinuing treatment altogether leads to severe refractory liver dysfunction; treatment should not be stopped during pregnancy.
- First-degree relatives must be investigated for WD once a single family member has been diagnosed with WD; genetic testing is most efficient.

Definition

Wilson disease is a genetic disorder of hepatic copper disposition. The abnormal gene is *ATP7B*, identified in 1993. The transmission pattern is autosomal recessive. The vast majority of affected individuals are compound heterozygotes.

Hepatology: Diagnosis and Clinical Management, First Edition. Edited by E. Jenny Heathcote.
© 2012 John Wiley & Sons, Ltd. Published 2012 by John Wiley & Sons, Ltd.

Pathogenesis

ATP7B encodes the Wilson ATPase, a metal-transporting P-type ATPase, which has two principal functions in the hepatocyte. The Wilson ATPase is essential for incorporation of copper into nascent ceruloplasmin, and it expedites biliary excretion of copper. Thus, when the Wilson ATPase is absent or non-functional because of mutations in *ATP7B*, copper accumulates in hepatocytes. One reason for the copper accumulation is that excess copper is not excreted into the bile, and another is that copper is not used for producing ceruloplasmin. Ceruloplasmin is thus released into the bloodstream without containing copper. Since most of the copper measured in the blood is actually within ceruloplasmin, serum copper measurements are *low* in WD. Given the hepatic copper overload, this finding seems paradoxical. If copper is released from the liver, for example with progressive liver injury for fulminant hepatic failure, the serum copper is elevated. The excess copper in the plasma compartment is not "free" copper; instead it is loosely bound to albumin and certain amino acids.

As WD progresses, small amounts of copper leach out of the liver and accumulate in other organs: the brain, renal tubules, heart, and synovia, among others. Copper accumulating in Desçemet's membrane of the cornea produces the Kayser–Fleischer ring. Self-limited episodes of copper released from the liver can cause transient hemolysis, resulting in mild jaundice.

Epidemiology

WD is found worldwide. The average prevalence is 30 affected persons per million. The corresponding carrier frequency is approximately 1 in 90. More than 500 mutations have been identified. No one single mutation is extremely common. Certain mutations are typical for individuals of specific ethnic or geographical backgrounds. In north-eastern Europe, H1069Q is found as at least one of the mutations in 35–75% of WD patients. A circumscribed set of mutations is found in certain other populations including Iceland, Korea, Japan, Sardinia, and the Canary Islands.

Clinical features

WD can present clinically as liver disease, neurological disease usually with a movement disorder of some kind, or psychiatric disease.[1] Some presymptomatic patients are identified through family screening once a proband has been diagnosed. Presymptomatic infants may be identified through universal newborn screening in countries where such programs are established. Hepatic disease is more common in younger patients and neuropsychiatric disease in somewhat older patients, but the demarcation is vague. Certainly, children do present with mainly neurological disturbances in WD.

The first clinical presentation of WD can occur at any age. Age at diagnosis ranges from approximately 4 to 70 years. Toddlers (1.5–3 years old) and seniors (>70 years old) have been diagnosed with WD.

Hepatic WD. Hepatic involvement takes numerous forms. The patient may feel well but have moderately abnormal liver biochemistries. Non-specific symptoms such as fatigue or anorexia may be present. Hepatic steatosis (fatty liver, typically found by liver sonography) is common in WD, affecting up to half of patients. Some patients present with an illness closely resembling autoimmune hepatitis, and a few patients have a self-limited clinical illness resembling acute hepatitis with elevated serum IgG and presence of non-specific autoantibodies. Many patients present with cirrhosis and portal hypertension: hepatosplenomegaly, ascites, low serum albumin, and coagulopathy. These patients must be distinguished from those who present with fulminant hepatic failure (WD–FHF). Features of WD–FHF include acute Coombs-negative intravascular hemolysis, rapid onset of renal failure, disproportionately low serum aminotransferases (usually <<1500 IU/L) from the onset of clinically apparent disease, subnormal or just normal serum alkaline phosphatase, in addition to severe coagulopathy and some degree of encephalopathy. WD–FHF is somewhat more common in females than males.

Neurologic WD. Patients with neurologic WD generally have some liver involvement although it may be asymptomatic. The most common clinical symptoms are speech defects, drooling, hand tremors, and gait disturbance.[2] Overall, neurologic WD follows two broad patterns: movement disorders or rigid dystonia. Movement disorders typically occur in younger patients and include tremors, poor coordination, and loss of fine motor control. Tremor resembling a familial tremor is often present. Spastic dystonic disorders resemble Parkinson disease with mask-like facies, rigidity, and gait disturbance. Pseudobulbar involvement, such as dysarthria, drooling, and swallowing disorder, is more common in older patients but may occur in children and adolescents. Intellect is normal.

Psychiatric WD. Personality changes may be apparent in patients with neurological WD, but an actual psychiatric disorder is present in the approximately 20% of WD patients who present with psychiatric WD. The spectrum of disorder is highly variable.[3] Depression is probably most common. Neurotic behaviors such as obsessive–compulsive behaviors or phobias have been reported; aggressive or antisocial behavior may occur. Affected patients tend to be older and the psychopathology may be subtle: progressive disorganization of personality with anxiety and affective changes such as labile moods and disinhibition. Psychotic disorders are uncommon.

Associated disorders

WD can affect numerous organ systems besides the liver and brain. These are summarized in Table 23.1.

The classic Kayser–Fleischer (KF) ring is due to copper accumulation in Desçemet's membrane. Well-developed KF rings are a golden brown color and

Table 23.1 Systems affected by Wilson disease

Liver	Fatty liver; resembling autoimmune hepatitis; cirrhosis, etc.; bilirubinate gallstones
Brain	Movement disorders resembling chorea; rigid dystonia; dysarthria; dysautonomia
	Psychiatric manifestations
Eyes	Kayser–Fleischer rings; sunflower cataract
Blood	Self-limited intravascular hemolysis
Kidney	Renal tubular dysfunction; Fanconi syndrome; kidney stones; hypokalemic muscle weakness
Joints	Arthralgia or arthritis; osteoporosis, osteopenia
Pancreas	Pancreatitis
Heart	Arrhythmias; cardiomyopathy
Endocrine	Hypoparathyroidism Testicular dysfunction Amenorrhea; spontaneous abortion; infertility

can be seen by direct inspection only if the iris is a pale color: thus slit-lamp examination is required. It is absent in half of the patients with hepatic WD and occasionally is absent in patients with neurologic WD. Although KF rings are generally specific for WD in children, they are not specific for WD in older patients. Copper deposited in the lens produces the sunflower cataract, which does not interfere with vision.

Hepatocellular carcinoma was thought to be exceedingly uncommon in WD, but accumulating data suggest that this is not the case. Hepatic and abdominal malignancies may be found in older patients despite adequate treatment.

Differential diagnosis

The patient who presents with obvious liver disease (or typical neurological disorder), exceedingly low serum ceruloplasmin, and KF rings is easy to diagnose as having WD. Unfortunately, these patients are quite uncommon. A high index of suspicion is valuable for diagnosing Wilson disease. The differential diagnosis for WD falls into three major categories: hepatic disorders, neurological disorders, and diseases associated with low serum ceruloplasmin. The latter include protein-losing enteropathy, nephrotic syndrome, and malnutrition, and the rare genetic condition aceruloplasminemia associated with neurological, retinal, and pancreatic degeneration due to iron accumulation in the brain, retina, and pancreas.

Evaluation of liver disease

Severity of liver disease needs to be determined. Many patients have comparatively mild liver disease without much scarring or vascular damage. Those who have decompensated cirrhosis with coagulopathy, low serum albumin, and some degree of jaundice may still respond to medical treatment. Patients with WD–FHF or treatment-refractory liver disease require liver transplantation.

Presence of *any* liver disease must be ascertained in the first-degree relatives of a newly diagnosed patient with WD. A clinical strategy for such investigations is given in Table 23.2. Genetic testing is the most efficient way to diagnose WD in first-degree relatives, if the proband's genotype is known. If a brother or sister is a potential donor for a living donor liver transplant, genotypic diagnosis is essential.

Laboratory features

Routine liver biochemistries are usually abnormal with mild to moderately elevated serum aminotransferases. Biochemical testing may miss very early disease. Serum aspartate aminotransferase (AST) may be higher than alanine aminotransferase (ALT) because of mitochondrial damage or hemolysis. With more advanced disease, serum albumin may be low. Since serum albumin is normal in true acute liver failure, hypoalbuminemia may be an additional clue to WD–FHF. Mild coagulopathy may be the last laboratory feature to improve on medical treatment.

Serum ceruloplasmin is usually subnormal. Approximately one-third of patients have serum ceruloplasmin below 100 mg/L; one-third have serum ceruloplasmin between 100 and 200 mg/L; the remaining third have normal serum ceruloplasmin. Ceruloplasmin by itself is not adequate for diagnosing WD and is of questionable value in screening for WD. The main reason for the inadequacy of ceruloplasmin as a diagnostic criterion now, as compared to 50 years ago, is that the automated test is performed by immunological, not enzymatic, methods. Thus it does not determine whether copper-containing ceruloplasmin is present. Recent studies suggest that in adults serum ceruloplasmin below 140 mg/L is specific and sensitive for the diagnosis of WD.[4]

In WD serum copper concentration is low, in parallel with the low serum ceruloplasmin. The non-ceruloplasmin-bound copper concentration is elevated. Although direct methods for measuring non-ceruloplasmin-bound copper are bring developed, this fraction is usually estimated from the proportion of copper known to be associated with ceruloplasmin. The estimate depends on the accuracy of the ceruloplasmin measurement and has not been validated as a diagnostic tool. In normal individuals, the non-ceruloplasmin-bound copper is approximately 50–100 μg/L. In WD, the non-ceruloplasmin copper is more than 200 μg/L, but it may be even 10 times higher in WD–FHF.

Measurement of basal 24-h urinary excretion of copper is highly informative for the diagnosis of WD. Recent studies show that the cut-off for suspecting WD should be 0.6 μmol/24 h (>40 μg/24 h). Using the higher conventional reference values severely limits the utility of this test. The penicillamine challenge

Table 23.2 Strategy for investigation of first-degree relatives of a person newly diagnosed with Wilson disease (WD)

	Molecular testing available	No molecular testing available
Brother or sister of patient	*Haplotype or mutation analysis* Identical haplotype or two mutations → WD: baseline testing then treatment Different haplotype or no mutations → diagnosis excluded Indeterminate, such as only one mutation found → baseline testing	*Baseline testing* **Serum for liver biochemistries, ceruloplasmin, INR, complete blood count** **Urine for 24-h urinary copper excretion (basal)** **Slit-lamp examination** All normal → diagnosis excluded Abnormal liver tests *or* subnormal ceruloplasmin *or* elevated 24-h urinary copper excretion (>0.6 μmol/24 h) → liver biopsy with measurement of hepatic copper: Hepatic copper <50 μg/g dry weight → diagnosis excluded Hepatic copper >250 μg/g dry weight → WD, treatment Hepatic copper 51–250 μg/g dry weight → get molecular testing
Child of patient (if free of symptoms, test at >2 years old)	*Haplotype or mutation analysis* Identical haplotype or two mutations → WD, baseline testing then treatment Different haplotype or no mutations → diagnosis excluded Indeterminate, such as only one mutation found → baseline testing (no slit lamp exam until child >4 years old)	*Baseline testing (as above)* All normal → diagnosis excluded Abnormal liver tests → repeat baseline testing in 6–12 months Subnormal ceruloplasmin *or* elevated 24-h urinary copper excretion (>0.6 μmol/24 h) → liver biopsy with measurement of hepatic copper *or* get molecular testing

test has proven less reliable than previously thought, and it may add no extra information beyond what can be gained through measuring basal excretion of copper, which reflects the total body copper load and, more directly, the non-ceruloplasmin-bound copper.

Hepatic tissue copper concentration is highly informative in most WD patients. Hepatic copper content greater than 250 μg per gram dry weight is *accepted* as diagnostic of Wilson disease; however, recent data indicate that 100 μg per gram dry weight might be a better diagnostic threshold. Indeed, the hepatic copper concentration is generally 10 or more times the value found in normal individuals. Providing a large enough sample of liver tissue is important for accurate measurement. With cirrhosis, copper may be variably accumulated in different nodules. Some heterozygotes have moderate elevations of liver tissue copper, without having clinical liver disease. Finding elevated hepatic copper concentration also is not specific for WD; patients with chronic cholestasis or diseases such as Indian childhood cirrhosis may have elevated hepatic copper. Liver copper can be measured in formalin-fixed specimens.

For WD–FHF a simple formula of routine laboratory tests has proven sensitive and specific: alkaline phosphatase/total bilirubin < 4 *plus* AST/ALT > 2.2, all in American units.[5] For WD in general, a diagnostic profile has been developed but remains incompletely validated; moreover, definite limitations to its diagnostic accuracy have been identified.

Investigations

Imaging the liver may show fatty liver, nodular transformation, or features suggestive of cirrhosis. Imaging the central nervous system may be informative and should be performed even in the absence of neurological disorder. Magnetic resonance imaging (MRI) is more sensitive than computed tomography (CT). Generalized cerebral atrophy may be present. Abnormalities of the putamen and pons are most frequently found in patients with a neurological presentation; in patients with an hepatic presentation abnormalities of the globus pallidus are common. Only the so-called "face of the giant panda" sign seems to be specific for neurological WD.

Liver biopsy may provide important diagnostic information besides tissue for copper quantification, and it permits staging of the liver disease.[6] A routine disposable needle can be used; the specimen should be aliquoted immediately for histology and copper quantification with minimal exposure to metals. Earliest histological findings include steatosis, focal hepatocellular necrosis, and/or apoptotic bodies, and glycogenated nuclei in hepatocytes. Mallory–Denk bodies may be found. With progressive parenchymal damage, possibly by repeated episodes of lobular necrosis, periportal fibrosis develops. Typically, cirrhosis is macronodular. Commonly used histochemical stains for copper may be negative in the early stages of WD because only copper aggregated in lysosomes is stained. On electron microscopy (EM), classic changes in mitochondria may be identified. Mitochondria vary in size, with increased matrix density and dark inclusions; however, the most striking change is dilatation of the tips of the mitochondrial cristae so that each crista appears cystic, shaped like a tennis racquet rather than a shelf. Mitochondrial changes occur early in WD. If WD is the leading possible diagnosis, a portion of the biopsy should be placed in universal fixative immediately for possible EM examination.

Genetic diagnosis is definitive. The gene *ATP7B* is found on 13q14.3. It is a large gene. Mutations tend to be missense, nonsense, and splice-site mutations, and large deletions are uncommon. Mutations that interfere with production of the Wilson ATPase cause severe liver disease,[7] but extensive genotype–phenotype correlations have been elusive, mainly because most WD patients are compound heterozygotes with one copy of two different mutations. Modern high-throughput analytic methods make it possible to analyze the entire gene fairly easily; haplotype analysis and other methods are also available. A small percentage of patients who have WD by clinical diagnosis nevertheless appear to have no detectable genetic abnormality, and current research is aimed at understanding genetic mechanisms in these patients. Primary genetic diagnosis may not yet function as the most efficient diagnostic investigation, but it is ideal for evaluating siblings.

Natural history

Untreated WD is fatal. It has a good prognosis if it is diagnosed promptly and treated effectively. Treatment is lifelong. The best outlook is for the person with presymptomatic WD who starts treatment before any clinical abnormality is apparent.[8] Patients presenting with early hepatic disease generally have a good prognosis so long as treatment is taken consistently and is well tolerated, but some patients with hepatic WD develop progressive liver disease despite treatment.[2] Patients who discontinue treatment entirely tend to develop refractory liver disease or new neurological involvement. Women who discontinue their medication for WD during pregnancy may develop severe hepatic deterioration or liver failure postpartum. Severe neurological disease may not resolve entirely on drug treatment, although substantial improvement usually occurs.[9]

Liver transplantation should be reserved for patients who present with severe, decompensated liver disease unresponsive to medical therapy or for those who present with WD–FHF. After liver transplant, chelation therapy is no longer required. The efficacy of liver transplantation to improve neurological WD is highly disputed, and on balance it appears ineffective. Some WD patients have significant difficulty complying with the medical regimen after liver transplantation.

Patients with WD need to make a concerted effort to maintain good general health. Being overweight or obese should be avoided. Because of the potential for further hepatic mitochondrial damage, they should avoid—or at least limit—alcohol. Like any patient with chronic liver disease, they should have vaccinations for hepatitis A and B. Since WD may predispose to osteoporosis, all patients need to be assessed for osteoporosis and they should adopt lifestyle habits that promote maintenance of healthy bones.

Therapy

Therapy, summarized in Table 23.3, is guided mainly by clinical experience as few randomized controlled trials have been performed.[1,10] Large retrospective studies have recently become available. Some clinical studies investigating one treatment or another are subject to selection bias. Heterozygotes do not require treatment.

Table 23.3 Treatment options for adults with Wilson disease (see text for children's treatment)

Drug	Dose	Neurological deterioration at start of treatment	Side effects	Monitor
D-penicillamine (chelator)	Initial: 1000–1500 mg/day in 2–4 divided doses Maintenance: 750–1000 mg/day in 2 divided doses Begin with incremental doses: 250 or 500 mg/day, increasing by 250 mg/day every 4–7 days to total dose Reduce dose for surgery to promote wound-healing and during pregnancy Also give pyridoxine 25–50 mg/day	10–25%	Immediate adverse reaction: fever, rash, proteinuria Lupus-like reaction Aplastic anemia Leukopenia Thrombocytopenia Nephrotic syndrome Degenerative changes in skin: elastosis perforans serpiginosa Retinal damage: serous retinitis Hepatotoxicity	24-h urinary copper excretion 200–500 µg/24h (3–8 µmol/24h) for efficacy Complete blood count for cytopenias Urinalysis for proteinuria
Trientine (chelator)	Initial: 750–1500 mg/day in 2–4 divided doses Maintenance: 750–1000 mg/day in 2 divided doses Reduce dose for surgery to promote wound-healing and during pregnancy	10–15%	Gastritis Aplastic anemia rare Sideroblastic anemia	24-h urinary copper excretion 200–500 µg/24h (3–8 µmol/24h) for efficacy Complete blood count Urinalysis
Zinc (blocks intestinal uptake of copper)	50 mg *elemental* t.i.d. away from meals; *minimum* dose in adults 50 mg elemental Zn b.i.d. (actual zinc salt affects mainly tolerability) No dosage reduction for surgery or pregnancy	Rare	Gastritis Pancreatitis Zinc accumulation Possible changes in immune function	24-h urinary copper excretion <75 µg/24h (<1.2 µmol/24h) for efficacy Liver tests for efficacy Creatinine for toxicity

D-penicillamine. The first effective oral treatment of WD was introduced in the 1950s: D-penicillamine, an oral chelator. It markedly increases urinary excretion of copper and induces hepatic metallothioneins; additionally, it inhibits collagen cross-linking and has some immunosuppressant properties. It has proven to be very effective for treating WD. Unfortunately, it has important adverse side effects. Approximately 10–25% of patients with neurologic WD have a deterioration of their neurological status when they start D-penicillamine. Various types of skin disorders can occur, including rashes, pemphigus, and elastosis perforans serpiginosa. Loss of taste, althralgias, and diarrhea have been reported. The very severe side effects of D-penicillamine include proteinuria, leukopenia, or thrombocytopenia. Aplastic anemia is a rare catastrophic complication, which does not always reverse when D-penicillamine is stopped. Nephrotic syndrome, systemic disease resembling lupus erythematosus, Goodpasture syndrome, and a myasthenia gravis-like syndrome have all been reported in patients receiving chronic treatment with D-penicillamine. Severe side effects require immediate discontinuation of D-penicillamine with substitution of alternate therapy. Some patients develop an early adverse reaction with fever, rash, and proteinuria (within 7–10 days of beginning treatment); this mandates changing to another treatment, usually trientine.

The usual adult maintenance dose of D-penicillamine is 1000 mg daily, divided into two daily doses. Compliance and efficacy should be checked measuring 24-h urinary copper excretion every 6–12 months; complete blood count and urinalysis should be monitored regularly throughout its use. Pyridoxine 25 mg daily should also be given because of possible adverse effects on pyridoxine metabolism associated with D-penicillamine administration. Children's dosing is 20 mg/kg as total daily dose plus pyridoxine.

Trientine. This chelator has been used since the early 1980s and differs chemically from penicillamine by the absence of sulfhydryl groups. Thus it is a good substitute for D-penicillamine. It is highly effective primary therapy in children and adults, and it should be used as first-line treatment whenever there is apparent predisposition to adverse effects of D-penicillamine. Trientine is well-tolerated in WD apart from occasional gastritis. It can cause iron-deficiency anemia, apparently by chelating dietary iron, or rarely sideroblastic anemia. Bone marrow suppression is extremely rare. Neurological worsening after beginning treatment with trientine has been reported in neurologic WD, but it appears less frequent than with D-penicillamine.

The usual total daily dose is 1000–1200 mg (depending on tablet size available) divided into two daily doses, preferably taken not at mealtime (for example, the typical regimen is before breakfast and at bedtime). Monitoring for effectiveness and safety is as for penicillamine (notably, measuring 24-hour urinary copper excretion every 6–12 months and checking the complete blood count). Children's dosing is 20 mg/kg as total daily dose.

Zinc. Zinc salts have been utilized for treating WD since the 1960s (Europe) and the 1980s (North America). In pharmacological doses, zinc interferes with absorption of copper from the gastrointestinal tract by inducing enterocyte metallothionein, which has greater affinity for copper than for zinc and thus preferentially binds copper present in the intestinal contents. Once it is bound, the copper does not get absorbed and it is lost in the feces due to normal turnover of enterocytes. Since absorbable copper enters the gastrointestinal tract from the diet and from internal secretions (except bile), it is likely that zinc treatment mobilizes endogenous copper. The actual zinc salt does not matter to the mechanism of action but may affect tolerability. The common side effect of gastritis can be minimized by using a salt other than sulfate. In general, zinc has few adverse side effects. Neurological deterioration is uncommon.[11] Zinc treatment has been well tolerated in adults and children. Recent data suggest that zinc is not entirely effective for controlling hepatic WD over the long term. A disadvantage of zinc is that t.i.d. dosing is required and zinc should be taken away from meals; these dosing requirements may make adherence to the regimen difficult.

The usual adult daily dose is 50 mg *elemental* zinc taken three times a day away from meals. Single daily dosing is ineffective; b.i.d. dosing may not be effective. Children's dose is 25 mg *elemental* zinc taken three times a day away from meals.

Tetrathiomolybdate (TTM). Ammonium tetrathiomolybdate remains an investigational drug especially suitable for treatment of severe neurological Wilson disease because, unlike D-penicillamine, it is not associated with early neurological deterioration. It is a strong chelator. Adverse effects have been reported including overly aggressive removal of copper, and the disposition of administered molybdenum is not entirely clear. TTM is not generally available for clinical use.

"Combination treatment". Currently there is much interest in combining a chelator with zinc in order to maximize therapeutic effect synergistically. Either D-penicillamine or trientine is combined with zinc.[12] This ends up as a q.i.d. regimen. The two types of treatment must be temporally dispersed throughout the day, with usually 5–6 hours between administration of either drug, or else there is the likelihood that the chelator binds the zinc and thus negates the efficacy of both therapeutic modalities. A typical, possibly preferred, regimen is zinc (50 mg *elemental*, or 25 mg *elemental* in children) given by mouth as the first and third doses, and trientine (500 mg, or 10 mg/kg in children) given by mouth as the second and fourth doses. This strategy is fundamentally an induction regimen suitable for patients who present with severe disease. Some will fail and require liver transplantation, which should be arranged as a back-up. If it is effective, then it should be continued for 3–6 months after which time the clinically stable patient can be transitioned to monotherapy, preferably with the chelator. Long-term adherence to this intensive regimen appears neither necessary nor practical.

Antioxidants. Since oxidant stress plays an important role in the disease mechanism of hepatic WD, antioxidants might be effective. Based on anecdotal evidence, at a dose of 400–800 IU daily, natural-source vitamin E may be useful adjunctive therapy.

Diet. WD *cannot* be treated by dietary intervention alone. Especially in the first year of treatment, copper-rich foods should be removed from the diet. These foods include organ meats, shellfish, nuts, chocolate, and mushrooms. In real life, this means eliminating chocolate, nuts, and shrimp. Vegetarians require formal dietary counseling because legumes are high in copper. Installing a device in the plumbing system to adsorb copper is necessary only if the drinking water has a high copper concentration, possible with well water, or the plumbing has been installed with copper pipes.

Liver transplantation. With early diagnosis and effective treatment, liver transplantation can usually be avoided in WD. Patients who do not respond to treatment or who present in WD–FHF require liver transplantation. It corrects the hepatic metabolic abnormalities and may improve extrahepatic copper handling. One-year survival is on the order of 80–90%, and most who survive the first year do well long term.[13] Living-donor transplantation is effective even if the donor is a heterozygote.[14] With WD–FHF, plasmapheresis, exchange transfusion, or albumin dialysis may stabilize the patient and minimize renal damage. These interventions extend the time available for actually obtaining a liver graft and, very rarely, may obviate the need for transplantation.

Special therapeutic challenges

Decompensated chronic liver disease. These patients may be diagnosed as having acute liver failure, especially if the criterion of encephalopathy is discounted. Many of these patients will respond to an intensive medical regimen, such as the combination regimen described above. *Automatic* liver transplantation may be inappropriate, although liver transplantation should be available as an urgent alternative and thus a consultation should be requested.

Pregnancy. Treatment must not ever be stopped just because a woman is pregnant; liver failure may develop. D-penicillamine is classified as a teratogen. Treatment can be *converted* to trientine or zinc for the duration of the pregnancy. Insufficient data are available to judge the safety of these drugs in pregnancy. The dose of either chelator should be decreased in the third trimester by 25–50%, but the dose of zinc need not be altered. Women with extensive liver disease should receive obstetric care by a team in a high-risk pregnancy program. With patients on D-penicillamine, breast feeding should be discouraged; little is known about the safety of either trientine or zinc for breast feeding.

Infants with WD identified by universal newborn screening. Copper is required for normal development of the central nervous system. The possible adverse effects of zinc overload on development are not known. Serum ceruloplasmin is physiologically low in early infancy. At the present time there is no standard regimen for treating infants with presymptomatic WD. Treatment with zinc is favored, perhaps starting when the child is a toddler. Very young children with clinically evident WD require treatment with a chelator.

Presymptomatic disease. Most of these patients are best treated with a chelator. For the patient, identified by family screening, who has absolutely no abnormalities (liver tests normal, imaging normal), zinc may be preferred; however, t.i.d. dosing may prove problematic.

Stable patients on chelator therapy. Zinc has a role in long-term maintenance therapy, although the specifics of that role are still being determined. Switching over to zinc can be considered in a patient who is clinically stable on a chelator after 1–5 years (typically 3–5 years) of treatment and has an excellent record of adherence to medical regimen. Liver biochemistries should be normal, as well as copper homeostasis. Close follow-up is still required, and if liver tests become abnormal, the chelator should be restarted. No patient with proven WD should be permitted to stop all treatment completely.

Case study 23.1

John is a 17-year-old male who is referred for evaluation of mildly abnormal liver biochemistries. He feels fine except that he gets really tired after soccer practice and his coach thinks his game is not as sharp as it used to be. He is an average student but lately his grades have been not as good as usual. His hand writing is tiny. He has always been healthy and there is no liver disease in the family. He denies drinking alcohol or using marijuana. On physical exam, he is well nourished and muscular. His height is on the 75th percentile, weight and waist circumference on the 50th percentile for age/gender. He is not jaundiced. The abdominal examination is unremarkable except that the spleen tip might be palpable. Neurological examination is normal. Laboratory tests show: normal full blood count, AST 110 IU/L, ALT 80 IU/L, ALP 353 IU/L, unconjugated bilirubin 33 μmol/L, conjugated bilirubin 8 μmol/L, GGT 50 IU/L, albumin 42 g/L, INR 1.2. IgG is within normal range; antinuclear antibody (ANA) and smooth muscle antibody (SMA) are undetectable; anti-HBs is positive (postvaccination); anti-HAV and anti-HCV are negative. Serum ceruloplasmin is 180 mg/L, serum copper 12.3 μmol/L; 24-h urinary copper is 1.0 μmol/24h. KF rings are negative. Hepatic sonogram: fatty liver, no sign of cirrhosis. Head MRI: hyperintensity in basal ganglia on T2 weighting. Liver biopsy: steatosis, occasional glycogenated nuclei, focal necrosis, normal portal bile ducts without inflammation or obstruction; prominent abnormal mitochondrial morphology on EM. He is diagnosed as having WD and treated successfully with trientine 500 mg by mouth twice a day. D-penicillamine is avoided because of the changes on head MRI and the subtle signs of neurological involvement.

> **Case study 23.2**
>
> Mary is a previously healthy 23-year-old woman who presents acutely ill, having collapsed at her work as a ceramics designer. Her known medical history reveals allergy to peanuts; she is taking no medications. On examination, she is acutely ill and lethargic and somewhat uncooperative. She appears pale and mildly jaundiced. There is hepatomegaly but no ascites. Laboratory tests show: Hgb 70 g/L, WBC 16 000, platelets normal; AST 1400 IU/L, ALT 600 IU/L, ALP 25 IU/L, unconjugated bilirubin 80 μmol/L, conjugated bilirubin 28 μmol/L, GGT 140 IU/L, albumin 26 g/L, INR 2.1. Anti-HBs is positive (postvaccination); anti-HAV IgM and anti-HCV are negative. Coombs test is negative. Hepatic sonogram is consistent with cirrhosis. Serum ceruloplasmin is 280 mg/L. Serum copper is ordered and a 24-h urinary copper is commenced, although nurses note that urinary output is poor. After obtaining a total bilirubin and converting all data to American units, you compute Korman's ratios (alkaline phosphatase/total bilirubin <4 *plus* AST/ALT >2.2, American units): ALP/TB = 3.3 and AST/ALT = 2.3. Treatment with albumin dialysis stabilizes her until liver transplantation can be performed. Afterwards Mary is back at work, feeling great, and is promoted to team manager. Post-transplant when she can cooperate for a slit-lamp examination, an ophthalmologist confirms that KF rings are present, but a year later slit-lamp exam shows that they are almost gone.

Multiple choice questions

1. Which of the following is *not* true of Wilson disease?
   - A. It is a rare monogenic disorder of hepatic copper handling.
   - B. Laboratory testing often reveals a subnormal serum copper concentration.
   - C. Occurrence is worldwide.
   - D. It is occasionally diagnosed in persons older than 60 years.
   - E. Inheritance pattern is X-linked recessive.

2. Treatment for Wilson disease:
   - A. Is usually unsuccessful
   - B. Is lifelong
   - C. Is relatively free of adverse side effects
   - D. Includes liver transplantation in almost every patient
   - E. Invariably requires corticosteroids

3. A key responsibility for the physician who diagnoses Wilson disease in an individual is to:
   - A. Provide a crash course on copper physiology to the patient
   - B. Ensure that a water purification system is installed in the household to exclude copper from the water supply

   C. Counsel against use of copper-wire IUD as birth control

   D. Take a complete family history and screen brothers and sisters for Wilson disease

   E. Refer the patient to a psychiatrist

Answers

1. E

2. B

3. D

References

1. Roberts EA, Schilsky ML. Diagnosis and treatment of Wilson disease: an update. Hepatology 2008; 47: 2089–111.
2. Merle U, Schaefer M, Ferenci P, et al. Clinical presentation, diagnosis and long-term outcome of Wilson's disease: a cohort study. Gut 2007; 56: 115–20.
3. Shanmugiah A, Sinha S, Taly AB, et al. Psychiatric manifestations in Wilson's disease: a cross-sectional analysis. J Neuropsychiatry Clin Neurosci 2008; 20: 81–5.
4. Mak CM, Lam CW, Tam S. Diagnostic accuracy of serum ceruloplasmin in Wilson disease: determination of sensitivity and specificity by ROC curve analysis among ATP7B-genotyped subjects. Clin Chem 2008; 54: 1356–62.
5. Korman JD, Volenberg I, Balko J, et al. Screening for Wilson disease in acute liver failure: a comparison of currently available diagnostic tests. Hepatology 2008; 48: 1167–74.
6. Stromeyer FW, Ishak KG. Histology of the liver in Wilson's disease: a study of 34 cases. Am J Clin Pathol 1980; 73: 12–24.
7. Thomas GR, Forbes JR, Roberts EA, et al. The Wilson disease gene: spectrum of mutations and their consequences. Nat Genet 1995; 9: 210–7.
8. Sternlieb I, Scheinberg IH. Prevention of Wilson's disease in asymptomatic patients. N Engl J Med 1968; 278: 352–9.
9. Medici V, Trevisan CP, D'Inca R, et al. Diagnosis and management of Wilson's disease: results of a single center experience. J Clin Gastroenterol 2006; 40: 936–41.
10. Wiggelinkhuizen M, Tilanus ME, Bollen CW, et al. Systematic review: clinical efficacy of chelator agents and zinc in the initial treatment of Wilson disease. Aliment Pharmacol Ther 2009; 29: 947–58.
11. Brewer GJ. Practical recommendations and new therapies for Wilson's disease. Drugs 1995; 50: 240–9.
12. Askari FK, Greenson J, Dick RD, et al. Treatment of Wilson's disease with zinc. XVIII. Initial treatment of the hepatic decompensation presentation with trientine and zinc. J Lab Clin Med 2003; 142: 385–90.
13. Emre S, Atillasoy EO, Ozdemir S, et al. Orthotopic liver transplantation for Wilson's disease: a single-center experience. Transplantation 2001; 72: 1232–6.
14. Tamura S, Sugawara Y, Kishi Y, et al. Living-related liver transplantation for Wilson's disease. Clin Transplant 2005; 19: 483–6.

Liver disease in pregnant women

CHAPTER 24

E. Jenny Heathcote

Division of Gastroenterology, Toronto Western Hospital, University Health Network, University of Toronto, Toronto, Ontario, Canada

---

Key points

- It is necessary to establish the stage of pregnancy, as some hepatic complications are semester specific.
- Collect information on prior obstetric history.
- Collect information on prior history of a hepatitis (e.g. chronic hepatitis B or C, autoimmune hepatitis), chronic cholestatic liver disease (e.g. Alagille syndrome, primary biliary cirrhosis/primary sclerosing cholangitis), and prior surgery to liver (e.g. Kasai procedure, liver transplant).
- Complete medication history is required. Evaluate alcohol intake and enquire about non-prescription drug use.
- Evaluation of liver disease severity includes:
  - symptoms and signs of liver failure: jaundice, vomiting, easy bruising, ascites, and encephalopathy;
  - evaluate for potential systemic effects, for example hypertension or hypotension, impaired renal function, anemia with or without gastrointestinal hemorrhage, and impaired cognition.

Assessment of liver disease in pregnancy

Most women with pregnancy-related liver diseases present acutely to the emergency room with nausea, vomiting, abdominal pain, jaundice, pruritus, and even drowsiness. The pattern of liver disease in pregnant women varies greatly both at presentation and in subsequent follow up. The trimester of their pregnancy needs to be established as this will suggest which liver disease may be present should their symptoms be pregnancy related.

Hepatology: Diagnosis and Clinical Management, First Edition. Edited by E. Jenny Heathcote.
© 2012 John Wiley & Sons, Ltd. Published 2012 by John Wiley & Sons, Ltd.

Both in the emergency room and the physician's office it is essential to collect historical details of prior pregnancies and to perform both a thorough history (including a list of all medications) and examination (including a check for easy bruising, spider nevi, jaundice, scratch marks (from pruritus), and abdominal and/or ankle swelling) (Box 24.1). Surprisingly though it may seem, some

---

Box 24.1 Investigation and management of a pregnant woman with possible liver disease

History
- Presenting symptoms: vomiting, edema, jaundice, pruritus
- Prior pregnancies (+outcome)
- Details from last antenatal clinic: blood pressure, urine protein, weight gain
- Prior diagnosis of cirrhosis (establish alcohol intake)
- Prior hepatobiliary surgery
- Recent risk factors for viral hepatitis

Physical
- Jaundice, bruising
- Systemic blood pressure
- Edema, ascites
- Hepatic fetor/flap/confusion
- Pruritus (±scratch marks)

Immediate investigation of a pregnant woman with possible liver disease
- Serial monitoring
  Blood pressure and blood sugar
  Urine analysis and output
  Blood urea, creatinine, and electrolytes
  CBC + film (? thrombocytopenia)
  Liver enzymes ALP, AST/ALT
  Liver function, bilirubin, (fractionate) INR, albumin
- Ultrasound of abdomen and Doppler examination of portal and hepatic veins
- Ascitic tap if fluid present (send for albumin content, culture, and WBC)

Immediate management of a pregnant woman with possible pregnancy-associated liver disease
- Establish i.v. access: saline/dextrose as needed
- Dipstick urine + microscopic examination
- Monitor serial Hb, blood glucose, platelets, BUN, INR, bilirubin, AST/ALT
- Arrange for immediate abdominal ultrasound with Doppler examination of portal veins
- Regular dialog with obstetrician and/or general surgeon

ALT, alanine aminotransferase; ALP, alkaline phosphatase; AST, aspartate aminotransferase; BUN, blood urea nitrogen; CBC, complete blood count; INR, international normalized ratio; WBC, white blood cell.

> **Box 24.2 Approach to liver disease in pregnancy**
>
> 1 Liver disease caused by pregnancy
> 2 Liver disease coincidental to pregnancy
> 3 Liver disease present prior to pregnancy

women don't know that they are pregnant—this therefore has to be taken into consideration if any premenopausal woman arrives at the ER with any of the above symptoms (i.e. need to avoid exposure to X-rays, CT scans). Full evaluation of cardiac, respiratory, as well as neurological status, is required. Examination of the abdomen should look for evidence of hepatomegaly and/or splenomegaly as well as ascites. Risk factors for recent exposure to viral hepatitis, for example new sexual partner (hepatitis B and/or D), recent travel (hepatitis A and E) or recurrent vaginal herpes simplex and prior medical (and surgical) history, may all be potentially relevant (Box 24.1).

For those who present with an acute onset of symptoms, physical examination must include a careful evaluation of the patient's mental status. If there is any evidence of impairment then regular (1 hourly) evaluation of their state of cognition is required. Adequate fluid and electrolyte replacement should be given to maintain systemic blood pressure, renal output, and blood glucose and electrolyte balance. Viability of the fetus must be closely monitored. The process of investigation depends both on the presenting symptoms and the timing of the clinical presentation (Box 24.2).

Liver diseases as a consequence of pregnancy

First trimester: hyperemesis gravidarium

Pregnant women who present with severe nausea and varying degrees of vomiting with consequent dehydration and weight loss, that is hyperemesis gravidarium, may be noted to have abnormal liver biochemistry, that is aspartate aminotransferase (AST) and/or alanine aminotransferase (ALT) (Table 24.1). This condition occurs in 1–20 per 1000 pregnancies and is more common in young obese mothers pregnant with their first baby or with multiple pregnancies; recurrence with subsequent pregnancies is common. Pre-existing diabetes is not unusual. Jaundice is rare but when present is all unconjugated (secondary to starvation). Elevation in AST and ALT is generally less than 250 IU/mL and values should return to normal with rehydration. Both fluid and electrolyte (phosphate, magnesium, and potassium) replacement must be attended to. Vitamin supplements, particularly thiamine must be administered. In severely compromised mothers, sublingual odansetron may reduce symptoms. Symptoms usually lessen with progression of the pregnancy.

Very, very rarely mothers with severe, continued vomiting and consequent malnutrition develop serious complications such as esophageal rupture, retinal hemorrhage, and Wernicke encephalopathy or central pontine myelinosis.

Table 24.1 Acute liver disease caused by pregnancy

Stage of pregnancy	Presentation	Treatment
First trimester	**Hyperemesis gravidarum** Associated with ↑ AST/ALT ± unconjugated hyperbilirubinemia Rare complications: esophageal rupture retinal hemorrhage central positive myelinosis	Generally responds well to fluid and electrolyte replacement Ondansetron
Second/third trimester	**Cholestasis of pregnancy** Generalized pruritus without a skin rash	Must treat with UDCA 1g/day
Third trimester	**Acute fatty liver** (mitochondrial injury) Nausea, vomiting, rarely jaundiced May coexist with eclampsia or HELLP Marked leukocytosis ± low platelets Hypoglycemia common—correct Acidosis (↑ lactate and uric acid, ↑ creatinine)	Deliver baby as soon as possible
	Toxemia of pregnancy Severe systemic hypertension Fluid retention Proteinuria AST >10 fold ↑ Unconjugated hyperbilirubinemia Thrombocytopenia Hepatic infarction (seen on ultrasound)	Immediate delivery
	HELLP syndrome Pre-eclampsia + hemolysis ↑ AST/ALT, >10 fold↑ Thrombocytopenia Hyperuricemia (>464 μmol/L associated with ↑ maternal and infant death) Hepatic infarction (seen on ultrasound) Maternal mortality 1.5–5% Fetal mortality 10–60%	Immediate delivery CT/MRI confirms

ALT, aspartate aminotransferase; AST, aspartate aminotransferase; HELLP, hemolysis, elevated liver enzymes and low platelet count; UDCA, ursodeoxycholic acid.

Second to third trimester
Cholestasis of pregnancy

Anywhere from midsecond trimester onwards some pregnant women may start to complain of generalized pruritus despite no evidence of background liver disease. Unless the pruritus becomes intense and disturbs their sleep, the mother remains well.

Typically, the pattern of abnormality of the biochemical tests reflecting cholestatic symptoms in pregnancy show a "mixed" picture with elevation of both serum transaminase and alkaline phosphatase levels although typically GGT remains normal (as is the case with other biliary transporter defects). A conjugated hyperbilirubinemia may be present. Prolonged cholestasis with jaundice results in malabsorption manifested by marked weight loss and a coagulopathy (the latter is correctable with parenteral administration of vitamin K). Elevated serum bile acid levels in the absence of any prior history of liver disease clinches the diagnosis (typically >10 μmol/L but in this condition levels exceed 40 μmol/L in symptomatic patients). Intrahepatic cholestasis of pregnancy is associated with increased rates of fetal loss from placental insufficiency. Treatment with ursodeoxycholic acid (UDCA, 1–2 g/day) is *mandatory* as it not only abrogates the pruritus but also reduces fetal loss—there are no untoward side effects of UDCA on the mother or fetus.

Pruritus spontaneously resolves within 2 weeks of delivery, unless there is background chronic cholestatic liver disease (the usual culprit being primary biliary cirrhosis (PBC)).

There is a genetic component to many causes of cholestasis including that related to pregnancy. Many different mutations of the bile acid transporters have been described—mutation in the *MDR3* gene (the patient is usually a heretozygote) seems to be what promotes cholestasis of pregnancy; thus the condition recurs with subsequent pregnancies. It is not associated with any permanent hepatic consequences although recurrent intraductal stones may develop in those with mutations in the *MDR3* gene.

Third trimester

There are three serious pregnancy-related conditions that affect the liver, fortunately they are rare (1 in 14 000) births. These are: acute fatty liver, pregnancy-related toxemia (systemic hypertension, proteinuria, and fluid retention), and the HELLP syndrome (hemolysis, elevated liver enzymes, and low platelet count). It may be particularly hard to distinguish these latter two conditions. Rarely, acute fatty liver may accompany one of the two other syndromes! However, the more common causes of acute jaundice must not be forgotten.

Acute jaundice with biochemical evidence of cholestasis

Bile becomes more lithogenic during pregnancy and gall bladder emptying is reduced—this promotes cholelithiasis, which is rarely problematic during pregnancy. If choledocolithiasis is suspected on the basis of an ultrasound examination of the biliary tree then once into the second trimester it is safe (in terms of exposure to radiation to the fetus) for the mother to undergo endoscopic retrograde cholangiopancreatography (ERCP) and stone removal. Cholecystectomy if required is also safe in pregnancy.

Acute fatty liver of pregnancy (AFLP)

The pregnant woman at about 34 to 36 weeks of pregnancy may suddenly complain of nausea accompanied by vomiting and abdominal pain complicated by hypoglycemia, lactic acidosis, and hyperammonemia. Jaundice is usually absent. It is more common in primipara, with twins, and/or male child (Box 24.3). These symptoms should prompt immediate admission to hospital where rehydration must be initiated promptly before hypoglycemia, lactic acidosis, and/or renal failure complicate the illness. If jaundice develops this often heralds subsequent hepatic encephalopathy and other serious complications such as disseminated intravascular coagulation, pulmonary emboli, ascites and rarely polydipsia and polyuria (diabetes insipidus) develops. About 50% of AFLP patients will have coexistent pre-eclampsia. Differential diagnosis includes viral hepatitis, drug-induced liver disease, and the HELLP syndrome.

The blood film often shows both thrombocytopenia and a leukocytosis. Other laboratory investigations are helpful in supporting the diagnosis, that is raised aminotransferases, bilirubin, and uric acid levels, with or without a prolonged prothrombin time. Monitoring of disease severity must include serial measurements of lactic acid, uric acid, and creatinine. Hypoglycemia and hyperammonemia reflect the severity of mitochondrial failure within hepatocytes.

Box 24.3 Swansea diagnostic criteria for diagnosis of acute fatty liver of pregnancy

Six or more of the following features in the absence of another explanation

- Vomiting
- Abdominal pain
- Polydipsia/polyuria
- Encephalopathy
- High bilirubin (>14 μmol/L)
- Hypoglycemia (<4 mmol/L)
- High uric acid (>340 μmol/L)
- Leukocytosis (>11 × 10⁶/L)
- Ascites or bright liver on ultrasound scan
- High AST/ALT (>42 IU/L)
- High ammonia (>47 μmol/L)
- Renal impairment (creatinine >150 μmol/L)
- Coagulopathy (PT >14 s or APTT >34 s)
- Microvesicular steatosis on liver biopsy

ALT, alanine aminotransferase; AST, aspartate aminotransferase; PT, prothrombin time; APTT, activated partial thromboplastin time.

Ultrasound of the liver does not help to make the diagnosis, although a sonographic pattern of fat deposition may be noted. Neither is a liver biopsy essential to make the diagnosis but should this be done the findings typically show a pattern of microvesicular fat within hepatocytes with a centrally placed nucleus (Plates 24.1–24.3). The patient needs to be closely observed in consultation with the obstetrician so that prompt delivery of the baby can be performed if there is *any* deterioration such as increasing coagulopathy, worsening renal function, hypoglycemia, increasing jaundice, and/or intractable vomiting. This disease carries with it a maternal mortality that ranges from 0 to 18% and a fetal mortality of 9 to 23%. Death of the mother is usually secondary to the complications of disseminated intravascular coagulation (DIC) with massive gastrointestinal hemorrhage. If a Cesarean section is performed this may be complicated postoperatively by an intra-abdominal hemorrhage. It is not unusual for a mother with AFLP to also have toxemia of pregnancy.

The etiology for AFLP may be related to a deficiency in long chain 3-hydroxyaceyl-coenzyme A dehydrogenase (LCHAD)—the baby is generally a homozygote and the mother a heterozygote for this inherited defect. The mother cannot metabolize the free fatty acids being delivered to her from the fetus. The child may develop hepatic failure and/or a myopathy.

The cure for AFLP in the mother is immediate delivery of the child. The latter should (if available) be tested for LCHAD deficiency. Early after delivery the baby may need steroid therapy to treat lung immaturity. The infant requires frequent feeds to prevent hypoglycemia and lifetime avoidance of fasting may be required. Additionally, the child requires supplements with carnitine. The mother may experience cholestasis (jaundice and/or pruritus) persisting for up to a month following delivery. Just occasionally, liver transplantation is necessary if the mother develops severe hepatic encephalopathy—hence all mothers thought to have AFLP should be transferred to a transplant centre if possible.

Pregnancy toxemias (hypertension-related liver diseases of pregnancy)

These must be suspected in a pregnant woman who after 20 weeks of gestation or within 48 h of delivery is found to have systemic hypertension, fluid retention, and proteinuria which defines pre-eclampsia if there is no other obvious cause for these findings.

The pathogenesis is presumed to be increased systemic vascular resistance due to excessive pressure responses to endogenous vasoconstrictors. This in turn leads to increased endothelial cell permeability, and deposition of platelets and fibrin in hepatic sinusoids, which causes both focal and diffuse hepatocellular necrosis with hemorrhage. Both are best seen on liver biopsy although this procedure is rarely necessary to make the diagnosis.

Evidence that the disease is hepatic in origin is obvious on routine blood testing as a marked elevation of serum aminotransferases (>10-fold elevation) and modest increase in serum alkaline phosphatase (ALP) is usual. Jaundice is rare unless disseminated intravascular coagulation has superseded, in which case there may be an unconjugated hyperbilirubinemia. The platelet count may be low. Ultrasound of the liver may show focal filling defects due to intrahepatic hematomas.

Strict control of systemic blood pressure is always required throughout pregnancy, but if the blood pressure goes out of control and there is also evidence of hepatic involvement (ALT 10-fold elevation) immediate delivery of the baby should be contemplated and supportive care maintained.

The HELLP syndrome

The HELLP syndrome (hemolysis, elevated liver enzymes, and low platelet syndrome; Box 24.4) is a rare variant of pre-eclampsia (occurring in 5–10%) when hemolysis and thrombocytopenia are added to the complex described above (i.e. elevated serum aminotransferase and ALP levels). Sometimes there may have been no overt preceding pre-eclampsia. The mother may be quite asymptomatic; others complain of right upper quadrant pain, nausea, and vomiting. Hypertension and proteinuria are present in 85%, INR values usually remain normal and elevated serum uric acid levels are the best marker of disease severity (>464 µmol/L associated with both maternal and infant mortality). Sometimes there may also be an overlap with AFLP. A falling platelet count is the marker of this "mixed" syndrome. The degree of elevation in the liver biochemical tests does not reflect the severity of liver disease, so as soon as the diagnosis is made immediate arrangements for delivery of the fetus is essential as the perinatal mortality ranges from 10–60% with a maternal mortality 1.5–5%.

On occasion, immediate liver transplantation is required—hence communication with a liver transplant center should be done as soon as the diagnosis has been established. Serial ultrasound examination of the liver is wise and arterial embolization with or without surgery instigated if hepatic infarcts are visualized radiologically. These procedures may avoid the often fatal complication of hepatic rupture. This complication has a 50% mortality rate in the mother, the risk being higher the lower the platelet count. Severity of HELLP syndrome may be classified (Box 24.4).

Box 24.4 Mississippi system guide to severity of the HELLP syndrome

AST >40 IU/L and LDH >600 IU/L *and*
  Class I: platelets <50 × 10⁹/L
  Class II: platelets 50–100 × 10⁹/L
  Class III: platelets 100–150 × 10⁹/L
HELLP, hemolysis, elevated liver enzymes, and low platelets; AST, aspartate aminotransferase; LDH, lactate dehydrogenase.
  (Data from Joshi D et al. Lancet 2010; 375: 594.)

There is an increased risk of this event in women who are heterozygotes for Factor V Leiden mutation.

Other causes of hepatic rupture in pregnancy include hepatic adenomas— hence the need to resect these prior to contemplating pregnancy (hepatic adenomas are associated with prior oral contraceptives use). A CT scan or MRI helps to identify the site and possibly the cause of the hepatic rupture. Hepatic angiography with or without embolization needs to be performed if blood pressure cannot be maintained.

Budd–Chiari syndrome

Although not specific to pregnancy the Budd Chiari syndrome is a condition that is promoted by any procoagulant state (pregnancy being one). It can occur any time during pregnancy or shortly after delivery because of the pregnancy-associated increases in the coagulant Factors VIII, IX, and XII and a physiologic decrease in protein S. Hepatic vein thrombosis may also occur at any time in patients with systemic lupus erythematosus (SLE) when a lupus anticoagulant and anticardiolipin antibodies are present, the latter being in part responsible for the spontaneous abortions which are known to complicate individuals with SLE.

Presenting symptoms in the pregnant woman are, typically, sudden increase in size of their abdomen (found to be fluid by identifying "shifting dullness") with or without right upper quadrant pain and/or jaundice. The diagnosis may be easily made by Doppler ultrasound, which will indicate no flow in the hepatic veins and this widely available, harmless procedure should be carried out when there is the slightest suspicion of the Budd–Chiari syndrome. Once the diagnosis is made with ultrasonography, anticoagulation with low-molecular-weight heparin must be started and maintained during pregnancy (warfarin is teratogenic). Inserting a stent through the blocked hepatic vein to make a direct connection to the portal veins (transjugular intrahepatic porto-systemic shunt (TIPS)), with the minimum exposure to radiation, is the current treatment of choice if the ascites does not respond to treatment with diuretics. If this technique cannot be performed for any reason then referral for liver transplantation may be required, depending on the degree of hepatic compromise (also see Chapter 21).

Acute onset of liver disease coincidental to pregnancy

Acute viral hepatitis is responsible for 50% of cases of jaundice developing during pregnancy (Table 24.2). High levels of estrogen as a consequence of pregnancy promotes cholestasis, thus any individual who acquires a "hepatitis" is more likely to develop jaundice if they are pregnant. If the cholestasis is profound, pruritus can develop.

It is important once the mother has been found to have biochemical evidence of a "hepatitis" to narrow down the differential diagnosis. A full blood count

Table 24.2 Acute liver disease coincidental with pregnancy		
Stage of pregnancy	**Presentation**	**Treatment**
Any trimester	**Viral hepatitis**	
	Acute onset of flu-like illness ± jaundice Hepatitis A and B ± D and C: outcome benign	Regardless of etiology vaccinate all the family (within 12 h) for hepatitis B (+hepatitis B immune globulin if mother tests HBsAg + ve) No known therapy
	Hepatitis E: 30% maternal and 50% fetal mortality	No known therapy
	Herpes simplex II hepatitis: vesicular lesions present in mother (in 70%)	Treat with acyclovir immediately upon diagnosis
	Cholestatic jaundice	
	Common bile duct stones	Ultrasound ± ERCP
	Cholestasis of pregnancy: pruritus: starts 2nd–3rd trimester	UDCA 1 g/day
	Drug induced e.g. sulfonamides	Stop drug
	Ascites	
	Budd–Chiari syndrome: Diagnostic portal vein ultrasound + Doppler Check blood and ascitic fluid for albumin, bacteria Check for esophageal varices	Heparin i.v. ± TIPS (No oral anticoagulants— teratogenic)

ERCP, endoscopic retrograde cholangiopancreatography; TIPS, transjugular intrahepatic porto-systemic shunt; UDCA, ursodeoxycholic acid.

is required to look for thrombocytopenia and the INR measured to make sure there is no evidence of liver failure. All pregnant women found to have a transaminitis need to be screened for viral hepatitis.

Acute hepatitis A. Acute hepatitis A (confirmed by detecting anti-HAV IgM) is almost always a benign, short lived hepatitis and has *no* effect on the fetus.

Other household contacts should be vaccinated against hepatitis A as soon as the infection in the mother is confirmed. Hyperimmune globulin for the household contacts is also advised.

Hepatitis B. Hepatitis B if acute is also usually a short-lived infection but serial testing for HBsAg must be done even if all symptoms and signs resolve, to exclude a silent chronic infection. Chronic infection with hepatitis B is generally the result of infection of the mother as a neonate or toddler, as acute hepatitis B in adults becomes chronic in less than 5%. In order to differentiate acute from chronic hepatitis B, HBsAg testing should be repeated during the pregnancy to establish whether viral clearance takes place. If IgM-positive antiHBs is detected, this supports acute, but does not rule out a flare up of chronic, hepatitis B. If the mother remains HBsAg positive during the third trimester her infant must receive both hepatitis B immune globulin and the hepatitis B vaccine within 12 hours of delivery—with follow up vaccination at 1–2 months and 6 months. Breast feeding is safe if the baby is vaccinated. If any mother has been in contact with hepatitis B when she is pregnant, prophylactic HBV vaccination is recommended and safe.

Hepatitis D. This only causes a "hepatitis" if the infection occurs simultaneously with an acute infection with hepatitis B or occurs on a background of established, chronic hepatitis B. If transmitted to the baby, coinfection with hepatitis D gives rise to severe liver disease after birth, but is preventable by instituting the same hepatitis B vaccination regimen for the newborn baby as described above for hepatitis B.

Hepatitis C. Mothers at high risk of acute hepatitis C are generally those using injection drugs under unsterile conditions. At least 50% of persons using illicit drugs administered by a needle are infected with hepatitis C within the first year of their addiction and 80% go on to develop a chronic infection. Treatment for hepatitis C cannot be given during pregnancy as ribavirin (one of the constituents) is teratogenic. Pregnancy rarely affects the course of chronic hepatitis C although there are reports of spontaneous viral clearance in a few mothers postdelivery. The mother may request that her baby be checked if this is agreed upon—only for HCV RNA (passive transfer of antibody is not indicative of infection). However, regardless of whether the HCV RNA test is negative or positive in the baby, first time (and perhaps repeat) testing should be performed only once the infant is a year old (see Chapter 14). Breast feeding is safe. Transmission of hepatitis C from mother to child may occur during delivery but this is a relatively rare event (up to 6%, mainly if the mother has a high viral load, which is always the case if she is coinfected with HIV). If it is decided that the mother has an acute hepatitis C she should be started on treatment shortly after delivery, that is within 1 year of her presentation with acute HCV. Ribavirin is not required, just pegylated interferon-α monotherapy for treatment of acute hepatitis C.

Hepatitis E. This is both a water-borne infection and a zoonosis. While rates of infection are highest in South Asia, acute hepatitis E has been reported in North America and Europe. Thus all pregnant women with an acute onset of a "transaminitis" must be tested for *all* forms of viral hepatitis as, unlike the other viral hepatides, hepatitis E can be very severe in pregnant women, with a maternal mortality of 30%. Whereas 50% of babies do not become infected, the others do and subsequently die of fulminant hepatitis, that is there is a 50% fetal mortality. There is no known treatment for hepatitis E.

Herpes simplex (type II). This too can be very severe, likely because of the change in cellular immunity that occurs with the pregnant state. The mother may have herpetic lesions (seen in 70%) in the vagina or on the cervix. Herpes hepatitis is usually accompanied by severe leukopenia and marked lymphopenia; ALT values are generally very high. Fulminant liver failure may develop. A liver biopsy is diagnostic, showing what are described as Chowdry type A inclusions in hepatocyte nuclei in addition to focal and confluent hemorrhagic necrosis with little inflammation. There needs to be a high index of suspicion in a pregnant woman who abruptly becomes unwell, who is found to have leukopenia, and a marked transaminitis. A positive search for overt herpetic lesions seals the diagnosis and acyclovir needs to be given immediately. This infection untreated is associated with a high fatality rate in the mother (and hence also the fetus).

Pregnancy in the individual with pre-existing cirrhosis

Cirrhosis present in fertile women may be the result of either childhood- or adult-acquired liver disease (Table 24.3). If a young cirrhotic woman becomes pregnant her mortality rate is around 10%! If the mother has esophageal varices, about 25% will bleed during pregnancy.

Cirrhosis acquired in early childhood is most likely due to a metabolic disorder (some inherited, others not, e.g. non-alcoholic fatty liver disease). Of the inherited disorders that may lead to cirrhosis early in life, the most common is Wilson disease. Autoimmune hepatitis and/or primary sclerosing cholangitis (PSC) are also chronic liver diseases that may be present in young women and cause cirrhosis even at a young age. The patient with Wilson disease must *not* stop their chelation therapy during pregnancy—otherwise an often-fatal reactivation may occur. Similarly the mother with autoimmune hepatitis must remain on her prescribed immunosuppressive regimen—usually prednisone with or without azathioprine, both drugs being safe in pregnancy. Often the degree of immune suppression required during pregnancy is less so that doses may be reduced but they should not be stopped altogether. Postdelivery flare up of AIH is common, usually within 3 months of delivery. Thus all mothers should have their liver biochemistry monitored 2–3 months following delivery—this may be a challenge if the weather is inclement!

Table 24.3 Pregnancy in individuals with known liver disease	
Cirrhosis	e.g. AIH, Wilson disease, PSC, PBC, steatohepatitis (obesity) Check varices 2nd trimester and treat prophylactically Maintain treatment for AIH or Wilson disease throughout pregnancy Ascites—tap to check for bacterial infection and albumin content
Chronic cholestatic liver disease	e.g. Inherited disorders that impair bile flow, biliary atresia with Kasai procedure, Alagille syndrome, PBC and PSC Pruritus worsens during pregnancy (treatment: cholestyramine, may also require plasmapheresis to control pruritus)
Prior liver transplantation	Maintain immunosuppressive regimen Fetal loss 30%, maternal 8–9%

AIH, autoimmune hepatitis; PBC, primary biliary cirrhosis; PSC, primary sclerosing cholangitis.

There are many other causes of cirrhosis that can affect young women, most are rare but sadly it may include alcohol-induced liver disease or non-alcoholic fatty liver disease. Cirrhosis of the liver is for the most part a clinically silent disease and so may be first diagnosed when a young woman presents to her physician pregnant. Pregnancy in those with cirrhosis (even if well compensated, i.e. clinically silent) carries with it a high risk of a poor outcome (mortality rate 10%). Variceal hemorrhage is the most common reason for acute hepatic decompensation in a pregnant woman with cirrhosis. If cirrhosis is known to be present prior to pregnancy, upper panendoscopy is suggested during the second trimester when the blood volume increases, to identify whether esophageal varices are present. Prophylactic measures include either banding of the varices and/or non-selective beta-blockade. However, use of the latter may be associated with fetal growth retardation and hypoglycemia. If variceal hemorrhage occurs early in the pregnancy, intervention with a TIPS may be safer than using intravenous vasoconstrictors.

Chronic cholestatic liver disease
Mothers with a chronic cholestatic liver disease, for example Alagille syndrome, biliary atresia with a Kasai procedure, PSC, or PBC, will often notice the development or worsening of any prior pruritus, at times so severe as to disturb sleep and cause agitation. Under such circumstances standard antipruritics such as cholestyramine are usually ineffective and plasmapheresis

may be the only way to alleviate their intolerable pruritus. There are a number of other childhood diseases that affect the normal flow of bile leading to cholestasis which may not have been associated with chronic pruritus and jaundice until they become pregnant. Thus all pregnant mothers who complain of pruritus should be investigated for an underlying chronic cholestatic liver disease. Good management of children given a diagnosis of biliary atresia or hypoplasia (Alagille syndrome) means that these children are now surviving into adulthood. Their liver function remains good so they have an almost normal chance of becoming pregnant. These mothers notice the onset or worsening of pruritus in the first trimester (and so should not be confused with "cholestatic disease" of pregnancy which never presents before 20 weeks). Both primary sclerosing cholangitis (PSC) and PBC can affect teenagers (or younger in the case of PSC) and as their primary pathology is biliary, pregnancy may precipitate new-onset pruritus.

Non-cirrhotic portal hypertension: cause of variceal hemorrhage

In any pregnant individual who is clinically well but in whom a low platelet count with or without splenomegaly is detected a check for varices is required. Often times the underlying process is relatively benign in that the thrombocytopenia is due to a portal vein thrombosis—easily diagnosed via ultrasonography plus Doppler examination. In such an individual the liver is normal and hepatic decompensation does not follow a variceal bleed even after a period of systemic hypotension. Other non-cirrhotic causes of variceal hemorrhage could relate to portal hypertension secondary to hepatic outflow block, that is Budd–Chiari syndrome.

Mother with a liver transplant

Maternal complications occur in 8–9% and fetal loss is as high as 30%. There is no evidence that liver transplant and the need for long-term immune suppression is associated with any increase in viable congenital malformations in the fetus. Mothers with a prior liver transplant are at high risk of gestation-associated systemic hypertension. Breast feeding should be avoided because the mother needs to maintain her antirejection therapies.

Case study 24.1

Mrs. JW was a 29-year-old Chinese woman who close to term presented with a 5-day history of right upper quadrant pain, nausea, and vomiting with jaundice and a low-grade fever. She had never been jaundiced prior to this event and gave no past history of hepatitis (born in China, emigrated to Canada 3 years prior to her admission). She had not taken any medications or over-the-counter medications/supplements during her pregnancy except for iron supplements. She gave no significant past history or family history of liver disease. She was admitted to her local hospital and underwent almost immediate Caesarian section in view of clinical evidence of fetal distress. She was successfully delivered of a live fetus and subsequently was found to have abnormal liver tests and worsening liver function and transferred to a liver transplant centre for further management.

Upon arrival at the tertiary care center she looked unwell, was jaundiced, but was not encephalopathic. She gave no history of past liver problems. She had no scratch marks or signs of chronic liver disease. In view of her recent abdominal surgery, it was hard to reliably detect ascites. Her temperature was 38.5°, pulse 120 beats/min and her BP at admission was 90/50 mmHg with a 20 mmHg postural drop.

Her blood work at the time of admission indicated that she was in liver failure: Hb 111 g/L, WBC 26.5×10^9/L, platelets 171×10^9/L, INR 3.32. Her bilirubin was 100 mmol/L, albumin 19 g/L, creatinine 215 μmol/L, AST 160 IU/L, ALT 88 IU/L, ALP 567 IU/L. The ultrasound of her liver showed normal echo texture, no focal lesions, normal portal venous flow, and no evidence of biliary dilatation. Gall bladder was hard to visualize (likely edematous). Her leukocytosis was secondary to a marked neutrophilia 23.1×10^9/L. D-dimers 4.00 μmol/mL (normal range <0.4). Fibrinogen 0.84 g/L (normal range 1.5–3.5). Serum ceruloplasmin normal, serum hapatoglobin low. Her IgM Hep A Ab was negative (Hep A IgG positive). Her HBsAg negative, antiHBs and antiHBc positive. Hep HCV Ab negative, Hep E Ab negative, HIV 1+2 screen negative, CMV IgG Ab positive, EBV VCA IgG Ab positive. Blood, rectal, and cervical swab, throat swab, and urine—no evidence of bacterial infection or herpetic lesions.

A transjugular liver biopsy was performed, which showed a high corrected "sinusoidal" pressure of 16 mmHg suggesting severe postsinusoidal portal hypertension.

Liver histology: small droplet fat (zone 2 and 3) and marked cholestasis (canalicular plugging). No hepatocellular necrosis. Oil Red O fat stain showed fat accumulation with hepatocytes, typical of acute fatty liver of pregnancy (Plate 24.2). She spontaneously recovered.

Multiple choice questions

1. A 23-year-old primipara in her first trimester presented to the office with nausea, recurrent vomiting, dizziness when suddenly standing, weight loss (remained obese!). She did not appear jaundiced and she had no bruising or petichael hemorrhages. Her blood pressure was 75/40 mmHg with a 15 mmHg postural drop and a pulse of 130 beats/min. Her abdomen was flat, uterus not palpable. She had no hepatic fetor or hepatic flap—she was fully alert. Which is *incorrect*?
   A. You request a full blood count, blood film examination, and INR.
   B. You check her serum Na, K, PO_4, and Mg.
   C. Her liver tests show transaminitis and a conjugated hyperbilirubinemia.
   D. Her symptoms improve with sublingual odansetron.

2. A 20-year-old Indian woman has come with her young husband to the hospital clinic because she feels unwell, has no appetite, occasional vomiting, and she is clearly in the advanced stages of pregnancy. She is a primipara. She is jaundiced and drowsy without any obvious hepatic flap. She has a 10 mmHg postural drop in her blood pressure and a marked tachycardia. She has no ascites or ankle edema. She has a gravid uterus near term; fetal heart sounds are barely audible. She has no prior history of liver disease and no one in her family has a current or past liver problem. She lives in a crowded dwelling with no running water. Which of the following is *incorrect*?
   A. Her CBC shows a moderate leukocytosis, her INR is 5.
   B. You screen her blood for HBsAg and antiHBc, HCV RNA and HCVAb, and HCV RNA and hepatitis E Ab (IgM)—the latter is positive.
   C. Later in the day the fetal heartbeat cannot be heard as the mother lapses into a coma and dies the following day.
   D. You can reassure the family that the mother's disease will not be transmitted to her baby.

Answers

1. C
2. D

Further reading

Alallam A, Barth B, Heathcote EJ. Role of plasmapheresis in the treatment of severe pruritus in pregnant patients with primary biliary cirrhosis: case reports. Can J Gastroenterol 2008; 22: 505–7.

Hay JE. Liver disease in pregnancy. Hepatology 2008; 47: 1067–76.

Joshi D, James A, Quaglia A, et al. Liver disease in pregnancy. Lancet 2010; 375: 594–605.

Khuroo MS, Kamili S, Khuroo MS. Clinical course and duration of viremia in vertically transmitted hepatitis E virus (HEV) infection in babies born to HEV-infected mothers. Viral Hepat 2009; 16: 519–23.

Lee NM, Brady CW. Liver disease in pregnancy. World J Gastroenterol 2009; 15: 897.

Murthy SK, Heathcote EJ, Nguyen GC. Impact of cirrhosis and liver transplant on maternal health during labour and delivery. Clin Gastroenterol Hepatol 2009; 7: 1367–72.

Radha Krishna Y, Saraswat VA, Das K, et al. Clinical features and predictors of outcome in acute hepatitis A and hepatitis E virus hepatitis on cirrhosis. Liver Int 2009; 29: 392–8.

Shekhawat PS, Matern D, Strauss AW. Fetal fatty acid oxidation disorders, their effect on maternal health and neonatal outcome impact of expanded newborn screening on their diagnosis and management. Pediatr Res 2005; 78: 86R.

Cystic disease of the liver

CHAPTER 25

Morris Sherman

Toronto General Hospital, University Health Network and University of Toronto, Toronto, Ontario, Canada

Key points

- Simple cysts are benign and do not cause symptoms. They do not need investigation or follow-up.
- Simple cysts can be multiple and not be part of a polycystic liver disease syndrome. The cysts do not cause symptoms and do not grow.
- Polycystic liver disease rarely causes liver failure. Symptoms are due to pressure, secondary infection, and very occasionally to the complications of portal hypertension. No treatment is required unless there are pressure symptoms.

Congenital cysts in the liver

A cyst is defined as a membrane-bound, fluid-filled structure. In autosomal dominant polycystic kidney disease (ADPKD) and polycystic liver disease (PLD), as well as in simple cysts, the epithelium lining the cyst is secretory, so that there is a tendency for cysts to enlarge over time. The cyst fluid has a composition similar to serum.

The inherited cystic diseases of the liver are all related to abnormal proteins in the cilia of the biliary epithelium (ciliopathy). The basic abnormality is defective cilial function, as a result of abnormal or absent membrane proteins. These are polycystin 1 and 2 (PC1 and PC2), hepatocystin, and fibrocystin/polyductin. PC1 is important in cell–cell adhesion. PC2 is probably a calcium channel protein. The precise functions of hepatocystin and fibrocystin/polyductin are unknown. The clinical phenotype varies, depending on the genetic abnormality. Similarly, whether the liver cysts are associated with kidney cysts also depends on the particular genetic abnormality (Fig. 25.1).

Hepatology: Diagnosis and Clinical Management, First Edition. Edited by E. Jenny Heathcote.
© 2012 John Wiley & Sons, Ltd. Published 2012 by John Wiley & Sons, Ltd.

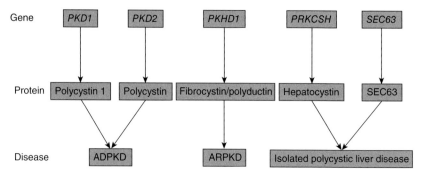

Fig. 25.1 Relationship between the genes, proteins, and diseases constituting congenital cystic conditions of the liver. ADPKD, autosomal dominant polycystic kidney disease; ARPKD, autosomal recessive polycystic kidney disease.

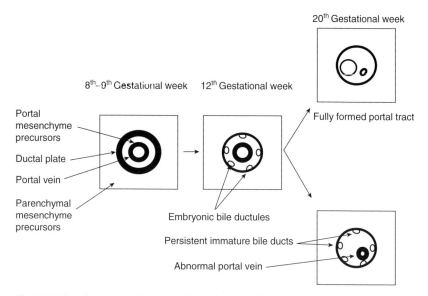

Fig. 25.2 Development of the normal bile duct and the ductal plate malformation.

Congenital liver cysts occur as part of several syndromes. In order to understand the relationships between different cystic diseases in the liver it is necessary to discuss the embryology of the development of the biliary drainage system (Fig. 25.2). The bile ducts develop from the ductal plate, a cylindrical tube of cells surrounding a portal vein branch. The interlobular and intralobular bile ductules are formed by progressive remodeling after about week 12 of gestation. Arrest of maturation and lack of remodeling leads to persistence of an excess number of embryonic biliary structures (ductal plate malformation).[1] This in turn results in the development of periportal fibrosis and dilatations in the bile ducts. Morphological studies demonstrate that the peripheral cysts of

ADPKD and PLD arise from these biliary microhamartomas, but the centrally located cysts of Caroli disease arise from dilatations of the peribiliary glands in the liver.

The liver cysts in ADPKD and PLD do not communicate with the biliary system. The cysts in Caroli disease do communicate with the biliary system.

Autosomal dominant polycystic kidney disease
Genetics
The prevalence of this entity is between 1:400 and 1:1000. The disease is characterized by progressive enlargement of cysts in the liver and kidney, leading to renal failure in about 50% of affected individuals. Most often the disease is caused by a mutation in the *PKD1* gene coding for PC1, with about 20% being due to mutations in the *PKD2* gene, coding for PC2. Liver cysts occur in about 60–75% of these patients. The frequency and severity of liver cystic disease is related to the severity of renal disease. Liver failure is rare, but can occur. The major hepatic manifestation is massive hepatomegaly as a result of large and enlarging cysts. The liver disease affects mostly females, and may have a relationship to female sex hormones.

Clinical
Polycystic liver disease causes symptoms because of the size of the liver. These may include early satiety, gastroesophageal reflux, mechanical back pain, and occasionally obstruction to the inferior vena cava, portal vein, or extrahepatic bile duct. Cysts may rupture, may bleed, or become infected but these are rare events.[2]

Diagnosis
The diagnosis of cystic liver diseases is usually made by ultrasonography. Computed tomography (CT) scanning provides similar information, but is usually easier for the non-radiologist to read.

Classification
Polycystic liver diseases are classified on the basis of number and size of the cysts and the amount of residual normal liver parenchyma between the cysts. Type I patients have a limited number (<10) of large cysts with large areas of non-cystic parenchyma. Type II PLD has diffuse involvement of liver parenchyma by medium-sized cysts with remaining large areas of non-cystic parenchyma. Type III patients have massive, diffuse involvement of liver by small and medium-sized liver cysts with little normal liver parenchyma between cysts. This classification holds for both ADPKD and PLD.

Treatment
In ADPKD, longevity is more related to kidney function than liver function, and renal failure is common, so that these patients end up on dialysis sooner or later. Liver function is seldom affected in these conditions, presumably

because regeneration preserves functional liver volume. Treatment of the liver cysts, therefore, is directed at symptomatic relief from pressure symptoms. Patients with type I cystic disease are most easily treated because they have a relatively small number of large and easily discernible cysts. Type II is also amenable to surgical treatment because ablation of a few large cysts may provide adequate relief of symptoms. However, type III, in which there are innumerable small and medium cysts, is less amenable to ablation of the cysts. These patients may receive benefit, albeit transient, from partial hepatectomy.[3] Therapy with somatostatin analogues theoretically could reduce the accumulation of cyst fluid, but the therapeutic use of, for example octreotide, has been met with only modest reduction in cyst volume (about 5%).[4]

Practice point. Patients with polycystic liver diseases do not develop liver failure but may develop portal hypertension.

Liver transplantation has also been performed for these patients, although it is important to weigh up the risks of surgery and long-term immunosuppression against the severity of symptoms. The cysts can be massive and multiple, so that symptoms cannot realistically be attributed to any specific cyst or cysts. However, destruction of the largest cysts can be associated with temporary relief of symptoms. This can be accomplished at laparotomy, laparoscopy, or percutaneously. At laparotomy or laparoscopy cysts can be de-roofed and allowed to drain into the peritoneum. Since the fluid is similar to serum it is rapidly re-absorbed, although ascites has been described. The cysts can also be drained percutaneously and a sclerosant introduced to destroy the secretory epithelium and hopefully prevent recurrence of the cyst. Since liver function is preserved, liver transplantation is seldom necessary except when the size of the liver severely compromises the patient's quality of life.

Treatment of symptomatic cysts can be surgical or by interventional radiology.

Infection of a cyst is rare, but serious, and has a mortality rate of about 2%. These require antibiotic and external drainage as for hepatic abscess.

Autosomal recessive polycystic kidney disease

Autosomal recessive polycystic kidney disease/congenital hepatic fibrosis (ARPKD/CHF) is caused by mutations in the *PKHD1* gene located on chromosome 6p12. *PKHD1* is a relatively large gene containing 66 coding exons, which demonstrates a complex splicing pattern. The gene codes for the protein fibrocystin, a hepatocyte growth factor receptor-like protein that functions on the primary cilia of renal and biliary epithelial cells (Fig. 25.1). Dysfunction of fibrocystin leads to abnormal ciliary signaling, which is normally required for regulation of proliferation and differentiation of renal and biliary epithelial cells.

This is a rare condition that occurs in about 1:40000 live births. Its primary manifestation is renal cystic disease, with progressive renal failure. However, it is associated with disease in other organs, including chronic lung disease, growth retardation, intracranial aneurysms, adrenal insufficiency, and hypertension. The hepatic manifestations of this condition are **Caroli disease**[5] and CHF. When both Caroli disease and CHF are present the condition is known as **Caroli syndrome**.

Caroli disease is characterized by multiple fusiform or cystic dilatations of the intrahepatic bile ducts that communicate with the biliary system. The major complications are related to recurrent bouts of cholangitis, and biliary stone formation. There is a risk of developing cholangiocarcinoma. In CHF, the portal tracts are abnormal, with multiple abnormally shaped embryonic bile ducts, often retaining the ductal plate conformation. The portal vein is abnormal. There is significant periportal and bridging fibrosis. The clinical manifestations are those of portal hypertension, including splenomegaly, thrombocytopenia, and variceal bleeding (and patients are thus frequently misdiagnosed as having cirrhosis). What they really have is "congenital hepatic fibrosis". They may also have had medullary sponge kidneys and nephrocalcinosis diagnosed in the past.

These patients often present *in utero*, with oligohydramnios, but when they present later in life the symptoms are related to the liver and/or kidney disease. About 30% of cases die in the perinatal period with respiratory difficulty. Generally, liver cysts are not observed in children, but develop over time.

There are four variants of Caroli syndrome, with slightly differing clinical presentations. These are the portal hypertensive presentation, a cholangitic presentation with multiple episodes of cholangitis, a mixed picture, and a latent pattern, in which presentation occurs late in life, often presenting with complications, such as cholangiocarcinoma. On examination the liver is firm and enlarged. The spleen and kidneys may be enlarged. It may be difficult to tell whether the organ being palpated is liver and spleen or the kidneys. In those with a predominantly cholangitic or mixed picture, the alkaline phosphatase and gamma glutamyl transpeptidase are usually markedly elevated. The bilirubin may also be elevated, particularly during episodes of acute cholangitis.

Diagnosis

The disease is usually first detected, often incidentally, by ultrasonography. This might show, in addition to the cysts, changes in the sizes of various liver lobes or segments, focal or more generalized intrahepatic biliary dilatation and stones (Caroli disease), or splenomegaly. There may be periportal thickening (congenital hepatic fibrosis), cavernous transformation of the portal vein, and enlarged cystic kidneys. Magnetic resonance imaging (MRI) (Fig. 25.3) or magnetic resonance cholangiopancreatography (MRCP) have been used to evaluate the liver and biliary tree in the setting of ARPKD/CHF.[6] Intrahepatic biliary ductal dilatation can be demonstrated on axial, coronal, and reformatted MR cholangiography images. A distinctive feature of CHF MR cholangiograms is that the ducts do not taper to the periphery of the liver as they do normally. Instead, they remain dilated throughout the parenchyma, often forming

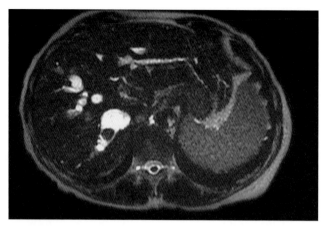

Fig. 25.3 Caroli disease. Note the fusiform dilatations of the biliary system, with a large stone present.

cisterns and small cysts at the periphery of the liver. MR cholangiography is also useful for detecting biliary system complications including stones and cholangitis and cholangiocarcinoma.

In congenital hepatic fibrosis, CT can also be used.

In ARPKD, MRI of the brain is also required because of the possibility of intracranial aneurysms.

Treatment
There is no specific therapy for Caroli disease. Occasionally, a single segment of the liver is the site of recurrent cholangitis, and that can be treated by seg-mentectomy. However, if the disease is diffuse the only treatment is liver transplantation. Patients with Caroli disease should be monitored for the development of cholangiocarcinoma. They may need long-term, cyclical antibiotic treatment if they have recurrent cholangitis.

Practice point. Patients with Caroli disease require monitoring with periodic MRI for the detection of cholangiocarcinoma.

Polycystic liver disease
This is an autosomal dominant condition, without renal manifestations. It is caused by a mutation in the hepatocystin gene (Fig. 25.1). The clinical manifestations are similar to the hepatic manifestations of ADPKD. There is no associated disease in other organs.

Simple cysts of the liver
These may be single or multiple, small or massive. They are found in up to 5% of the general population. These are not associated with any known genetic

mutation, but presumably arise as a result of isolated ductal plate malformations. They do not communicate with the biliary system. The cysts are not loculated, but adjacent cysts may be separated by a thin wall, giving the appearance of loculation. These cysts are more common in women, and tend to be discovered later in life, as the cysts enlarge over time. These are almost invariably asymptomatic, but occasionally very large cysts can cause pressure symptoms that require treatment. These can be treated in a manner similar to polycystic disease. Such patients are good candidates for percutaneous aspiration of cyst fluid and ablation of the cyst lining by absolute alcohol or other sclerosant.

Acquired cysts of the liver

Hydatid disease of the liver

Hydatid disease is caused by *Echinococcus granulosis*, a small tapeworm about 3–6 mm in length. These live in the intestine of the definitive host, usually a dog, but also wild canines and cats. The intermediate hosts are man, sheep, and cattle.

Epidemiology

Human echinococcosis is endemic in rural areas of the world. These include the Mediterranean, Eastern Europe, South America, the Middle East, Central and East Asia, and East Africa. The burden of illness is considerable with an estimated loss of nearly 300 000 disability adjusted life years/year. There is a significant mortality in untreated patients, which is about 2–4%.

Pathogenesis

Gravid proglottids hatch either in feces, or in the intestinal lumen. The definitive host is infected by ingesting the viscera of an infected animal. The embryo burrows through the intestinal wall into a blood vessel, and is carried to the liver. Most embryos remain in the liver, but some may end up in lung, spleen, kidneys, or other organs. Most embryos are destroyed by the host, but some may survive. Within a few days these grow to produce cysts filled with clear fluid and surrounded by an acellular laminated layer, which in turn is surrounded by host tissues and fibrosis. There is an inner germinal layer from which new scoleces are formed. Over time, the cyst may grow or may die and become calcified.[7] Daughter cysts may be present within or adjacent to, and connected to, the "mother" cyst. Cysts may also rupture, or involute and disappear.[8]

Ultrasound surveys have shown that cysts may grow 1–50 mm per year or may persist without change for years.

Classification

In 1995, the WHO developed a standardized classification that could be applied in all settings. This grouped the cysts into three groups: active (CE1 and 2), transitional (CE3), and inactive (CE4 and 5). CE1 is a single cyst. CE2 includes daughter cysts or multiple cysts. CE4 and 5 are involuting cysts that have lost their cystic appearance, but the cyst wall is still visible. CE3 retains the cystic structure, but the cyst walls are no longer convex and may be irregular.

Diagnosis

The diagnosis of hydatid cyst requires demonstration of a slowly growing or static cystic mass(es) diagnosed by imaging techniques, anaphylactic reactions due to ruptured or leaking cysts, or an incidental finding of a cyst by imaging techniques in asymptomatic carriers or detected by screening strategies (Fig. 25.4). Furthermore, there should be at least one typical organ lesion detected by imaging techniques (e.g. ultrasound, CT, plain film radiography, MRI), specific serum antibodies to echinococcosis assessed by high-sensitivity serological tests, confirmed by a separate high-specificity ELISA using cyst antigens, histopathology or parasitology compatible with cystic echinococcosis (e.g. direct visualization of the protoscolex or hooklets in cyst fluid), or detection of pathognomonic macroscopic morphology of cyst(s) in surgical specimens.

For epidemiological purposes, cases are classified as: "possible" if there is a clinical or epidemiological history, and imaging findings including ring calcification on plain X-ray or CT scan or serology positive for cystic echinococcosis; as a "probable" case if there is a combination of clinical history, epidemiological history, imaging findings, and serology positive on two tests; and as a "confirmed" case if the previous conditions are met together with either (1)

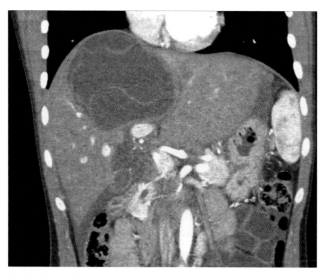

Fig. 25.4 Hydatid cyst. Note the internal septa of the endocyst breaking away from the exocyst.

demonstration of protoscoleces or their components, using direct microscopy or molecular biology, in the cyst contents aspirated by percutaneous puncture or at surgery, or (2) changes in ultrasound appearance, for example detachment of the endocyst in a CE1 cyst, thus moving to a CE3 stage, or solidification of a CE2 or CE3, thus changing to a CE4 stage, after administration of albendazole (at least 3 months) or spontaneously.

Hydatid cysts can be identified by several different imaging modalities. Ultrasound is often the first study to raise the question of hydatid disease. The diagnosis can be confirmed by CT or MRI. The major diagnostic issue is whether the cyst is viable or not. Viable cysts require treatment, whereas dead cysts do not. Viable cysts are often loculated, and daughter cysts may be seen. Thus, the differential of a multiloculated cyst without calcification in the liver must include hydatid cyst. All cysts that are not clearly dead (e.g. CE5) need to be assessed for viability. Positive serology for *Echinococcus* cyst antigens does not confirm viability.

Aspiration of cyst contents for diagnosis carries with it a risk of peritoneal seeding of scoleces. These may then grow and cause intestinal obstruction. Therefore, aspiration should be done surgically, or, if done percutaneously, must be accompanied by injection of a scolicide after aspiration, and preferentially, under cover of systemic therapy.

Practice point. Patients with hydatid disease who require treatment should be pretreated with albendazole prior to resection or aspiration. Aspiration must be accompanied by instillation of a scolicide into the drained cyst cavity.

Presence of calcification is not reliable as an indicator of non-viability. Calcification is more frequent in CE4 and CE5, but it may be observed at all stages.

Treatment[9–11]

Asymptomatic cysts do not necessarily require resection. Surgery is the first choice for complicated cysts. In the liver, it is indicated for removal of large CE2–CE3 cysts with multiple daughter vesicles, single liver cysts, situated superficially, that may rupture spontaneously or as a result of trauma, infected cysts, cysts communicating with the biliary tree, and cysts exerting pressure on adjacent vital organs. Single large cysts can be treated percutaneously by aspiration and injection of hypertonic saline or absolute alcohol. Aspiration also provides an opportunity to sample the cyst fluid for scoleces. All active cysts should also be treated with drug therapy. The drug of choice is albendazole, or mebendazole. Addition of praziquantel may improve the efficacy of treatment. The ideal duration of treatment is unknown, but should be at least several months. Efficacy of therapy is determined by reduction in cyst size.

Cystadenoma and cystadenocarcinoma[12,13]

Intrahepatic biliary cystadenoma is a rare cystic liver tumor that may also occur in the extrahepatic bile ducts. It occurs more frequently in women over 40 than in men and is a tumor of adulthood. It is usually single, and because it grows without causing symptoms is usually only discovered at a large size. Most present either incidentally or with symptoms related to tumor compression of adjacent organs caused by their large size. Most are benign, but there is a significant risk of the development of malignancy in the cyst wall (cystadenocarcinoma).

The pathology is that of a multiloculated cyst or cysts lined by a columnar or cuboidal epithelium that contains mucous-producing cells. There may be papillary projections into the lumen. Cystadenocarcinoma is macroscopically similar, but the lining epithelium shows features of malignant cellular changes with invasion of the cyst stroma.

Practice point. Cysts that have nodules in the wall are suspicious for cystadenoma.

Presentation

With the frequent use of abdominal imaging these lesions may be identified at an earlier stage than previously. However, in the absence of imaging the most common presentation is due to compression of adjacent organs. Thus there may be compression of the common bile duct, the portal vein or the inferior vena cava. Less common presentations include intracystic hemorrhage, rupture, and fever from secondary bacterial infection.

Diagnosis

The characteristic findings on imaging are that the cyst is multiloculated, with internal septae, thickened and irregular walls, with nodules, papillary projections, calcification, and arterial enhancement in the cyst wall. Imaging studies are the key to diagnosis, and are characteristic. Cyst aspiration might demonstrate mucinous fluid, but is not accurate for the diagnosis of malignancy. The diagnosis of malignancy requires sampling of the cyst wall, but since malignancy may be focal and is often macroscopically similar to the non-malignant tissue, sampling of the cyst wall has a high false-negative rate.

Treatment

Theoretically, these lesions can be treated by aspiration. However, because of the malignant potential they should be removed. Enucleation of the cyst is a recognized treatment, but resection is preferred owing to the possibility of malignant transformation, the high rate of recurrence, and the possibility of progressive symptomatic enlargement, secondary infection, and sepsis.

An algorithm for the classification of liver cysts is present in Fig. 25.5.

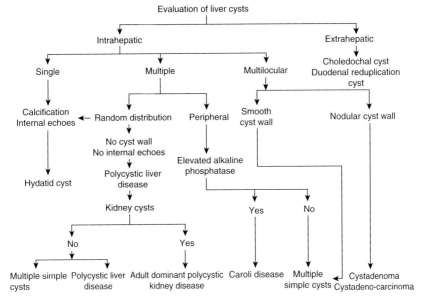

Fig. 25.5 Algorithm for the evaluation of cysts in the liver. This algorithm will cover most cysts found in the liver but occasionally cysts may not be typical, in which case the use of this algorithm may not lead to the correct answer.

Case study 25.1

A 50-year-old woman has an ultrasound because of vague left-sided upper quadrant pain. She is diagnosed with irritable bowel syndrome. In the course of investigation an ultrasound reveals two cysts in the liver. This was her first ever abdominal ultrasound. She was born and grew up in rural Greece. No family members have a history of liver cysts. The two cysts are adjacent to each other and about 4.5 cm in diameter. The two cysts are separated by a thin septum, which has a small nodule on one side. There is no calcification.

The differential includes two adjacent simple cysts, hydatid cyst and adjacent daughter cyst, and cystadenoma or cyst adenocarcinoma. Hydatid serology is negative, making hydatid disease unlikely. Cyst aspiration reveals serous fluid with no malignant cells. Six months later a repeat ultrasound shows that the nodule on the cyst wall is slightly larger. CT scan shows some vascularity in the nodule. A diagnosis of cystadenocarcinoma is made and a partial hepatectomy is performed. The diagnosis is confirmed pathologically.

Multiple choice questions

1. A 61-year-old immigrant man from Greece is being investigated for multiple myeloma. In the course of investigation he has an abdominal CT scan which shows several cysts in the liver. The cysts do not have walls and the surfaces of the cysts are smooth. Some of the cysts appear to be septated. Further investigation should include:
   A. CT scan
   B. No further follow-up
   C. Hydatid serology

2. A 65-year-old female refugee from Afghanistan is seen because of a palpable mass in the liver. An ultrasound shows a large cyst, with some adjacent smaller cysts. The cysts are walled and there are internal echoes. The ultra-sonographer suspects hydatid disease. What else is in the differential diagnosis?
   A. Multiple single cysts
   B. Polycystic liver disease
   C. Cystadenoma

3. A CT scan in this patient shows that there are cysts in both lobes of the liver. The largest cyst lies just under the capsule of the liver and straddles both the left and right lobes. There is a thin strip of liver between the cyst wall and the peritoneal cavity, indicating that rupture may be imminent. The appropriate treatment is
   A. Resection only
   B. Albendazole followed by resection
   C. Albendazole only
   D. Albendazole followed by cyst drainage and injection of a scolicide

Answers

1. B. These are multiple simple cysts. Although he is from a hydatid endemic area the radiological appearances are not consistent with hydatid disease.
2. C.
3. D. The position of the cyst and the multiplicity of cysts make resection unlikely to eradicate disease. Albendazole is required to "sterilize" the cysts prior to puncture and to decrease the likelihood of peritoneal infection should cyst contents spill into the peritoneum. Aspiration will initially deal only with the largest cyst causing symptoms. If necessary the other cysts can be dealt with at a later stage.

References

1. Desmet VJ. Congenital diseases of intrahepatic bile ducts: variations on the theme "ductal plate malformation". Hepatology 1992; 16: 1069–83.

2. Qian Q, Li A, King BF, et al. Clinical profile of autosomal dominant polycystic liver disease. Hepatology 2003; 37: 164–71.

3. Que F, Nagorney DM, Gross JB Jr, et al. Liver resection and cyst fenestration in the treatment of severe polycystic liver disease. Gastroenterology 1995; 108: 487–94 .

4. Caroli A, Antiga L, Cafaro M, et al. Reducing polycystic liver volume in ADPKD: effects of somatostatin analogue octreotide. Clin J Am Soc Nephrol 2010; 5: 783–9.

5. Caroli J. Diseases of intrahepatic bile ducts. Isr J Med Sci 1968; 4: 21–35.

6. Zeitoun D, Brancatelli G, Colombat M, et al. Congenital hepatic fibrosis: CT findings in 18 adults. Radiology 2004; 231: 109–16.

7. WHO/OIE. Manual on Echinococcosis. Echinococcosis in Humans and Animals: A Public Health Problem of Global Concern. World Organization for Animal Health (Office International des Epizooties) and World Health Organization, 2001.

8. Romig T, Zeyhle E, Macpherson CN, et al. Cyst growth and spontaneous cure in hydatid disease. Lancet 1986; 1: 861.

9. WHO Informal Working Group on Echinococcosis. Guidelines for treatment of cystic and alveolar echinococcosis in humans. Bull WHO 1996; 74: 231–42.

10. Brunettia E, Kern P, Vuitton DA, et al. Expert consensus for the diagnosis and treatment of cystic and alveolar echinococcosis in humans . Acta Tropica 2010; 114: 1–16.

11. Smego Jr RA, Bhatti S, Khaliq AA, Beg MA. Percutaneous aspiration injection—reaspiration drainage plus albendazole or mebendazole for hepatic cystic echinococcosis: a meta-analysis. Clin Infect Dis 2003; 37: 1073–83.

12. Dixon E, Sutherland FR, Mitchell P. Cystadenomas of the liver: a spectrum of disease. Can J Surg 2001; 44: 371–6.

13. Lewis WD, Jenkins RL, Rossi RL, et al. Surgical treatment of biliary cystadenoma. A report of 15 cases. Arch Surg 1988; 123: 563–8.

An internist's approach to radiologic examination of the liver

CHAPTER 26

Anthony E. Hanbidge[1] and Korosh Khalili[2]

[1]Department of Medical Imaging, University of Toronto; Abdominal Imaging, Toronto Western Hospital; Joint Department of Medical Imaging University Health Network, Mount Sinai Hospital and Women's College Hospital, Toronto, Ontario, Canada
[2]Department of Medical Imaging, University of Toronto, Toronto, Ontario, Canada

---

Key points

- Imaging is essential when evaluating the patient with suspected hepatobiliary disease.
- Ultrasound is the first choice when imaging the majority of these patients.
- Ultrasound is widely available, portable, inexpensive, and does not use ionizing radiation.
- Ultrasound will frequently answer the clinical question alone or will direct the next most appropriate imaging investigation.
- Computed tomography, magnetic resonance, endoscopic retrograde cholangio-pancreatography, endoscopic ultrasound, and image-guided biopsy may be necessary beyond ultrasound, either alone or in combination for certain diagnoses.

Radiologic examination in liver disease

Acute hepatic failure

Acute hepatic failure is an uncommon but devastating syndrome that leads to death or a need for liver transplantation in greater than 50% of cases.[1] There are numerous causes with viral hepatitis, drug toxicity, and idiosyncratic reactions amongst the most common. Frequently, imaging of the liver will be normal in these cases but should be performed to investigate the possibility of an acute event such as hepatic vein or portal vein thrombosis. Acute fatty liver of pregnancy and diffuse tumor infiltration of the liver by hepatocellular carcinoma (HCC), metastases, leukemia, or lymphoma may also rarely present with acute hepatic decompensation and will be suggested by imaging.

Hepatology: Diagnosis and Clinical Management, First Edition. Edited by E. Jenny Heathcote.
© 2012 John Wiley & Sons, Ltd. Published 2012 by John Wiley & Sons, Ltd.

Acute hepatic vein thrombosis (Budd–Chiari syndrome) is a rare condition that occurs with or without thrombosis of the inferior vena cava (IVC). The typical patient in the developed world is a young adult woman taking the birth control pill. Other causes include coagulation abnormalities, trauma, pregnancy, and tumor extension from HCC, renal cell cancer, adrenal cortical cancer, and leiomyosarcoma of the IVC. There are also congenital causes and obstructing membranes. The clinical course is dictated by the acuity of onset, degree of occlusion, and the presence of a collateral circulation to drain blood from the liver. These patients are generally well evaluated by ultrasound with Doppler. In the acute phase, the liver is enlarged and ascites is invariably present. The caudate lobe is often spared and hypertrophy will occur over time due to its independent venous drainage through the emissary veins directly into the IVC. Evaluation of the hepatic veins may show acute thrombosis or possibly stricturing, fibrosis, or complete obliteration. Doppler ultrasound will document flow direction in patent segments of the hepatic veins and IVC, and will also document the development of venous collaterals. Portal blood flow may also be affected and can be slowed or reversed. Computed tomography (CT) and magnetic resonance imaging (MRI) may give a more global picture of the liver, including vascular anatomy and may aid in treatment planning.

Assessment of steatosis, fibrosis, and cirrhosis

Imaging is part of the work-up of patients found to have elevated liver enzymes during medical assessment. Ultrasound is the most appropriate initial imaging investigation. Diffuse fatty infiltration of the liver is suggested by increased echogenicity of the liver relative to the kidney. If severe there will be poor penetration of the liver with poor visualization of the hepatic vessels and diaphragm. Often there are areas of focal fatty sparing, which help support the diagnosis. The interpretation of fatty infiltration with ultrasound remains subjective, even in experienced hands, and it is not possible to quantify the degree of fatty infiltration beyond mild, moderate, or severe.

Fatty infiltration of the liver can also be diagnosed with CT scan as reduced attenuation of the liver relative to the spleen. Unenhanced images are the most accurate. Again, it is possible to grade the infiltration as mild, moderate, or severe but it is not possible to accurately quantify the degree of fatty infiltration with routine CT, particularly with milder degrees of fatty infiltration. Research is being conducted on the benefits of dual energy CT in quantifying the degree of fatty infiltration but to date the results are not promising.[2]

Chemical shift MR imaging and MR spectroscopy are the most accurate non-invasive methods to detect fatty infiltration of the liver and to date are the most sensitive non-invasive methods of quantifying the degree of fatty infiltration, particularly in patients with milder involvement.[3] MR is not as widely available as the other modalities and MR spectroscopy is not available at every center. However, chemical shift MR imaging is routinely used as a first-line fat quantification method in specialized centers for specific clinical settings, such as in live liver donor assessment.

Patients with elevated liver enzymes may be found to have unsuspected changes of cirrhosis. Also, patients with known risk factors for chronic liver disease are at risk of developing cirrhosis and imaging may be performed to detect changes of cirrhosis and portal hypertension. In general, early stages of cirrhosis are difficult to diagnose but once cirrhotic changes are confidently identified imaging has a high specificity. Morphologic changes of cirrhosis can be confidently detected with ultrasound, CT, and MRI. The common signs of cirrhosis include surface nodularity of the liver (better appreciated in the presence of ascites), nodularity of the hepatic vein/parenchymal interface, heterogeneous liver parenchyma and lobar redistribution with typically atrophy of segments 4, 5, 6, 7, and 8, and hypertrophy of segments 1, 2, and 3. Signs of portal hypertension are also important and if detected are highly suggestive of cirrhosis in the correct clinical context. Findings include ascites, splenomegaly, patency of the parumbilical vein, dilation of the portal vein, loss of phasicity in flow in the hepatic veins, and once advanced reversed flow in segments of, or the entire, portal venous system. Ultrasound with Doppler is excellent at demonstrating these features but if in doubt CT and MR will give a more global picture of the liver morphology and may demonstrate additional features including siderotic nodules in the liver and, in the case of MRI, Gamna–Gandy bodies in the spleen. Liver biopsy remains the gold standard for early stages of cirrhosis. It is, however, an invasive procedure, which can be associated with significant morbidity and rarely mortality making it less acceptable to patients. The accuracy may also be as low as 80% because of specimen size and fragmentation, sampling error, and interobserver variability.

There is currently much interest in developing elastography as a non-invasive method of detecting and grading fibrosis. The principle of these methods is to non-invasively measure liver stiffness as a predictor of fibrosis. Both ultrasound and MR elastography hold much promise[4,5] and when used in conjunction with serological markers are clinically useful in reducing the number of liver biopsies. With transient elastography (FibroScan, Echosens, France) an ultrasound transducer is located at the end of a vibrating piston that produces a vibration of low amplitude and frequency, which generates a shear wave that passes through the skin and liver tissue. The ultrasound then detects the propagation of the shear wave through the liver at a depth of 2.5 to 6.5 cm from the skin surface by measuring its velocity. The shear wave velocity is directly related to tissue stiffness with a higher velocity equating to higher tissue stiffness, corresponding to an increasing severity of fibrosis; its great advantage is it can be done in the clinic.

MR elastography uses a similar principle but instead of ultrasound, magnetic resonance is used to follow the propagation of the shear wave through the liver, ultimately producing a computer-generated, color-coded elastogram of the liver showing the stiffness in various areas of the organ. Higher tissue stiffness corresponds to increasing severity of fibrosis.

Portal vein thrombosis is an important complication of cirrhosis and can result in sudden hepatic decompensation. The thrombosis may be bland or result from tumor infiltration from hepatocellular carcinoma. As in Budd–Chiari syndrome, ultrasound with Doppler is an excellent initial means of evaluation and can distinguish between benign and malignant thrombus in cirrhotic patients. Pulsatile arterial flow from within the thrombus has 95% specificity for the diagnosis of malignant thrombus.

Hepatic cirrhosis can be mimicked by several conditions. Congenital hepatic fibrosis, nodular regenerative hyperplasia, hepatic schistosomiasis, diffuse hepatic metastasis, and so-called pseudocirrhosis of the liver can all morphologically appear as cirrhosis. Congenital hepatic fibrosis is often manifest by complications of portal hypertension, but despite abnormal hepatic morphology and occasional regenerative nodules which may mimic malignancy, it is not associated with liver failure or hepatocellular carcinoma. It is associated with medullary sponge kidneys, cystic renal diseases, and Caroli disease. When chemotherapy leads to regression of certain hepatic metastases, especially breast carcinoma, a residual fibrotic scar with adjacent liver hyperplasia is seen. If the metastatic disease was diffuse, the regressed disease appearance mimics cirrhosis, and is called "pseudocirrhosis".

Surveillance for hepatocellular carcinoma

Surveillance for HCC has been shown to improve survival, particularly in individuals chronically infected with hepatitis B or in any cirrhotic patient, and is advocated by the American, European, and Asian–Pacific societies for the study of liver diseases.[6–8] Populations at risk that benefit from surveillance have been defined, with some differences for each region; however, all advocate use of ultrasound primarily as the imaging surveillance technique. Surveillance frequency is recommended at 6-month intervals. Due to the difficulty in detection of malignancy in a diseased liver and operator dependence of ultrasound, it is important to perform surveillance at centers with established expertise.

The algorithm for work-up of nodules found on surveillance depends on their size (Fig. 26.1). Nodules under 1 cm can be followed by ultrasound in 3–6 months for 18–24 months. Practically speaking, such nodules can be followed on routine surveillance, provided that it is at no longer than 6-month intervals. A nodule measuring 1 cm or more is considered significant and requires contrast-enhanced imaging work-up. While any of contrast-enhanced CT, MRI, or ultrasound is advocated as the initial work-up scan, our preference is MRI since it consistently covers the whole of the liver (compared to contrast-enhanced ultrasound (CEUS) in some patients), does not use ionizing radiation (compared to CT scan), and may provide slightly improved specificity due to additional means of tissue characterization unique to MRI.

A nodule is considered malignant when it demonstrates, relative to the adjacent liver, higher enhancement in the arterial phase (i.e. arterialized) and lower enhancement in the venous or equilibrium phases (i.e. relative washout).[7] In a known cirrhotic patient or individual with chronic viral hepatitis, this pattern is considered sufficiently specific for HCC and treatment can commence without tissue biopsy. Otherwise, the scan is equivocal and a second

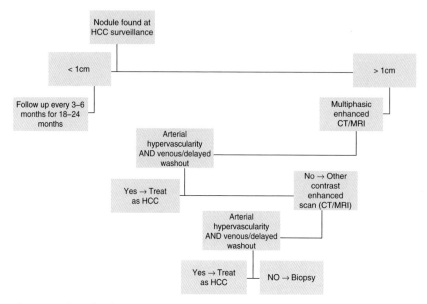

Fig. 26.1 Algorithm for management of nodules found at HCC surveillance. Modified from Bruix J, Sherman M. Management of hepatocellular carcinoma: an update. Hepatology 2011; 53: 1020–2.

contrast-enhanced scan is recommended (e.g. CT or CEUS).[7,9] If both scans are equivocal then biopsy is advocated, which is almost always by ultrasound guidance. Follow-up by imaging is reserved for nodules that cannot be biopsied due to inaccessible location or "indeterminate" biopsy results. In the course of imaging work-up, additional nodules are sometimes found, which were not visible on ultrasound. These too need to be followed by the imaging modality that discovered them if their enhancement characteristics are not typical for malignancy.

The recommended follow-up of nodules by imaging is for a period of 18–24 months.[7] If a nodule is unchanged in size and enhancement characteristics during this interval or resolves, it is considered benign and the patient can return to routine surveillance. Also, when a nodule seen on surveillance is shown to be benign in its work-up (e.g. hepatic lobulation, hemangioma, or enhancing similar to the background liver in all phases) the patient can return to routine surveillance by ultrasound.

Assessment of liver masses

Liver masses are often well characterized by imaging, and biopsy is rarely required. Contrast enhancement is required for CT, MRI, and ultrasound to substantially improve both sensitivity and specificity of imaging. The dual vascular supply of the liver is used to advantage with multiphase studies using intravenous contrast bolus injection; the arterial and portal vein supply of

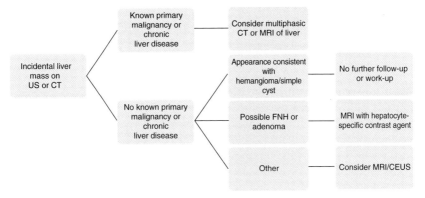

Fig. 26.2 Algorithm for the work-up of incidental masses found on abdominal ultrasound or CT scan.

masses relative to the liver is thus used to characterize lesions. A scan prior to injection (unenhanced phase) determines the relative attenuation of the mass and also allows measuring relative enhancement upon contrast instillation. After injection of contrast material into a peripheral vein it first enters the liver through the hepatic artery (arterial phase). Relatively more contrast material enters the liver when enhanced blood returns from the gut through the portal vein (portovenous phase). After about 3 min, the concentration of contrast in the vascular system has equalized (equilibrium phase) and imaging at this late phase reflects the relative vascular volume, which indirectly indicates the fibrotic component of lesions.

The incidental liver mass is commonly discovered when an unenhanced ultrasound or single (often portovenous) phase CT of the abdomen is performed for unrelated reasons (Fig. 26.2). Incidental asymptomatic masses are almost always benign and care should be taken not to perform extensive imaging or follow-up unless deemed necessary. Also, contrast-enhanced MRI and ultrasound are preferable when working up such lesions in order to minimize ionizing radiation of CT scan. The initial imaging scan often can characterize cysts and hemangiomas with relative high specificity and in patients without a history of prior malignancy or of chronic liver disease, further imaging work-up or follow-up is not necessary. The contrast enhancement pattern of hemangiomas is highly specific and can make the diagnosis when the initial imaging with ultrasound is equivocal. The hepatobiliary phase of hepatocyte-specific MRI contrast agents is highly specific for focal nodular hyperplasia (FNH) and is primarily recommended when these common lesions (in 3% of the population) are to be differentiated from hepatocellular adenoma.

The staging of patients with a known malignancy is usually by protocol and CT is often preferred to MRI when the remainder of the abdomen is also being assessed and ionizing radiation is of less concern. Hypervascular primaries (especially neuroendocrine tumor, melanoma, renal cell carcinoma, and gastrointestinal stromal tumor) require multiphase scans to improve specificity and assess response to treatment. Sensitivity for small (<1 cm) metastases is improved with MRI during the hepatobiliary phase of hepatocyte-specific MRI contrast agents and may be considered when hepatectomy is contemplated.

Right upper quadrant pain: acute cholecystitis, cholangitis, hepatitis, hepatic abscess, and parasitic liver disease

Acute abdominal pain is a common symptom, leading to emergency department visits in the developed world and acute cholecystitis accounts for 5% of these visits. Ultrasound is the preferred imaging modality to diagnose acute cholecystitis.[10,11] The sensitivity and specificity when adjusted for verification bias is approximately 88% and 80%, respectively, poorer than hepatobiliary iminodiacetic acid (HIDA) nuclear medicine scan's sensitivity and specificity of 97% and 90%, respectively, but has the advantage of being more practical and time efficient. In contrast to HIDA scan, it can also document complications of acute cholecystitis such as gangrenous change and perforation and can often diagnose an alternate cause of pain if the gallbladder is normal. Ultrasound also has a very high sensitivity and specificity of 97% and 95%, respectively, for diagnosing gallstones in cases of suspected biliary colic.

Ultrasound is also the preferred initial imaging test in cases of suspected choledocholithiasis or in cases of suspected cholangitis. It is readily available and can be performed at the bedside in acutely ill patients. Ultrasound is very sensitive (99%) and accurate (93%) at demonstrating biliary dilation. Once it is established that biliary dilation is present, ultrasound will also frequently demonstrate the level and cause of biliary obstruction. Ultrasound has a sensitivity of 55 to 85% in detecting common bile duct (CBD) stones but has a high specificity (89–91%), so if confidently identified then these patients can be referred for definitive treatment, most often with endoscopic retrograde cholangiopancreatography (ERCP) after they have been fluid resuscitated and given antibiotic coverage. If biliary obstruction is present and stones are suspected but cannot be demonstrated then magnetic resonance cholangiopancreatography (MRCP) can be performed, once the patient is stable, prior to referral for drainage. If MRCP is not readily available unenhanced CT may have a complementary role with ultrasound increasing overall sensitivity.[10,11] In cases of cholangitis, ultrasound may also demonstrate thickening of the walls of the bile ducts.

Ultrasound is also the preferred imaging modality for cases of "suspected" acute hepatitis. Often the liver will appear normal but increased periportal edema manifesting as increased periportal echoes are in keeping with this diagnosis. Gallbladder wall edema may also be present but again is not specific and can be seen in many other conditions including heart failure and acute pancreatitis. Gallbladder wall edema can also be present in cases of acute cholecystitis but it is neither sensitive nor specific for this diagnosis so the presence of gallbladder wall edema alone should not lead to surgery to remove the gallbladder as a fatality may ensue should the patient have an acute hepatitis. The most important role of ultrasound in the setting of acute hepatitis is to rule out other causes of acute derangement of liver function such as tumor infiltration of the liver, biliary dilation, or an acute vascular condition, namely Budd–Chiari syndrome or acute portal vein thrombosis.

Pyogenic hepatic abscess is difficult to visualize by ultrasound in the early phase and only when matured does the classical heterogeneous fluid-filled (and sometime gas-filled) cavity become easily visible. Similarly, ultrasound has low sensitivity for small peribiliary pyogenic abscesses (seen in complicated cholangitis) or small mycobacterial or fungal infections commonly in immunodeficient patients. In all these scenarios, contrast-enhanced CT scan is preferable to ultrasound, where inflammatory hyperemia can be shown (Fig. 26.3). Differentiation of amebic from pyogenic abscess may not be reliable by imaging; the former is considered when a large subdiaphragmatic collection is seen in the right lobe, and there has been travel to an endemic region. While large hepatic abscesses need to be drained percutaneously, most early or small hepatic abscesses resolve with antibiotic therapy. Thrombosis of portal vein branches, usually subsegmental and peripheral, due to portal vein septicemia is a common finding in hepatic infections and does not require specific treatment. It is also commonly seen following colonic surgery, presumably due to transient portal bacteremia, and is subclinical.

Parasitic hepatic infections can have specific imaging appearances, which may lead to definitive diagnosis in endemic regions. Ultrasound has been successfully utilized as a diagnostic and prognostic tool in echinococcal and schistosomiatic infections. Early in the course of infection, a hydatid cyst mimics simple hepatic cysts, but after a few weeks there is a perceptible wall to the cyst which represents the combination of the parasitic entity (exo- and endocyst) and the inflammatory hepatic reaction (pericyst) (Fig. 26.4). Echogenic mobile material (hydatid sand), folding internal septae (due to separation and in-folding of endocyst), internal fat, and daughter cysts are more advanced and telling findings. Ultrasound appearance of chronic schistosomiasis infection results from chronic inflammation and fibrosis in the periportal regions related to the lodging of the parasitic eggs, which travel up the portal venous system from the colon. Echogenic bands surrounding the central portal veins in cases of *Schistosoma mansoni* and echogenic lines extending from portal triads to the capsule of the liver in cases of *Schistosoma japonicum* are often diagnostic. Splenomegaly and other signs of portal hypertension are also present.

Various parasites may affect the biliary tree in differing ways. Biliary ascariasis may present with typical symptoms of ascending cholangitis. The diagnosis is made when the long, sometimes moving, worms are visualized within the large bile ducts and gallbladder. In the acute phase of infection, lasting 3–5 months, *Fasciola hepatica* infestations also may present with right upper quadrant pain, hepatomegaly, and prolonged fevers.[12] This represents the migration of the parasite through the liver capsule and parenchyma. Multiple, small peripheral hepatic lesions may be identified on imaging, with telltale linear tracks better seen on CT scans, along with hepatomegaly and hilar adenopathy. The chronic phase of infection, lasting up to 10 years, relates to chronic infestation of the biliary tree by the liver fluke. Intermittent bouts of jaundice and

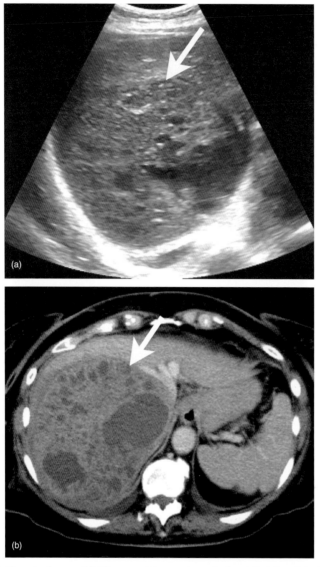

Fig. 26.3 Hepatic abscess. (a) Ultrasound image through the right lobe of the liver shows a large multiseptate, mostly solid-appearing mass (arrow). (b) The corresponding CT scan depicts the multiple loculations of an abscess (arrow). (c) Axial CT scan in a different patient demonstrates a multiloculated, gas-containing mass (arrow). The presence of gas is uncommon but highly specific for a pyogenic abscess.

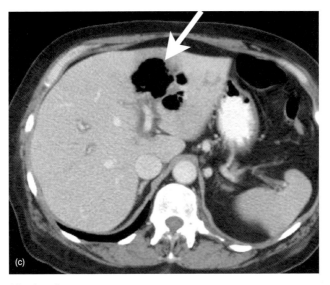

Fig. 26.3 (*Continued*)

fever mark this phase where imaging, especially sonography, may reveal debris and mobile flat worms within the central bile ducts and gallbladder. *Clonorchis sinensis* and *Opisthorchis viverrini* infestations, seen in East and South-east Asia, are asymptomatic early on, and tend to present clinically in the chronic phase. As opposed to *Fasciola hepatica* infestation, the central bile ducts are usually of normal caliber, but there is chronic, multisegmental or diffuse dilatation of small and medium-sized bile ducts where the flukes live for decades. Debris may be seen within the gallbladder and affected peripheral ducts where the dilatation may persist after treatment. Cholangiocarcinoma and recurrent pyogenic cholangitis have been associated with these liver flukes (Fig. 26.5).[12]

Painless obstructive jaundice

When the history, clinical examination, and serological tests suggest an obstructive cause for a jaundiced patient, ultrasound is the first recommended imaging scan. For patients with acute symptoms suggestive of cholangitis, please refer to section above on right upper quadrant pain. Ultrasound scans determine whether there is dilation of the biliary tree, and if so they can suggest the level of obstruction and provide clues as to the cause. Advances in ultrasound technology now allow detection of mild central intrahepatic bile duct dilatation, in addition to the CBD, and the absence of dilation should prompt re-evaluation for non-obstructive causes of jaundice, for example acute hepatitis of any etiology. The CBD normally measures up to 0.6 cm in diameter, but may be larger in elderly patients or those with prior cholecystectomy.[12]

The most common error in the management of obstructive jaundice is ERCP and stent placement *prior* to completion of non-invasive imaging. The stent interferes with visualization of tumors and the procedure may cause acute

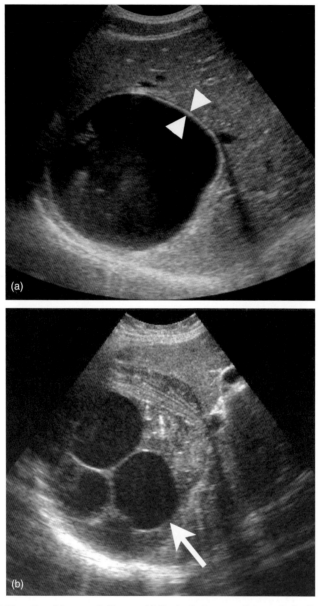

Fig. 26.4 Hepatic echinococcal disease. (a) Sagittal ultrasound through the liver shows a large cyst. The presence of the perceptible cyst wall (arrowheads), which develops after the early phase of infection, differentiates hydatid cysts from simple liver cysts. (b) A different patient with more advanced disease has a large, complex cyst in the right lobe with several internal daughter cysts typical of echinococcal disease.

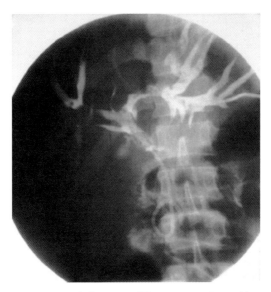

Fig. 26.5 Recurrent pyogenic cholangitis in Vietnamese patient with sepsis and cholestasis. A cholangiogram demonstrates chronically dilated bile ducts with multiple filling defects representing pigment stones. Reproduced from Abdalian R, Heathcote EJ. Hepatology 2006; 44: 1063 with permission from VG Wort.

pancreatitis or lead to cholangitis and peribiliary abscesses, all of which may result in the incorrect staging of patients with malignancy. When obstruction is at the level of the hepatic hilum, common causes include hilar cholangiocarcinoma, IgG4-associated sclerosing cholangitis, malignant adenopathy, and metastatic disease to the bile ducts. Distal causes of biliary obstruction include pancreatic adenocarcinoma, autoimmune (IgG4-associated) pancreatitis, and chronic pancreatitis.

When a mass is seen as the cause of obstruction, further imaging by contrast-enhanced CT or MRI is recommended for characterization and staging. The choice between CT and MRI depends on the level and suspected cause of obstruction, availability of MRI, and local expertise. It is usual to start with CT for hilar and pancreatic causes of obstruction, and MRI for ampullary causes. However, it is not uncommon to resort to both tests and/or dedicated focused ultrasound evaluation by an experienced physician in complicated cases. The assessment of biliary tree and pancreas requires multiphase, multiplanar scans to allow assessment of pancreatic and liver parenchyma and the vasculature, and generally higher spatial resolution than liver scans due to the small size of bile and pancreatic ducts. MRI should also include MRCP sequences for evaluation of bile and pancreatic ducts. Due to the invasiveness and cost of endoscopic ultrasound (EUS), it should be used for patients who are determined as operable based on CT/MRI staging. In such patients, EUS may add further diagnostic information and biopsy may be performed if deemed necessary.

Cast study 26.1

A 73-year-old woman presented to her family physician with a 3-week history of progressive painless jaundice, and a 4-month history of 5 kg weight loss. Her serum bilirubin was found to be 183 μmol/mL. She was referred for an abdominal ultrasound which showed dilatation of the intrahepatic biliary tree and common bile duct, the latter measuring up to 1.3 cm in diameter. The duct terminated in a 2.6-cm mass in the pancreatic head, which was also causing pancreatic ductal dilatation (Fig. 26.6). The patient underwent staging MRI of the abdomen, which showed the tumor to be confined to the pancreatic head with no evidence of adjacent vascular involvement or metastatic disease. A pancreatoduodenectomy (Whipple's resection) was performed, the specimen was positive for pancreatic ductal adenocarcinoma with 1/12 nodes involved. She received adjuvant chemotherapy (gemcitibine). She has recovered well with no evidence of disease recurrence 6 years after her surgery.

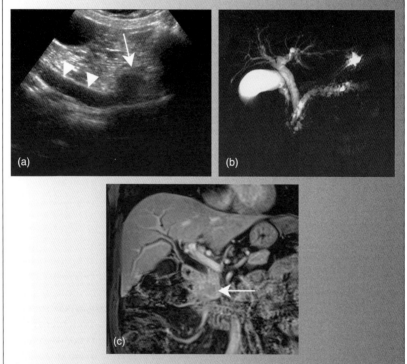

Fig. 26.6 A 73-year-old woman with jaundice. (a) Ultrasound shows a dilated common bile duct (arrowheads) terminating in a mass in the head of the pancreas (arrow). (b) On staging MRCP image, markedly dilated common bile duct and pancreatic ducts are seen. (c) Coronal-enhanced MRI shows the small mass with no involvement of adjacent vessels.

Cast study 26.2

A 22-year-old woman with a 4-year history of systemic lupus erythematosus was noticed by her physician to have hepatosplenomegaly and a mildly elevated bilirubin (mostly conjugated). Ultrasound with Doppler (Plate 26.1a–c) showed no features of cirrhosis but note was made of monophasic flow in the hepatic veins, suggesting possible venous outflow obstruction. More careful assessment showed the right hepatic vein to be narrowed and thick walled with no flow. A collateral vein drained the right lobe via the middle hepatic vein. This middle hepatic vein shared a common confluence with the left hepatic vein to the inferior vena cava. High venous blood flow velocities were demonstrated at this common confluence, suggesting a web or stricture. Hepatic venography via a jugular approach (Fig. 26.7a) showed a narrowing at the hepatic venous confluence with a pressure gradient and collateral venous channels in the liver. Angioplasty of this narrowing (Fig. 26.7b) was performed at the time of venography. The patient was subsequently anticoagulated and has remained well from a liver perspective for 6 years.

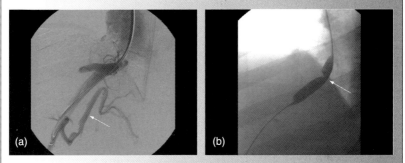

Fig. 26.7 A 22-year-old woman with chronic Budd–Chiari syndrome. (a) Injection of the middle hepatic vein at the time of venography shows a collateral vein (arrow). (b) A stricture at the common confluence of the middle and left hepatic veins with the IVC causes "waisting" (arrow) of the inflated angioplasty balloon.

Multiple choice questions

1. Multiphase CT scan of a 3-cm heterogeneous mass in a cirrhotic liver showing higher enhancement in the arterial phase and lower enhancement in the venous or equilibrium phase is considered diagnostic of:
   A. Hemangioma
   B. Hepatic adenoma
   C. Focal nodular hyperplasia
   D. Hepatocellular carcinoma

2. The most appropriate management for a 2-cm echogenic liver mass discovered on ultrasound performed to look for gallstones in a 40-year-old woman with no history of liver disease or primary malignancy is:
   A. Multiphase CT scan
   B. MRI
   C. Follow-up ultrasound in 6 months
   D. No further investigation or follow-up

3. Ultrasound shows biliary dilation caused by choledocholithiasis in a 70-year-old man with right upper quadrant pain. The next most appropriate imaging investigation is:
   A. MRCP
   B. Multiphase CT
   C. ERCP
   D. Scintigraphy with HIDA

Answers

1. D
2. D
3. C

References

1. Ostapowicz G, Fontana RJ, Schiødt FV, et al. Results of a prospective study of acute liver failure at 17 tertiary care centers in the United States. Ann Intern Med 2002; 137: 947–54.
2. Mendler MH, Bouillet P, Le Sidaner A, et al. Dual-energy CT in the diagnosis and quantification of fatty liver: limited clinical value in comparison to ultrasound scan and single-energy CT, with special reference to iron overload. J Hepatol 1998; 28: 785–94.
3. Ma X, Holalkere NS, Kambadakone RA, et al. Imaging-based quantification of hepatic fat: methods and clinical applications. Radiographics 2009; 29: 1253–77.
4. Carrion JA, Navasa M, Bosch J, et al. Transient elastography for diagnosis of advanced fibrosis and portal hypertension in patients with hepatitis C recurrence after liver transplantation. Liver Transpl 2006; 12: 1791–8.
5. Huwart L, Sempoux C, Salameh N, et al. Liver fibrosis: noninvasive assessment with MR elastography versus aspartate aminotransferase-to-platelet ratio index. Radiology 2007; 245: 458–66.
6. Bruix J, Sherman M, Llovet JM, et al. Clinical management of hepatocellular carcinoma. Conclusions of the Barcelona-2000 EASL conference. European Association for the Study of the Liver. J Hepatol 2001; 35: 421–30.
7. Bruix J, Sherman M. Management of hepatocellular carcinoma: an update. Hepatology 2011; 53: 1020–2.
8. Amarapurkar D, Han KH, Chan HL, et al. Application of surveillance programs for hepatocellular carcinoma in the Asia-Pacific Region. J Gastroenterol Hepatol 2009; 24: 955–61.

9. Khalili K, Kim TK, Jang HJ, et al. Optimization of imaging diagnosis of 1–2 cm hepatocellular carcinoma: an analysis of diagnostic performance and resource utilization. J Hepatol 2010; 54: 723–8.

10. Stoker J, van Randen A, Laméris W, et al. Imaging patients with acute abdominal pain. Radiology 2009; 253: 31–46.

11. Hanbidge AE, Buckler PM, O'Malley ME, et al. From the RSNA refresher courses: imaging evaluation for acute pain in the right upper quadrant. Radiographics 2004; 24: 1117–35.

12. Khalili KW. The biliary tree and gallbladder. In: Diagnostic Ultrasound. Rumack CM, Wilson SR, Charboneau W, Johnson A, eds, St Louis: Elsevier-Mosby, 2005.

Index

3TC 265, 273–5, 276–8

A2 50–62
AAT deficiency 6, 35, 37–8, 66–79, 99–100, 121–2, 124–7, 255–7, 282, 285–6, 300, 307, 312, 330, 335–6, 344, 345–6
abacavir (ABC) 275, 277–8
abdomen 4–5, 9, 11–19, 28, 36–8, 43, 46–8, 64–79, 117, 221–2, 233, 239–41, 248–50, 284, 295, 316–17, 324–5, 370–2, 402–5
    see also ascites; imaging; pain; physical examinations; spider nevi; symptoms
    discomfort 4–5, 15, 17–18, 36–8, 221–2, 233, 239–41, 248–50, 284, 295, 316–17, 324–5, 370–2, 402–5
    prominent wall veins 9, 18–19, 47–8
absolute/relative contraindications, liver transplants 122–31
abstinence needs, alcohol 54–6, 59, 85, 226–34, 269–71
acamprosate alcohol treatment 230–1
acanthosis nigricans 247–8, 253, 260
acarbose 237
aceruloplasminemia 355
acetaminophen 21, 23, 33–4, 36–40, 54–6, 122, 128–9, 132–3, 134, 138–40, 236–7, 239, 241–2, 270–1, 294–5
    antidotes 138, 140
    safe uses 54–6, 241
acidosis 370–2
acne 284
acquired cysts of the liver 389–93
    see also cystic diseases
acute alcoholic hepatitis 11

acute brain injuries, hepatic encephalopathy (flapping tremor) 114, 115, 135–6
acute cellular rejection (ACR) 142, 144–5, 154–5
acute cholecystitis 15, 402–5
acute fatty liver of pregnancy (AFLP) 370, 371, 372–3, 396–7
acute hepatitis 5, 21, 23, 47, 163–84, 185, 208–25, 233, 238–9, 367, 369, 375–8, 402–5
    see also hepatitis...
acute liver disease 2–16, 21–4, 35–8, 39–40, 43, 47, 121–2, 124–31, 132–41, 163–84, 185, 208–25, 233, 235–43, 298–9, 345, 348–9, 367, 369, 370–2, 375–8, 396–7, 402–5
    see also fulminant hepatic failure
    management approaches 23–4, 121–2, 124–31
    symptoms 2, 3, 4, 5–6, 9, 11, 14–16, 21–3, 35–8
acute liver failure (ALF) see fulminant hepatic failure
acute respiratory distress syndrome (ARDS) 136
acute tubular necrosis (ATN) 88, 135–7
acute viral hepatitis 5, 21, 23, 39–40, 47, 163–84, 208–25, 233, 367, 369, 375–8, 402–5
    see also hepatitis...
acyclic phosphonates 195
acyclovir 137, 180, 181, 376, 378
adefovir (ADV) 195, 198–9, 201–2, 272–4
adenoviruses 37–8, 146, 162–3, 182
ADPKD see autosomal dominant polycystic kidney disease

Hepatology: Diagnosis and Clinical Management, First Edition. Edited by E. Jenny Heathcote.
© 2012 John Wiley & Sons, Ltd. Published 2012 by John Wiley & Sons, Ltd.

Index compiled by Terry Halliday